# Contents

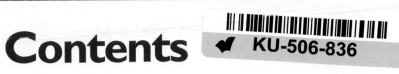 

About the author...........................................................................................................................ii

Foreword......................................................................................................................................iii

**Section 1- Malignancies**

Chapter 1: Malignant melanoma.................................................................................................1

Chapter 2: Malignant melanomas and seborrhoeic wart ...........................................................5

Chapter 3: Mimickers of malignant melanoma...........................................................................7

Chapter 4: Keratoacanthoma /Basal cell caricinoma/Squamous cell carcinoma.........................13

Chapter 5: Cutaneous T-cell lymphoma...................................................................................17

Chapter 6: Skin manifestations of breast cancer.......................................................................21

Chapter 7: The nipple.............................................................................................................25

**Section 2 - Moles and Other Skin Lesions**

Chapter 8: Brown pigmented lesions........................................................................................29

Chapter 9: Telangiectasia........................................................................................................33

Chapter 10: Viral warts...........................................................................................................39

Chapter 11: Genital warts.......................................................................................................43

**Section 3 - Rashes**

Chapter 12: Diagnosis spots and vesicles.................................................................................49

Chapter 13: Plaque psoriasis...................................................................................................55

Chapter 14: Lichen planus.......................................................................................................61

Chapter 15: Interigo...............................................................................................................67

Chapter 16: Scaly feet/Keratoderma.......................................................................................71

Chapter 17: Hand dermatitis /Tinca manuum ..........................................................................75

Chapter 18: Insect bites/Bullous pemphigoid............................................................................77

**Section 4 - Pruritus**

Chapter 19: Urticaria..............................................................................................................81

Chapter 20: Erythema multiforme............................................................................................87

Chapter 21: Atopic eczema......................................................................................................89

Chapter 22: Compulsive itch....................................................................................................95

Chapter 23: Scabies...............................................................................................................101

Chapter 24: Infestations.........................................................................................................105

Chapter 25: Genital...............................................................................................................109

**Section 5 - Specific areas of the body**

Chapter 26: Tinea Corporis....................................................................................................113

Chapter 27: Nails 1- A pointer to disease ...............................................................................119

Chapter 28: Nails 2 - The traumatized nail..............................................................................123

Chapter 29: Red faces............................................................................................................127

Chapter 30: Red and spotty faces...........................................................................................133

Chapter 31: Acne vulgaris......................................................................................................137

Chapter 32: Facial swelling.....................................................................................................143

Chapter 33: Alopecia 1: Non-scarring.....................................................................................149

Chapter 34: Alopecia 2: Scarring............................................................................................155

Chapter 35: Lip lesions..........................................................................................................161

Chapter 36: The tongue.........................................................................................................167

Chapter 37: Abnormalities of the ear lobe ..............................................................................173

Chapter 38: Spots around the eyes.........................................................................................177

**Section 6 - Drug Reactions**

Chapter 39: Adverse reactions to topical steroids....................................................................181

Chapter 40: Drug induced reactions of the skin .......................................................................185

Test your knowledge answers.................................................................................................191

Index.....................................................................................................................................201

# About the Author

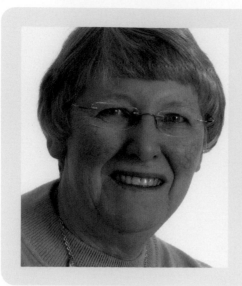

Dr Jean Watkins' career journey began when she qualified in medicine at the Royal Free Hospital, London, in 1955. She became a trainee in a large estate at St Paul's Cray before moving to another estate in Downham, Kent, as a partner in a general practice. By 1974, she was ready to move on to the challenge of a rapidly growing new town estate at Thamesmead.

Following an interest in photography she began to realise the value of documenting pictures of patients in teaching students and trainees. Hence she built up the collection of images that has enabled this book to be produced.

These days, Dr Watkins is retired but is an active member of the Practice Nursing Editorial Board and, in April 2004, was awarded a Fellowship of the Royal College of General Practitioners.

## Acknowledgements

*I would like to thank Liam Benison for his initial help and support in setting up the series, together with his team, for the continuing help and support that has followed*

cology

Diagnosis

kins

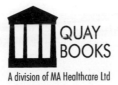

QUAY
BOOKS
A division of MA Healthcare Ltd

Quay Books Division, MA Healthcare Ltd, St Jude's Church,
Dulwich Road, London SE24 0PB

British Library Cataloguing-in-Publication Data
A catalogue record is available for this book

© MA Healthcare Limited 2010
ISBN-10: 1 85642 4014 ; ISBN-13: 978 1 85642 4011

Printed by CLE, Huntingdon, Cambridgeshire
Designer: Carolyn Allen (Fonthill Creative - 01722 717057)
Associate Publisher: Thu Nguyen

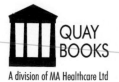

QUAY BOOKS

A division of MA Healthcare Ltd

# Foreword

Skin problems are one of the most common reasons for people to seek help from a nurse or GP in general practice. Up to 15% of GP consultations are for skin disorders (Royal College of General Practitioners, 2007). General practice nurses have undertaken responsibility for treating skin problems for many years, but the advent of nurse prescribing has now furnished them with the power to complete dermatology consultations independently. Courtenay et al (2007) have estimated that practice nurses prescribe more often and for a wider range of dermatological products than nurses working in other healthcare settings.

As this book demonstrates, the range of skin conditions that can affect patients in primary care is great, and diagnosis and management is very often a complex matter that requires consideration of personal and family history, home, work or school environments, and a variety of possible differential diagnoses.

The typical presentation, diagnosis and treatment of common conditions such as eczema and psoriasis may be familiar to many primary care professionals, but long-term management can pose many difficult assessment decisions for the practice nurse and GP. Lesions such as melanomas must be diagnosed with particular care and urgent action taken when required. It is also important to be aware of skin lesions that might indicate any underlying conditions such as diabetes or infections that may be playing a role.

Careful attention to a patient's psychological wellbeing is also important. The discomfort and irritation of skin conditions and their social consequences can have profound effects. For example, Finlay and Coles (1995) found that 49% of patients with psoriasis were prepared to spend 2–3 hours a day on treatment if it gave them normal skin for the rest of the day.

Skin conditions are usually obvious to other people, whether to partners and family, or to everyone in a person's life, including friends, colleagues, acquaintances and strangers. They can result in embarrassment, impair intimate relationships, and provoke social ostracism and bullying from the external world. The International Study of Life with Atopic Eczema (ISOLATE) found that some people with eczema experience discrimination in the workplace (Medical News Today, 2004).

Profound internal psychological effects are prevalent, such as low self-esteem, anxiety and depression (Lewis-Jones, 2006). In a long-term condition such as eczema, the psychological impact can begin very early in life, as Sausenthaler et al (2009) have demonstrated, and last throughout life.

While some skin problems may be long lasting and require long-term treatment, the effect of others may be disfiguring and psychologically disturbing for an individual, but have no serious physical consequences. The question is then whether to treat or not. The impact and treatment of skin conditions is highly dependent on the individual and his/her social circumstances.

An array of treatment options is available for many skin problems, and treatment choice needs to be appropriate to the individual. Patient adherence may be difficult to achieve and difficult to assess where it is a matter of using quantities of topical creams, ointments and lotions rather than a simple pill. Moreover, the relapsing pattern of long-term skin conditions is hard to predict and often difficult to treat when flare-ups occur.

Only 24% of patients with eczema or their caregivers could manage flare-ups effectively, according to the ISOLATE study, which investigated the management of 2002 patients or caregivers with eczema in eight countries (Zuberbier et al, 2006). These researchers found that patients or caregivers waited on average 7 days before treating a flare-up. Stress and anxiety can play a substantial role in the appearance of symptoms and the effectiveness of treatments.

This book comprises edited and updated versions of articles from a long running and highly popular series published in Practice Nursing journal on the differential diagnosis of dermatological conditions. This series was born in 2002, when an earlier series of dermatological case studies was expanded into a format that allowed for discussion and practical recommendations on diagnosis and management in greater detail.

Dr Jean Watkins has developed an interest and expertise in dermatology during a long career as a GP, and is particularly aware of the psychological impact of skin disorders. In this book she takes a practical approach to the assessment, diagnosis and management of a wide variety of skin conditions. This book will interest GPs and general practice nurses alike. It is complemented by images from Dr Watkins's own library, taken over the course of her career. It will provide a useful, practical guide to help GPs and practice nurses improve the quality of life of patients suffering with skin disorders.

**Liam Benison**
*Editor/Publisher, Practice Nursing*

## References

Courtenay M, Carey N, Burke J (2007) Independent extended nurse prescribing for patients with skin conditions: a national questionnaire survey. *Journal of Clinical Nursing* **16**(7): 1247–55

Finlay AY, Coles EC (1995) The effect of severe psoriasis on the quality of life of 369 patients. *Br J Dermatol* **132**(2): 236–44.

Lewis-Jones S (2006) Quality of life and childhood atopic dermatitis: the misery of living with childhood eczema. *Int J Clin Pract* **60**(8): 984–92

Medical News Today (2004) Eczema patients face a lifetime of isolation, bullying and discrimination. 21 November. www.medicalnewstoday.com/articles/16646.php (accessed 23 July 2010)

Royal College of General Practitioners (2007) Skin problems. Curriculum Statement 15.10. *RCGP*, London: p.6

Sausenthaler S, Rzehak P, Chen CM, Arck P, Bockelbrink A, Schäfer T, Schaaf B, Borte M, Herbarth O, Krämer U, von Berg A, Wichmann HE, Heinrich J; LISA Study Group (2009) Stress-related maternal factors during pregnancy in relation to childhood eczema: results from the LISA Study. *J Investig Allergol Clin Immunol* **19**(6): 481–7

Zuberbier T, Orlow SJ, Paller AS, Taïeb A, Allen R, Hernanz-Hermosa JM, Ocampo-Candiani J, Cox M, Langeraar J, Simon JC (2006) Patient perspectives on the management of atopic dermatitis. *J Allergy Clin Immunol* **118**(1): 226-32

# Malignant melanoma

There is an increasing public awareness of the dangers of sun exposure and possibility of developing malignant melanoma. Thinning of the ozone layer, global warming and constant media reminders of the risks of exposure to the sun are bringing patients to the surgery at the first sign of a mole or blemish on the skin.

It is often difficult to diagnose moles and decide whether a patient needs urgent referral or general advice. The job of the clinician is to separate, as far as possible, those lesions about which we should be unconcerned, from those that require further investigation or treatment. This chapter looks at those diagnostic features that should lead health professionals to suspect malignancy, as well as identifying the patients most likely to suffer from such problems.

Health professionals need to recognize problems and arrange appropriate, urgent intervention. They must also help to educate patients, particularly those at greatest risk, on how to prevent the development, and/or spot the signs of melanoma early on, at a stage when treatment will usually offer an excellent prognosis.

## Aetiology

Malignant melanoma arises in the pigment producing melanocytes in the basal layer of the epidermis as the result of over-stimulation by ultraviolet light. It has the potential to metastasize via the lymphatics and the circulation with fatal results (du Vivier, 2002). Malignant melanoma is rare before puberty, and tends to occur after the age of 20–30 years. The incidence and mortality of malignant melanoma is increasing world-wide (Muir et al, 1987). It has been predicted that the rate will rise with the increasing thinning of the ozone layer (Mackie and Rycroft, 1988). The incidence of malignant melanoma in the UK is about 10 per 100 000, with approximately twice the number of women with the condition compared to men

| Table 1.1. When to suspect malignant melanoma |
|---|
| *Any one of three major features or three out of four minor ones should raise suspicion of a melanoma:* |

**Major features**
- Change in size
- Irregular shape
- Irregular colour

**Minor features**
- Largest diameter greater than 7 mm
- Inflammation
- Oozing
- Change in sensation

From: Roberts et al, 2002.

(Buxton, 2003). A number of different factors lead to the possibility of development of malignant melanoma. The incidence of melanoma is highest in countries which enjoy the most sun throughout the year. At greatest risk, are people with, fair hair and fair skin that tends to burn easily after exposure to ultraviolet light, which may be either from sun exposure or the use of sunbeds. The risk of damage to the skin is cumulative over the years, and increased where there has been actual sunburn (Whiteman and Green, 1994) (*Figure 1.1*).

Genetic factors also play a part. For example, those with fair skin are at increased risk. Patients with a strong family history of malignant melanoma are also at greater risk (Roberts et al, 2002). Gene testing is not currently advised, however. Where there are three or more members of the family with malignant melanoma, they should be referred for counselling. Patients should also be referred if two or more members of the family have atypical mole syndrome with multiple pigmented naevi, mainly on the trunk (*Figure 1.2*), particularly if the pigmented naevi increase in number during adolescence, as the risk of

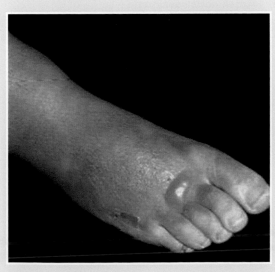

*Figure 1.1. Sunburn of the foot, increases the risk of development of melanoma.*

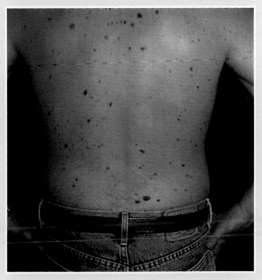

*Figure 1.2. Atypical mole syndrome.*

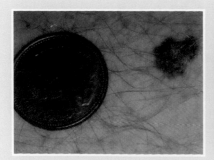

Figure 1.3. Superficial spreading
malignant melanoma.

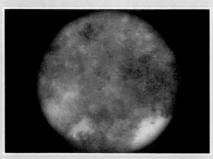

Figure 1.4. Dermatoscopic view of superficial
spreading malignant melanoma.

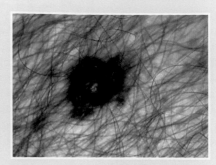

Figure 1.5. Nodular malignant
melanoma.

malignant melanoma is greater in such cases (Roberts et al, 2002). Mole mapping may be appropriate in these cases so that changes can be more easily recognized (NLH Question-Answering Service, 2006). Although malignant change in pre-existing moles is rare, the darkly pigmented, often hairy bathing trunk naevus, that is present at birth and may cover quite an extensive area, has a 3–7% risk of change to a melanoma and should be watched with care (Kantor, 2004).

## Diagnostic features

The British Association of Dermatologists (BAD) has produced a check-list of features that may suggest melanoma or malignant change in an existing pigmented lesion (Roberts et al, 2002) (*Table 1.1*). There are five main types of malignant melanoma: superficial spreading melanoma, nodular melanoma, acral lentiginous melanoma, amelanotic melanoma and lentigo maligna melanoma.

## Types of melanoma

### Superficial spreading melanoma

Superficial spreading melanoma is the most common type of melanoma, Figure 1.3 shows the classic features of an irregular outline and a small patch of inflammation in a mole that had changed and increased in size since a holiday in the sun. The use of a dermatoscope will help confirm anxieties if the features of disordered pigmented pattern, multiple brown dots, pseudopods (kinked projections at the edge of superficial spreading melanoma), scar-like depigmentation and multiple colours are seen. In some, a blue veil is seen throughout the surface. At least one of these features should be seen if the lesion is a malignant melanoma (Menzies et al, 2000) (*Figure 1.4*).

### Nodular melanoma

Nodular melanoma most commonly found in middle-aged men on the chest and the back. It presents as a dark, rapidly growing nodule that shows invasive, vertical growth from the beginning and has therefore, potentially, a poorer prognosis (*Figure 1.5*).

### Acral lentiginous melanoma

An acral lentiginous melanoma is mainly seen on the soles of the feet, palms of the hand and under the nails, and accounts for 8% of cases of melanoma (Goldstein and Goldstein, 2001). It is the most prevalent type of melanoma to occur in the skin of black and Asian people. A raised dark area is surrounded by a paler, lentiginous area (*Figure 1.6*).

In cases of patients with subungual melanoma, it is important to look for Hutchinson's sign, in which there is associated pigmentation of the adjacent nail fold (Buxton, 2003).

### Amelanotic melanoma

This anaplastic melanoma develops from melanocytes, without the formation of melanin (*Figure 1.7*). It is a

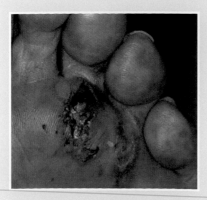

Figure 1.6. Acral malignant melanoma
on sole of foot.

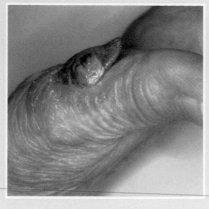

Figure 1.7. Amelanotic malignant melanoma.

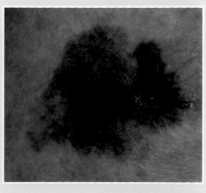

Figure 1.8. Lentigo maligna with in situ
malignant melanoma.

reminder not to ignore a lesion because it is not pigmented because amelanotic melanomas do occur. When in doubt about a lesion, it should be excised with adequate margin or biopsied. This elderly woman noticed that the lesion on her thumb had increased in size over the previous 6 months. Histology confirmed the diagnosis of an amelanotic melanoma.

### Lentigo maligna melanoma

Lentigo maligna lesions (also known as Hutchinson's freckle) are commonly seen on sun-exposed areas such as the face (*Figure 1.8*). The flat, pigmented brown or black lesion, with an irregular edge, gradually increases in size. In time, it may invade the basement membrane and this part of the lesion becomes thickened and nodular. It is then described as a lentigo maligna melanoma. A biopsy was taken from the thickened part of this lesion and confirmed as an *in situ* malignant melanoma.

## Prognosis

Success in the treatment of malignant melanoma is dependent on its site and thickness (Breslow thickness) (*Table 1.2*), therefore, early diagnosis and excision with sufficient margin is crucial.

The prospect for patients with more advanced disease is poor. This patient (*Figure 1.9*), who had been applying hydrocortisone ointment to an undiagnosed lesion, not only had wide local spread, but also inguinal lymph gland involvement. Open biopsy of the glands may be recommended to confirm such spread, and block dissection may be considered if computed tomography (CT) scan or ultrasound of the liver is found to be clear. Even so, the prognosis is not good. Although trials of adjuvant systemic therapy are continuing, there is not currently a standard approach (Roberts et al, 2002).

Where there is obvious metastatic disease, as in the patient in *Figure 1.10*, who has secondary nodules on the chest wall, gross weight-loss and several other melanomas, palliative care is all that is available. It may be worth removing solitary metastases, and although radiotherapy may be used for bone or skin metastases, short term symptomatic control is all that can be hoped for. New research continues in the search for other treatments for malignant melanoma with some hopes for a successful vaccine, new chemotherapy strategies and other drugs which hold out some promise for the future (Gore and Marais, 2005).

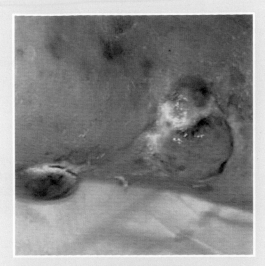

**Figure 1.9. Avanced malignant melanoma with local spread**

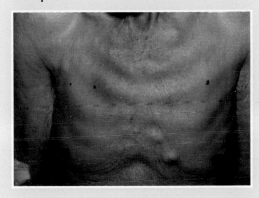

**Figure 1.10. Metastatic malignant melanoma with secondary nodules.**

## Prevention of melanoma

Prevention is obviously better than cure. There is now much more awareness of the risks associated with sun damage to the skin, and it is a message that is crucial to remember. On visiting Australia and New Zealand, for example, it is evident that there is a greater national awareness. It is normal practice to be equipped with a hat and cover-up clothes, particularly for children, and to adequately and frequently apply sun lotion. Schools also have strict policies and appropriate uniforms for outdoor sports and activities. If such practices are coupled with a good awareness of any skin changes that could indicate a malignant melanoma at an

## Table 1.2. Prognosis of malignant melanoma

| Breslow thickness | Excision margins | 5-year survival rate | Follow-up |
| --- | --- | --- | --- |
| *In situ* | 2–5 mm | 95–100% | Once after complete excision of primary lesion |
| <1 mm | 1 cm | 95–100% | Once after complete excision of primary lesion providing the specialist is satisfied |
| 1–2 mm | 1–2 cm | 80–96% | 3 monthly for 3 years Then 6 monthly for 2 years |
| 2.1–4 mm | 2–3 cm | 60–75% | 3 monthly for 3 years Then 6 monthly for 2 years |
| >4 mm | 2–4 cm | 50% | 3 monthly for 3 years Then 6 monthly for 2 years |

early stage, together with a greater input for those at greatest risk, this early intervention should also save lives. The BAD guidelines on prevention, state that:

- Individuals, particularly children, should not get sunburnt
- White skinned individuals should limit their total cumulative sun exposure throughout life
- Suspicious and changing moles should be seen by a doctor and undergo complete excision or be dealt with by the specialist
- A patient with a suspicious mole should be seen by a specialist within 2 weeks of receipt of a referral letter.
- All excised moles should be examined histologically to confirm the diagnosis and be complete removed with a sufficiently wide margin.

## Test Your Knowledge

This elderly woman went to stay with a friend for a holiday by the sea about 4 weeks previously. The friend first noticed the 'mole' on her leg while they were sitting on the beach. Since that time, it had increased in size, and by the time she saw her GP it measured about 1 cm across. It caused her no pain but did itch slightly. The doctor referred her urgently to the hospital for a further opinion as he suspected that is was a malignant melanoma.

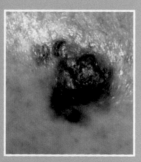

### Questions

1. What features of this lesion would lead you to suspect the diagnosis of malignant melanoma?
2. What action should be taken in a case such as this?
3. What further advice would you give to the patient and how could you discuss any future management with her?

## Conclusion

Practice nurses are advised to follow the guidelines of the BAD (Roberts et al, 2004) when assessing potential malignancy, taking into account the differential diagnoses and those at greatest risk. It is also important to advise patients of the preventive measures that should be taken to avoid melanoma.

## References

Buxton P (2003) Black spots in the skin. In: *ABC of Dermatology*. 4th edn. BMJ Publishing Group Ltd, London: 69

du Vivier A (2002) Malignant melanoma. In: *Atlas of Clinical Dermatology*. 3rd edn. Churchill Livingstone, London: 215–6

Goldstein B, Goldstein A (2001) Diagnosis and management of malignant melanoma. *Am Fam Physician* **63**(7): www.aafp.org/afp/20010401/1359.html (accessed 17 April 2007)

Gore M, and Marais R (2005) Institute of Cancer Research Annual Report 2005 www.icr.ac.uk/about_us/annual_research_report/5869.pdf (accessed 21 July 2010)

Kantor J (2004) Bathing trunk nevus. *University of Pennsylvania Health Service Encylopedia* www.pennhealth.com/ency/article/001453.htm (accessed 19 April 2007)

Mackie RN, Rycroft M (1988) Health and the ozone layer: skin cancers may increase dramatically. *BMJ* **297:** 369–70

Menzies S, Crotty K, Ingvar C et al (2000) Two step procedure for diagnosis of pigmented lesions. In: An Atlas of Surface Microscopy of Pigmented Skin Lesions: *Dermoscopy*. 2nd edn. McGraw-Hill Companies Inc, Australia: 153–4

Muir CS, Waterhouse J, Mack T (1987) Cancer Incidence in five continents. International Agency for Research on Cancer, Lyons

NLH Question-Answering Service (2006) What is the evidence that annual mole mapping detects early malignant melanomas? 18 May. www.clinicalanswers.nhs.uk/index.cfm?question=2911 (accessed 23 April 2007)

Roberts D, Anstey A, Barlow R (2002) *UK Guidelines for the Management of Cutaneous Melanoma*. British Association of Dermatologists, London

Whiteman D, Green A (1994) Sunburn and melanoma. *Cancer Causes Control* **5**(6): 564–72

# Malignant melanomas and seborrhoeic warts

People today are often reminded to look out for moles. They are warned of the risk of malignant melanoma and reminded that early diagnosis may make the difference between a 'cure' and a disastrous outcome. Not surprisingly patients frequently attend the surgery requesting action or reassurance. Sometimes it is easy to reassure patients that their 'mole' is not a melanoma. In other cases, the true nature of the 'mole' is more doubtful. However, the presence of certain signs can help the practice nurse be more confident about the diagnosis and help her decide whether to refer the patient immediately to the GP or give advice. Two types of mole that are difficult to distinguish are seborrhoeic warts and malignant melanomas.

## Seborrhoeic wart

Seborrhoeic warts, also called seborrhoeic keratosis or basal cell papilloma, are benign lesions, which usually occur in patients over 40 years of age. Seborrhoeic warts are regular in shape, outline and colour, but may be black, brown, yellow or pale. They have a greasy, granular or crumbly, 'stuck-on' appearance and do not ooze or bleed. They sit above the skin surface.

Seborrhoeic warts rarely cause serious long-term problems. They may be a cosmetic concern for the patient, and the occasional seborrhoeic wart causes problems by catching on clothes. The lesion can be treated by cryotherapy with liquid nitrogen if the patient wishes, but larger warts may need to be treated by curettage and cautery or, occasionally, excision.

*Figure 2.1* shows Bill's seborrhoeic wart. Bill is a 70 year-old man who has been aware of the mole on his back for many years. He thinks it has begun to enlarge in the last few months. It causes him no problems, does not itch, feel sore, weep or bleed. On examination the main lesion is uniformly black and has a waxy appearance. In the secondary underlying lesion there is more variation in colour. Both lesions have a regular outline and a 'stuck-on' appearance. The entire mole is about 20 x 15 mm in diameter.

## Superficial spreading malignant melanoma

Malignant melanoma is a serious condition that requires immediate referral and urgent treatment. Lesions are irregular in shape and colour, usually at least 7 mm in diameter, and may ooze, crust or bleed. They are more common in young adults. It is more likely to occur on skin exposed to the sun, e.g. the face, the lower leg in women who wear skirts, and on the back in men. Exposure often occurs during childhood.

A malignant melanoma needs urgent treatment with wide excision, and its complete removal needs to be confirmed by histological examination. After excision, the patient must be followed up to check that the melanoma does not recur and that the patient does not develop any other lesions.

The prognosis for malignant melanoma depends on the thickness of the lesion. If the lesion is less than 1.49 mm thick, the outlook is excellent, with a 5-year survival of 90%. Lesions 1.5 mm–3.49 mm thick are disease free 5 years after excision in 67% of cases. Only 38% of lesions thicker than 3.49 mm are disease free 5 years after excision.

*Figure 2.2* shows a malignant melanoma of the superficial spreading type in an 83-year-old man. Tom's daughter noticed this mole on the sole of his foot when he was sunbathing on the beach. This is an unusual position for malignant melanoma to occur. The lesion causes Tom no pain or discomfort and does not itch, crust or bleed. On examination the lesion shows several shades of brown and its edges are irregular. It measures about 10 mm across.

## Advice

Because Tom's mole has only just been noticed and is irregular in shape and colour, the practice nurse decides it

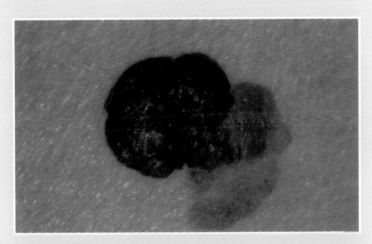

*Figure 2.1. Bill's seborrhoeic wart.*

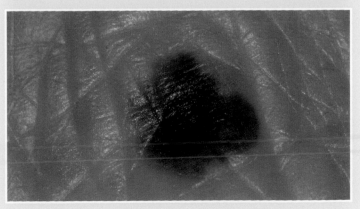

*Figure 2.2. Tom's superficial spreading malignant melanoma.*

## Table 2.1. Differential diagnosis

| Seborrhoeic wart | Malignant melanoma |
| --- | --- |
| Benign | Malignant |
| The patient is usually over the age of 40 years, but lesions may occur at a younger age. Common in the elderly | More common in young adults but may also occur in the elderly |
| The patient is likely to have several other similar lesions | One lesion will often look different from any other 'moles' |
| Regular shape and outline | Irregular, asymmetrical shape |
| Regular colour: either black, brown, yellow or pale | Irregular colour. Occasionally a lesion is non-pigmented |
| The lesion has a greasy, crumbly or granular, 'stuck-on' appearance. On the face they are often rather flat. Does not ooze or bleed | The lesion may ooze, crust or bleed |
| The bulk of the lesion is above the skin surface, i.e. is often present for many years | May have been present for –6 months with recent change in size. Usually ≥ 7 mm in diameter |
| May itch | May itch |

is probably a melanoma that has appeared recently and is increasing in size. She asks Tom to wait to see the GP for referral to a surgeon. Then she answers Tom's questions before he returns to the waiting room. She explains that the main factor associated with the development of malignant melanoma is exposure of white skin to sunlight. Problems are most likely to occur in people who burn easily in the sun, especially if they do not tan. People with fair or red hair and blue eyes are at greater risk. Those with large numbers of normal moles (i.e. more than 100) or with a family history of malignant melanoma are also at greater risk. Patients should be advised to monitor their moles for one that changes and stands out from the rest. Patients with multiple moles might be encouraged to photograph them, so that they can compare their appearance over time.

The practice nurse advises Tom always to wear a hat and T-shirt and liberally apply a 15+ sunscreen whenever he is likely to be exposed to the sun, especially during the warmer months. She explains this is necessary before and after his melanoma is removed, and that he should take particular care if visiting hot climates. She asks him to make a follow-up appointment once lesion is removed.

### Differential diagnosis

Several features distinguish a malignant melanoma from a seborrhoeic wart (*Table 2.1*). In cases where the diagnosis is uncertain, the lesion can be biopsied or excised, and sent for histology to confirm the diagnosis and the completeness of excision.

### Reference
Mackie RM (1989) *Malignant Melanoma. A Guide to Early Diagnosis.* Upjohn, London

# Test Your Knowledge

This 'mole' was noticed on 34-year-old Gianni's left forearm when he had vaccinations for his trip to Kenya. He had been aware of it, but had not worried because it caused him no trouble. It does not itch, crust or bleed, but has grown slightly in size in the last 3 months. It measures 10 × 7.5 mm and has a slightly raised, irregularly pigmented edge.

### Questions
1. What is the possible diagnosis?
2. What are the first three things you would do to help Gianni?

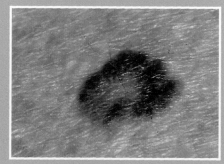

# Mimickers of malignant melanoma

Discussion in the media and greater public understanding of malignant melanoma has created a steady stream of patients coming to the surgery worried about a mole that may have appeared or recently changed. Anxieties are increased if the mole is pigmented. Faced with such a patient the practice nurse needs to decide whether or not any action is required.

In some cases the diagnosis may be obvious; in others there may be doubt. Sometimes the lesion is unsightly and the patient will ask for it to be removed for cosmetic reasons. For others, biopsy or excision of the lesion may be necessary.

The presenting lesions must be assessed carefully before giving advice, reassurance or any medication. It is important to avoid a situation in which a patient returns some time later with an advanced-stage melanoma that has been overlooked and may then be difficult to treat (*Figure 3.1*). This chapter considers some of the benign lesions that may raise doubts about the correct diagnosis.

## Melanocytic naevi

Melanocytic naevi are made up of clusters of melanin-bearing melanocytes (British Association of Dermatologists, 2005). These benign, asymptomatic, pigmented lesions may be termed congenital or acquired. They are extremely common but their cause remains unknown (Calmont, 2006).

### Congenital melanocytic naevi

Congenital melanocytic naevi are present at birth and may be present anywhere on the body. They may vary in size and be pigmented, smooth, warty, lobular or sometimes have raised mamillary projections (*Figure 3.2*). They are usually more than 1 cm in diameter. With growth they increase in size and in time, become darker, raised and may be hairy (*Figure 3.3*). Occasionally they may be large, covering extensive areas (giant hairy pigmented naevus).

### Acquired melanocytic naevi

Acquired melanocytic naevi are normally less than 1cm in diameter and evenly coloured.

### *Junctional melanocytic naevi*

Most junctional type naevi develop in childhood and throughout the first three decades of life. However, they seem to decrease with age. It is thought that they may be associated with excess exposure to the sun. They are small, flat or slightly raised and brown in colour, and may become raised and hairy later in life.

### *Compound melanocytic naevi*

A compound melanocytic naevus is raised, pigmented and sharply defined, round or oval, with a smooth or warty surface (*Figure 3.4*).

### *Blue naevus*

A blue naevus is a heavily pigmented melanocytic naevus that lies deeper in the lower dermis and so takes on a blue colour, owing to the refracting qualities of the skin (*Figure 3.5*). It is thought to be the result of a failure of melanocytes to reach the dermo-epidermal junction from the neural crest (du Vivier, 2002: 201). It presents as a symptomless, smooth, round papule or nodule that is usually less than 0.5 cm in diameter. It may occur anywhere on the body but is commonly seen on the face, scalp, hands and feet.

### *Halo naevus*

A halo naevus is seen relatively frequently in children and young adults. A circulating antibody and T cells attack the pigment cells in the mole and its surrounding skin, causing it to fade and eventually disappear (*Figure 3.6*). The mole itself is usually benign but very occasionally the same phenomenon may occur in association with a melanoma. Careful examination of the lesion should therefore be made (DermNet NZ, 2007).

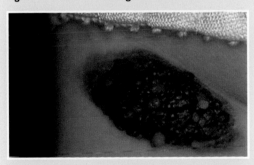

*Figure 3.1. Advanced malignant melanoma.*

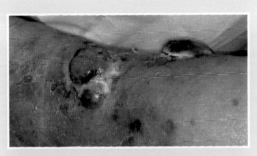

*Figure 3.2. Congenital melanocytic pigmented naevus with mamillary projections.*

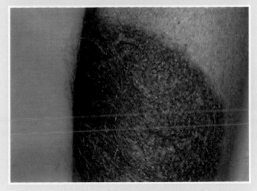

*Figure 3.3. Hairy, congenital melanocytic naevus.*

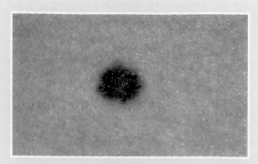

Figure 3.4. Benign warty, melanocytic compound naevus, confirmed by biopsy.

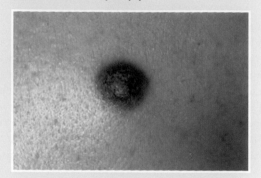

Figure 3.5. Blue naevus.

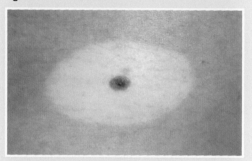

Figure 3.6. Halo naevus.

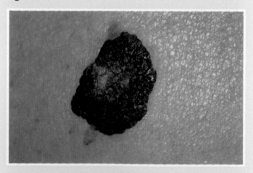

Figure 3.7. Basal cell papilloma.

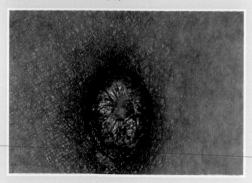

Figure 3.8. Inflamed basal cell papilloma.

## Management

Before reassurance can be offered, the rest of the skin should be examined to exclude any other suspicious lesions, especially the areas that have been at risk of sun exposure and sunburn. The risk of malignant change in most naevi is low but the patient should be encouraged to seek help in the event of change in any mole, particularly in relation to change in size, irregularity of outline and colour, itching or crusting.

In the case of large congenital moles where the risk of malignancy may be as high as 4–20% (De Raeve et al, 2005), excision, if this is feasible, may be suggested to avoid future change. Sun protection should be advised either in the form of a high factor sun-screen and/or covering clothes. The dermatoscope is a useful tool for those properly trained in its use, and will often help identify worrying moles that might need biopsy and/or excision (Menzies et al, 2003). A few moles will require removal for cosmetic or comfort reasons.

## Basal cell papilloma

Basal cell papillomas, or seborrhoeic warts, are benign lesions that are extremely common in the elderly although, not infrequently, they are seen in the younger people who may have suffered sunburn in childhood. The sudden appearance of large numbers of basal cell papillomas can be associated with an underlying malignancy (duVivier, 2002), or they may be particularly prolific in those with an inherited tendency (DermNet NZ, 2006).

They may start as brown spots but then gradually thicken. The well-defined lesions have a roughened, often fissured surface and 'stuck-on' appearance (*Figure 3.7*). The colour may range from yellow to brown or black. Basal cell papillomas are usually symptomless but may sometimes itch or become inflamed (*Figure 3.8*).

## Management

Removal may be considered if there is any doubt about the diagnosis, or if the patient wishes, because it rubs against clothes or for cosmetic reasons. The following methods of treatment are available:

- Cryotherapy (or laser therapy), as long as there is no doubt about the diagnosis
- Curettage and cautery
- Shave biopsy.

## Dermatofibroma

The cause of this benign, fibrous skin lesion is unknown but sometimes it seems to follow some minor injury such as a thorn prick or insect bite. Once developed, it persists for years. It is of no significance but occasionally raises concern if it mimics the appearance of a melanoma. Dermatofibromas present as firm nodules but often are coloured yellow or brown (*Figure 3.9*). If squeezed, a dimple appears in the overlying skin (DermNet NZ, 2006).

## Management

If the diagnosis is certain or if the lesion is cosmetically acceptable, no action is required but excision and histological examination should be carried out if there is any concern.

## Black heel syndrome

Black heel syndrome may occur in keen sports players and develops as the result of bleeding into the stratum corneum owing to shearing of the small capillaries when the skin rubs against footwear. It manifests as a blackened area on the foot at a shearing site (*Figure 3.10*), and may mimic a melanoma. However, if the lesion is pared with a scalpel, flecks of blood can be seen in the skin or it should be possible to distinguish it by the use of a dermatoscope.

*Management*

Once convinced about the diagnosis, no treatment is required for this condition, which should quickly settle. The patient can be advised to wear padded insoles in the shoes to protect the foot from further damage

## Venous lake

Venous lakes, or cavernous lakes, occur most often in men over the age of 50 years and are thought to be related to sun damage. Clinically they are symptomless and unimportant, except insofar as they may mimic the more serious problems of melanoma or basal cell carcinoma.

They appear as well-defined, single or multiple, soft, purple papules with a smooth surface that may reach up to 1 cm in diameter. They occur in sun-exposed areas of the head and neck as well as the vermillion border of the lower lip (*Figure 3.11*). The lesion can be blanched by compression with a glass microscope slide and it may be possible to differentiate the lesion from other more serious problems if viewed under the dermatoscope. This will show a homogeneous red-blue or black colour and no pigment network structures (Wang and Wang, 2005).

Management options are:

* Biopsy or excision if the diagnosis is in doubt
* Surgery: cryosurgery, electrosurgery or excision if removal is required for cosmetic reasons
* Laser treatment has been used but is liable to leave scarring.

## Pigmented basal cell carcinoma

Basal cell carcinoma is a common problem, especially in the fair-skinned, fair-haired, blue-eyed community who have had more than their ration of sun exposure. Checks on the size, colour, texture and appearance of these lesions will give clues to the diagnosis. The various features of basal cell carcinoma can be studied elsewhere (Halachmi, 2006).

In some cases, a basal cell carcinoma may be pigmented and raise concerns of a melanoma. In the case shown in *Figure 3.12*, the well-marginated, ulcerated lesion showed a pigmented area within it that raised doubts about the diagnosis.

In other cases there may be irregular pigmentation in a well-defined nodule, with telangiectatic vessels running across the surface.

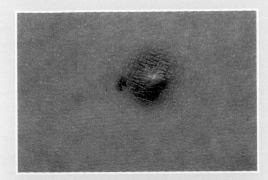

*Figure 3.9. Dermatofibroma.*

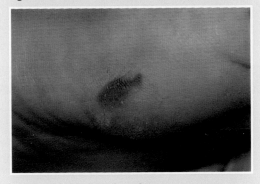

*Figure 3.10. Black heel syndrome.*

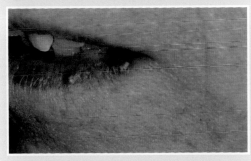

*Figure 3.11. Venous lakes.*

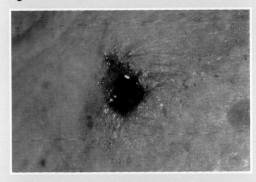

*Figure 3.12. Pigmented basal cell carcinoma.*

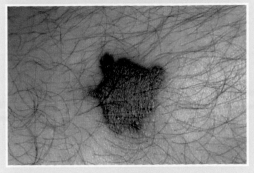

*Figure 3.13. Kaposi's sarcoma.*

### Management

Excision and histological examination of the lesion is the approach in most instances. The lesion in *Figure 3.12* was confirmed as a completely excised basal cell carcinoma.

Other approaches such as curettage and electrocautery or cryotherapy to destroy remaining cells are possible, but these interventions carry a risk of recurrence. They also have the effect of eliminating the opportunity to make an accurate diagnosis of the lesion.

In the case of more extensive lesions or where there is spread elsewhere in the body, radiotherapy is an option (Halachmi, 2006).

## Kaposi's sarcoma

This once rare, malignant tumour of connective tissue is now seen more often, in association with immunosuppression and AIDS. It develops very rapidly and affects the skin or other organs such as the gastrointestinal tract and the lungs.

Blue-red macules develop on the skin, and they become purple as they form plaques (*Figure 3.13*). They may occur anywhere on the skin but tend to appear first on the feet and limbs. Internal lesions may lead to melena, haematemesis or haemoptysis.

### Management

The underlying condition must be dealt with. Biopsy of a skin lesion will confirm the diagnosis and an endoscopy may be required to assess the state of the gastrointestinal tract. In the case of AIDS, antiviral therapy may help shrink the lesions. Alternative approaches are radiotherapy, cryotherapy or chemotherapy (Nanda, 2006).

## Table 3.1. The differential diagnosis of lesions that mimic malignant melanoma

| Lesion | Possible causes | Presentation | Management Choices |
|---|---|---|---|
| Congenital melanocytic naevi | Unknown | • Present at birth, <br> • Pigmented, smooth, warty, <br> • lobular, mamillary projections, <br> • Usually >1 cm diameter | • Exclude other lesions <br> • Sun protection <br> • Biopsy if diagnosis in doubt <br> • Excision as required <br> • Cryotherapy <br> • Curettage and cautery or shave biopsy |
| Acquired melanocytic naevi | • Unknown <br> • Sun exposure | • Develop in children and young adults <br> • Flat, raised, pigmented, sometimes hairy <br> • Usually <1 cm | *As congenital melanocytic naevi* |
| Compound melanocytic naevi | Unknown | Sharply defined, round or oval, pigmented Smooth or warty surface | *As congenital melanocytic naevi* |
| Blue naevus | Developmental anomaly | • Smooth round, blue papule <br> • Usually face, scalp, hands or feet | • None required <br> • Excision as required |
| Halo naevus | Probable autoimmune phenemenon Circulating antibody and T-cells attack the pigment cells | • Children and young adults <br> • Pallor of skin around resolving mole | • None required <br> • Biopsy/excision if diagnosis in doubt |
| Basal cell papilloma | • Degenerative change <br> • Genetic <br> • Sun damage | • Brown, yellow or black spots that thicken <br> • Rough, fissured, 'stuck-on' appearance | • Unnecessary unless required by patient <br> • Cryotherapy or laser <br> • Curettage and cautery or shave biopsy |
| Dermatofibroma | • Unknown <br> • Minor injury, e.g. insect bite | • Firm, yellow or brown nodule <br> • Dimples when squeezed | • None required <br> • Biopsy if diagnosis in doubt |
| Black heel syndrome | Trauma | • Blackened area on foot <br> • Flecks of blood when skin pared | Padded insoles in shoes |
| Venous lake | Sun damage | • Smooth purple nodules that blanch on compression <br> • Single or multiple, up to 1 cm in diameter <br> • Head and neck, lower lip | • Biopsy if in doubt <br> • Cryosurgery, electrosurgery or excision <br> • Laser (may scar) <br> • Sun protection |
| Pigmented basal cell carcinoma | Sun damage | Well marginated ulcer or well-defined nodule with overlying telangiectasia, pigmented | • Complete excision if possible <br> • Curettage and cautery or cryotherapy <br> • Radiotherapy |
| Kaposi's sarcoma | Association with immunosuppression | Blue or red macules, especially on feet and limbs | • Biopsy to confirm diagnosis <br> • Endoscopy to assess gastrointestinal tract <br> • Assess AIDS status <br> • Antiviral therapy, radiotherapy, cryotherapy or chemotherapy |

## Conclusions

There are a variety of moles and skin presentations that may mimic malignant melanoma (*Table 3.1*) and it is important to make a careful assessment and diagnosis of a patient's presenting lesions before giving any advice, reassurance or medication. Some of the conditions that mimic malignant melanoma have relatively benign or cosmetic consequences, but others are more serious and require careful attention and treatment.

## References

British Association of Dermatologists (2005) Melanocytic naevi. www.bad.org.uk/public/leaflets/melanocytic.asp (accessed 19 June 2007)

Calmont T (2006) Nevi, melanocytic. http://emedicine.com/derm/topic289.htm (accessed 19June 2007)

De Raeve L, Danau W, De Backer A et al (2005) Prepubertal melanoma in a medium sized congenital naevus. www.springerlink.com/content/h83x13774h3rm13h/ (accessed 19June 2007)

DermNet NZ (2006) Dermatofibroma. www.dermnetnz.org/lesions/dermatofibroma.html (accessed 19June 2007)

DermNet NZ (2007) Halo moles. www.dermnetnz.org/lesions/halo-mole.html (accessed 19June2007)

DermNet NZ (2006) Seborrhoeic keratoses. www.dermnetnz.org/lesions/seborrhoeic-keratosis.html (accessed 19 June 2007)

du Vivier A (2002) Benign tumours of the skin. In: *Atlas of Clinical Dermatology*. 3rd edn. Churchill Livingstone: 130–2

Halachmi S (2006) Basal cell carcinoma. Medline Plus. Medical Encyclopaedia.www.nlm.nih.gov/medlineplus/encyarticle/000824.htm (accessed 19June 2007)

## Test Your Knowledge

A 51-year-old women attended the surgery concerned about a mole on her right shoulder. She said that it had been present for many years, but that in recent weeks it had seemed to increase in size and become darker. Her general health was otherwise good and on examination there was no evidence of enlargement of any lymph nodes.

### Questions

1. From the clinical appearance of the lesion, what might you consider to be the most likely diagnosis in this case, and which features would you feel might suggest this?
2. What action would you take?
3. What advice would you give to this patient about future management?

Menzies S, Crotty K, Ingvar C et al (2003) *An Atlas of Surface Microscopy of Pigmented Skin Lesions, Dermascopy.* 2nd edn. McGraw-Hill Companies Inc, Australia

Nanda R (2006) Kaposi's sarcoma, Medline Plus. Medical Encyclopaedia. www.nlm.nih.gov/medlineplus/ency/article/000661.htm (accessed 19June 2007)

Wang J, Wang K (2005) Venous lakes. www.emedicine.com/derm/topic451.htm (accessed 19June2007)

# Keratoacanthoma/ Basal cell carcinoma/ Squamous cell carcinoma

Keratoacanthoma (KA), basal cell carcinoma (BCC) and squamous cell carcinoma (SCC) often have similar presentations and an accurate diagnosis is required for effective treatment. They are relatively common skin tumours in older people. Chronic overexposure to the sun or x-rays predispose people to these problems, which usually develop in sun-exposed areas, e.g. the face (particularly the nose, cheeks and ears) the backs of the hands and forearms. People with fair hair and blue eyes are more susceptible.

Industrial exposure to carcinogens such as tar, mineral oils or soot and ingestion of arsenic, which used to be in some of the older 'tonics' puts people at higher risk. Transplant recipients and the immunosuppressed are also at risk. An accurate clinical diagnosis is difficult in some cases because these three conditions display similar features (*Table 4.1*).

## Keratoacanthoma

Patients who present with KA often have a history of some minor injury to the area before the development of a KA. KAs arise from a single hair follicle and only occur on hair bearing skin. The lesion starts as a small spot, which rapidly increases in size over a few weeks. The papule develops into a red or flesh-coloured, well-defined nodule that stands proud from the surrounding normal skin. It has a central, keratin-filled crater with a surrounding collarette of tissue (*Figure 4.1*).

A KA may reach a size of 2 cm or more in diameter before it begins to involute and heal, leaving a pitted scar. The whole process may take about 4–12 months. Occasionally, the lesion may transform into a SCC.

It may be impossible to make a positive diagnosis of KA histologically. The pathological report usually returns a diagnosis of SCC, even though the lesion is, in fact, a KA and would resolve spontaneously. A short history of a few weeks suggests a KA.

Treatment of some kind is usually recommended because of the uncertainty of diagnosis, the appearance of the lesion and the fact that spontaneous resolution is likely to leave an unsightly scar.

There are three choices of treatment available: these are curettage and cautery, excision, and radiotherapy.

**Curettage and cautery** is the treatment of choice but should be done before spontaneous regression has begun. Once scar tissue has started to form it may be difficult to curette. The lesion may recur if it is not completely removed or it was in fact a SCC.

**Excision** under local anaesthetic is an option. However, it leaves the patient with a scar.

**Radiotherapy** may involve several visits to the hospital and subsequent scarring.

## Basal cell carcinoma

There are several different types of BCC (or rodent ulcer). The nodulo-ulcerative type is the one most likely to be confused with KA.

**Nodulo-ulcerative BCC** (*Figure 4.2*) is the most common type of BCC. It presents with a small, painless, translucent, skin-coloured papule that slowly enlarges over months or years. There follows central necrosis that may leave a crusting ulcer that may bleed and fail to heal. It has a rolled, pearly edge that can best be demonstrated by stretching the lesion with the fingers placed on either side of it.

## Table 4.1. Comparison of keratoacanthoma, basal cell carcinoma and squamous cell carcinoma

| | Keratoacanthoma | Basal cell carcinoma | Squamous cell carcinoma |
|---|---|---|---|
| **Rate of growth** | Rapid: a few weeks | Slow: months or years | Slower: months |
| **Appearance** | Flesh coloured, well defined nodule, central, keratin-filled crater | Small, painless, skin coloured, translucent, papule. Later, central necrosis and crusting ulcer | Thickened area of skin becomes indurated plaque fixed and nodular. Later ulcerated and crusted |
| **Edges of lesion** | Collarette of tissue | Raised, rolled pearly edge | Firm, often everted and irregular in shape |
| **Biopsy** | Inconclusive | Confirms BCC | Confirms SCC |
| **Untreated outcome** | Involution with residual scar | Locally invasive | Metastasizes to lymph nodes If untreated, may be fatal |
| **Treatment of choice** | Currettage and cautery | Local excision | Local excision |
| **Other treatments** | Local excision Radiotherapy | Radiotherapy Currettage and cautery Cryotherapy | Radiotherapy Currettage and cautery |

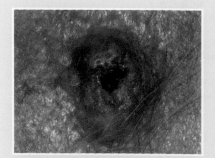

Figure 4.1. Keratoacanthoma.

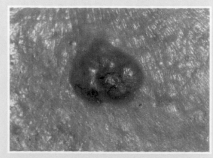

Figure 4.3. Cystic basal cell carcinoma.

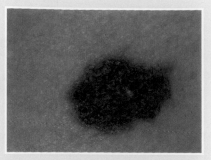

Figure 4.5 Superficial basal cell carcinoma.

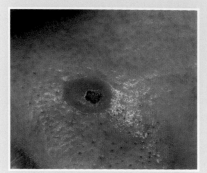

Figure 4.2. Nodulo-ulcerative
basal cell carcinoma.

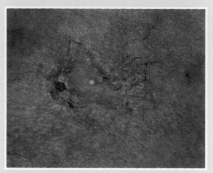

Figure 4.4. Cicatricial (morphoeic)
basal cell carcinoma.

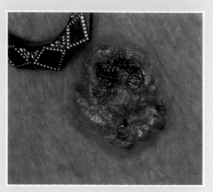

Figure 4.6. Pigmented basal cell carcinoma.

**Cystic BCC** (*Figure 4.3*) starts as a nodular BCC but cystic features persist. The nodule becomes more tense and translucent with obvious telangiectasia.

**Cicatricial (morphoeic) BCC** (*Figure 4.4*) looks like an enlarging scar as the yellow or white plaque gradually enlarges. Ulceration, crusting and fibrosis may follow. The edge of the lesion may be ill-defined but a raised, rolled edge may be seen.

**Superficial BCC** (*Figure 4.5*) may develop as several lesions, usually on the trunk. A pink or brown scaly plaque gradually increases in size. If untreated, it may reach as much as 10 cm in diameter. A fine 'whipcord' edge can usually be demonstrated.

**Pigmented BCC** (*Figure 4.6*) has the characteristic features of BCC, but the edges are pigmented. This sometimes leads to confusion with a malignant melanoma.

BCC rarely metastasizes but is locally invasive. It may, if untreated, gradually infiltrate underlying structures with serious consequences. Biopsy of the lesion should confirm a diagnosis of BCC.

Intervention of some kind should be offered to the patient. There is a 95% cure rate for BCC (Leppard and Ashton, 1998). Four treatment options are available: local excision, radiotherapy, curettage and cautery and cryotherapy.

**Local excision** is usually the treatment of choice. If the tumour is removed together with 1–2 mm of normal skin around it, the results should be satisfactory. If a large area is involved, a plastic surgeon may be required to ensure a good cosmetic result.

Particularly difficult areas are around the eyes or nose when Moh's micrographic surgery may be needed to ensure complete excision while preserving the surrounding tissues as much as possible. The excised lesion should be sent to pathology to confirm the diagnosis and whether complete excision of the lesion has been achieved.

There are three available treatment options: radiotherapy, curettage and cautery, and cryotherapy.

**Radiotherapy** should be preceded by biopsy to confirm the diagnosis. Good results may be achieved, but the treatment may involve a number of visits to the hospital as well as subsequent unpleasant local reactions and later scarring.

**Curettage and cautery** may be more appropriate for very elderly people or for those with numerous small lesions, but there is a higher recurrence rate.

**Cryotherapy** should be reserved for the housebound elderly patient. The recurrence rate following cryotherapy is high and the treatment is fairly unpleasant.

## Squamous cell carcinoma

SCC (*Figure 4.7*) is most common in areas of sun-exposed skin but may occur at other sites such as the genitalia, mucous membranes and in the mouth. Chimney sweeps in the 19th century sometimes developed carcinoma of the scrotum. It may arise in a solar keratosis, in an area of Bowen's disease, in previously irradiated skin or in otherwise normal skin.

SCC may appear as a thickening of the skin, become an indurated plaque and later become fixed and nodular. The surface later becomes crusted and ulcerated. The edge is firm and often everted and irregular in shape. It grows more rapidly than a BCC but not as quickly as a KA.

SCC may metastasize to the lymph nodes and have fatal results. A biopsy of the lesion confirms the diagnosis. There are three available treatment options: local excision, radiotherapy, and curettage and cautery.

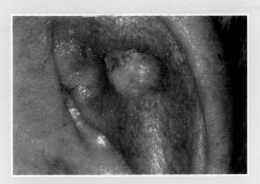

*Figure 4.7. Squamous cell carcinoma.*

**Local excision** with a margin of normal skin 2–3 mm around the lesion is normally sufficient. If larger areas are involved, a skin graft may be required.

**Radiotherapy** may be preferable if the tumour is too large to consider excision. Many treatments will be required over a period of 2–3 weeks but the results are normally good.

**Curettage and cautery** may be preferable for elderly patients if surgery is likely to prove difficult.

## Reference

Leppard B, Ashton R (1998) *Treatment in Dermatology*. Radcliffe Medical Press, Oxford: Vol A–D: 27

## Further reading

du Vivier A (1993) Solar damage and skin cancer. In: *Atlas of Clinical Dermatology*. 2nd edn. Gower Medical Publishing, London: 9.11–22

New Zealand DermNet (2002) Keratoacanthoma. www.dermnetnz.org (accessed 20 August 2002). New Zealand Dermatological Society

Rook A, Wilkinson DS, Ebling FJG (1986) *Textbook of Dermatology*. 3rd edn. Blackwell Scientific Publications, Oxford: Vol 2: 2149–51, 2169–77, 2186–90

# Test Your Knowledge

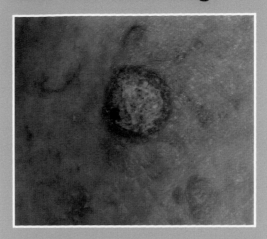

This 84-year-old woman presents with a crusting lesion on her right cheek. She first noticed a small spot about 18 months earlier. It gradually increased in size. It is not painful but is now causing problems because it bleeds if she scratches or knocks it. She has lived in India for many years and claims to be a 'sun-worshipper'. She has blue eyes and when younger had fair hair. She has always tended to burn in the sun.

## Questions

1. What is the likely diagnosis and what is there about the appearance of the lesion that might make you suspect this?
2. What treatment would you recommend?
3. What examinations would you do or arrange?

# Cutaneous T-cell lymphoma

Cutaneous T-cell lymphomas (CTCLs) are uncommon conditions that rarely present in the surgery. The fact that nurses are unlikely to have experienced such a problem previously may make it difficult to recognize the significance of symptoms that should be taken seriously, and therefore delay a correct diagnosis. This chapter will mainly focus on mycosis fungoides, which is the most common type of CTCL. Symptoms of this low-grade lymphoma often respond to treatment, but in the long run, it is incurable and a fatal outcome may follow. Studies have shown that the prognosis and mortality are related to the stage at which the condition is diagnosed (Pinter-Brown, 2006). It is, therefore, important to be aware of the warning signs that could enable an early diagnosis and early intervention, and benefit the patient.

Mycosis fungoides is the most common manifestation of CTCL but other, rarer conditions do occur, such as parapsoriasis, primary cutaneous anaplastic large cell lymphoma, lymphomatoid papulosis, Sézary syndrome (in which there is spread of the lymphoma to the rest of the body and its organs), and adult T-cell leukaemia/lymphoma (DermNet NZ, 2006).

## Mycosis fungoides
### Aetiology
The cause of CTCL is unknown, although there are a few theories suggesting exposure to substances such as Agent Orange, or viruses could play a part. However, nothing has been proven as yet. Changes in T-cells, which 'home to the

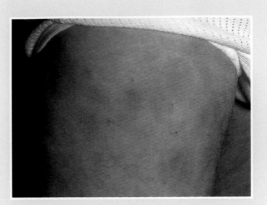

**Figure 5.1. Early mycosis fungoides with dry patchy rash.**

skin', allow abnormal neoplastic proliferation of the T-cells' lymphocytes with a T-subtype, leading to a malignant lymphoma. In some cases these malignant cells will travel to the lymph nodes and blood (Pinter-Brown, 2006). In essence, this is a systemic disease in which, at an early stage, clinical signs are limited to the skin. Some cases never progress further.

Mycosis fungoides is a rare condition that affects only 4 per 1 million people. It most commonly presents between the ages of 40–60 years, although it has occasionally been seen in children and younger people. It is more common in men and those with black skin (Cancer Research UK, 2006).

## Table 5.1. Presentations of cutaneous T-cell lymphoma

| Stage | Symptoms | Differential diagnosis | Treatment |
|---|---|---|---|
| **First stage** | • Single or multiple round or oval patches<br>• Dry, pink or red<br>• On the trunk and limbs<br>• Hyper/hypopigmentation in dark skinned<br>• Follicular mucinosis | • Psoriasis, eczema<br>• Skin biopsy necessary to confirm diagnosis of mycosis fungoides<br>• Full blood count and differential diagnosis | If rash does not respond to the normal treatments for eczema and psoriasis—consider the possibility of mycosis fungoides.<br>Biopsy may need to be repeated before a positive result is obtained |
| **Plaque stage** | • Rash more widespread<br>• Asymmetrical, odd shapes, central clearing, variety of colours<br>• Wrinkled and scaly<br>• Telangiectasia | | Other available treatments:<br>• Topical steroids<br>• UVL/PUVA<br>• Topical Nitrogen mustard<br>• Chemotherapy |
| **Tumour stage** | • Thickened, palpable, lesions—red or purple<br>• Mushroom-like lesions | | • Radiotherapy<br>• Interferon<br>• Oral retinoids |
| **Lymphadenopathy** | • Without malignant change in earlier cases<br>• Lymphoma cells in glands in more advanced disease. | | • Photophoresis |
| **Sézary syndrome** | • Extensive skin lesions<br>• Involvement of other organs | | |

PUVA = psoralen and ultra violet light; UVL = ultra violet light

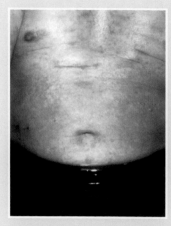

**Figure 5.2. Patient with chronic superficial eczema.**

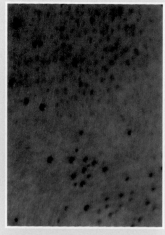

**Figure 5.4. Mucinous folliculitis in mycosis fungoides.**

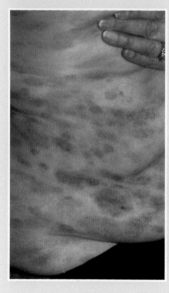

**Figure 5.3. Psoriasis.**

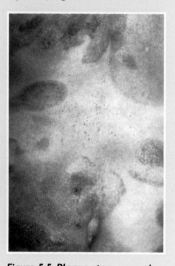

**Figure 5.5. Plaque stage mycosis fungoides.**

## Presentation

The signs of mycosis fungoides change with the progress of the disease (*Table 5.1*).

### First stage

Initially the patient may notice round or oval, dry, pink or red, single or multiple patches, usually on the trunk and limbs (*Figure 5.1*). At this stage there are unlikely to be problems of itching. These patches are barely palpable and may be misdiagnosed as eczema (*Figure 5.2*) or psoriasis (*Figure 5.3*). In those with dark skin, hyper- or hypopigmented patches may be visible. The rash may remain static, enlarge or disappear spontaneously.

Another feature that may present with the condition is follicular mucinosis. Mucin is deposited in the hair follicles and may form small cysts (*Figure 5.4*). Mycosis fungoides will not respond to the standard treatment of eczema or psoriasis and, therefore, such lack of response could alert the health professional to the possibility of a lymphoma.

### Plaque stage

As the disease progresses the rash becomes more widespread on the trunk and limbs. The rash is asymmetrical with odd shapes, central clearing and coloured a variety of reds and purples (*Figure 5.5*). The surface of the lesions is wrinkled and scaly and the patient is likely to complain of itching. Telangiectasia and atrophy of the skin may also be features.

### Tumour stage

Further progress of the disease is indicated by the development of thickened palpable, red or purple lesions that may be very itchy and ulcerate (*Figure 5.6*). At this late stage, large, mushroom-like lesions may develop (*Figure 5.7*). Occasionally, tumours are the first sign of the disease.

### Lymph node involvement

Spread to the lymph nodes with the development of a lymphadenopathy may occur. In the earlier stages the lymph glands may be enlarged without malignant change, but later lymphoma cells may be found in the nodes.

### Sézary syndrome

Sézary syndrome occurs at the late stage when large areas of skin are affected and abnormal lymphocytes are found in the blood and other organs such as the liver, lungs or bone marrow are involved. In these cases, all of the skin is affected and becomes bright red, thickened, scaly and itchy. The prognosis is poor at this stage of the disease, with a survival of only 2–4 years.

## Investigations

Skin biopsy should be taken to confirm the diagnosis of mycosis fungoides. This may not always prove positive and may need to be repeated several times in months or years before a conclusive diagnosis can be made. Histological changes, in the early stages, are not necessarily clear and may be difficult to separate from other conditions, especially eczema.

A full blood count is usually normal in mycosis fungoides, but if the lymphocyte count is raised or Sézary cells seen, it would indicate more serious problems.

In advanced cases, computed tomography (CT) or magnetic resonance imaging (MRI) scans are needed to assess the spread of the disease to other organs.

## Management

Cases of mycosis fungoides should be supervised by a hospital specialist. Depending on the stage of the condition and its response to treatment, the following options are available:

- Topical steroids
- Ultraviolet light (UVL)
- PUVA (psoralen and UVL)
- Topical nitrogen mustard
- Chemotherapy
- Radiotherapy
- Interferon
- Oral retinoids
- Photophoresis
- Surgical excision of localized lesion plus control with other treatments.

These treatments may be successful in improving symptoms, mortality rates and the prognosis of mycosis fungoides. This patient with a large tumour on her hand responded well to radiotherapy on the area (*Figure 5.8*).

## Parapsoriasis

### Aetiology

Parapsoriasis, or digitate dermatosis, is the term used to describe the problems of raised, scaly plaques that are similar to the plaques of psoriasis. Large plaque and small plaque parapsoriasis occur and are caused by T-cell predominant infiltrates in the skin (Wong, 2007).

Small plaque parapsoriasis rarely progresses and is a benign problem. In 10% of cases, large plaque parapsoriasis CTCL will develop later (Wong, 2007). It is an uncommon condition that usually occurs in middle-aged men.

### Presentation

The patient develops a rash of well-defined pink, red or brown, slightly scaly patches mainly on the trunk, backs of the thighs or inner aspects of the limbs. The lesions may tend to be either less than 5 mm in diameter (small plaque parapsoriasis) or greater than 6 mm (large plaque parapsoriasis).

Another variety of this problem is known as digitate dermatosis, in which the rash is streaked in finger-like processes (*Figure 5.9*). The rash itself causes few problems, apart from its appearance, and the prognosis for this condition is good with a 5-year survival rate of over 90% and long-term survival similar to that of the general population (Wong, 2007).

### Investigations

Skin biopsy should be performed to exclude the possibility of mycosis fungoides, as well as immunophenotyping and gene rearrangement studies (*Table 5.2*). A full blood count and differential is helpful as a high lymphocyte count or Sézary cells would suggest mycosis fungoides or CTCL.

### Management

In cases of small plaque parapsoriasis, treatment is only required to alleviate symptoms. Emollients may therefore help problems of scaling, and response may be better if topical steroids are used. It is recommended that large

## Table 5.2. Definitions

**Immunophenotyping**

An analytical method for dividing lymphomas and leukaemias into subgroups on the basis of differences in cell surfaces and cytoplasmic antigens. The antigenic differences are detected with monoclonal antibodies and flow cytometry.

**Gene rearrangement studies**

Examination of the ordered rearrangement of gene regions on the human genome which occurs normally during development, but may also cause disease such as cancer.

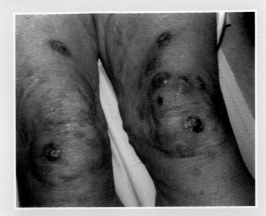

**Figure 5.6. Thickened, palpable red or purple lesions at the tumour stage of mycosis fungoides.**

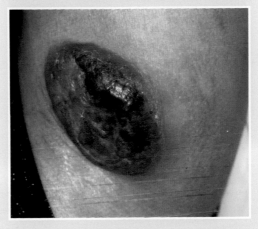

**Figure 5.7. Mushroom-like lesion in the axilla of a patient with tumour stage mycosis fungoides.**

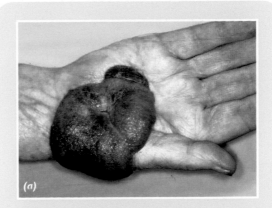

*(a)*

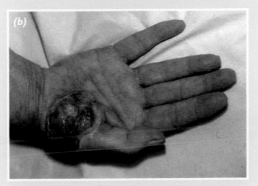

*(b)*

**Figure 5.8. (a) Tumour stage mycosis fungoides on the hand. (b) Tumour has regressed following radiotherapy.**

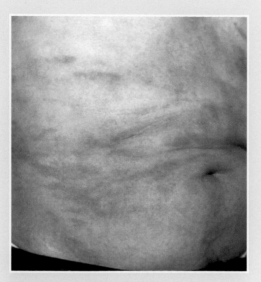

*Figure 5.9. Digitate dermatosis.*

plaque parapsoriasis should be treated, as this may prevent progress of the condition to mycosis fungoides. Choices are high potency topical steroids or phototherapy. Six-monthly follow-up should be recommended. Any deterioration in the condition could suggest progression of the disease and the development of mycosis fungoides. Further biopsy would be necessary. In any case, the patient should be under the care of a dermatologist.

### References

Cancer Research UK (2007) Cutaneous T-cell lymphoma. http:// tinyurl.com/29bemk (accessed 7 September 2007)

DermNet NZ (2006) Cutaneous T-cell lymphoma. http://tinyurl. com/2puhme (accessed 7 September 2007)

Pinter-Brown LC (2006) Mycosis Fungoides. *Emedicine*. http:// tinyurl.com/2wflx8 (accessed 7 September 2007)

Wong HK (2007) Parapsoriasis. *Emedicine*. http://tinyurl. com/2orw5k (accessed 7 September 2007)

### Further reading

Schwartz R (2010) Cutaneous T-cell Lymphoma *Emedicine* www. emedicine.medscape.com/article/202677 (accessed 22 July 2010)

## Test Your Knowledge

This young man had a widespread rash affecting his trunk and limbs (*Figure 11*). It had started about 2 months earlier, after he had had a throat infection. Initially he developed numerous 'drop like', deep red, slightly itchy papules on his body. They gradually increased in size to form these sore, red plaques. A diagnosis of guttate psoriasis, developing into an acute plaque psoriasis was made. He was referred for treatment with ultraviolet light. He responded well and the rash cleared.

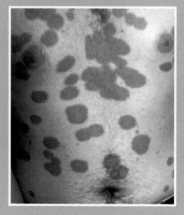

### Questions

1. What particular features of this rash would make the diagnosis of mycosis fungoides unlikely?
2. What other signs might you look for if you suspected the possibility of mycosis fungoides?
3. Should there be any doubt about the diagnosis, what action would you take?

# Skin manifestations of breast cancer

Breast cancer is the most common form of cancer in the UK, with 1 in 9 women developing the condition (Cancer Research UK, 2008). Cases in men are more rare and account for only 1% of all cases (Cancer Research UK, 2008).

Despite the high prevalence of breast cancer, in the past 20 years the 5-year survival rates for breast cancer have improved from 52% in 1971–1975 to 80% in 2000–2003 (Cancer Research UK, 2005). From the early 1990s to the present day, the 20-year survival rate has increased from 44% to 64%, with the greatest improvement in those presenting after the age of 50 years (Cancer Research UK, 2005). Further research has also shown that the earlier the diagnosis is made, the better the outcome and subsequent survival (Cancer Research UK, 2005).

Health professionals should be aware and alert to any symptoms that might suggest the condition, as early as possible. A patient may present with concerns or worrying changes might be noticed during some routine examination by a practice nurse or GP. The patient should be quickly referred for further investigation and treatment in order to maximize their chances.

By understanding the outward signs of the condition alongside other problems that may affect the breast area, health professionals will be better placed to deal with any concerns, whether cancerous or not. Practice nurses and GPs must be aware of the patient's anxieties and find ways of supporting him/her. The patient needs help to understand and manage the condition and should be advised what to expect at a visit to the breast clinic.

## Aetiology

In general terms, breast cancer results from a combination of environmental and hereditary factors. Genetic mutations or inherited defects in DNA-repair genes such as BRCA1 and BRCA2 may be a factor in between 5–10% of breast cancer cases (National Cancer Institute, 2005). The risk of developing breast cancer increases with:

- Age
- A family history of breast cancer in a first-degree relative
- Having a first child after the age of 30 years
- Not breastfeeding
- Early menarche and late menopause
- Radiation to the chest
- Intake of oestrogens, as in hormone replacement therapy (HRT) taken for more than 5 years (Vickers, 2005)
- Taking the contraceptive pill (only a slight increase in risk which returns to normal levels 10 years after stopping it) (Joint Formulary Committee, 2008: 7.3.2.1).

## Breast examination

Regular self-examination of the breasts, together with an annual examination by a professional, increases the chances of detecting breast cancer at an early stage and therefore a better prognosis for the patient (BreastCancer.org, 2008).

Women should be taught to check their breasts regularly each month, preferably after a period when the breasts are less likely to be swollen, tender or lumpy. By familiarizing themselves with what their breasts normally feel like, women will be able to recognize a change in the size or shape of the breast, changes in the nipple area or other

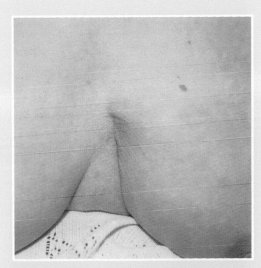

*Figure 6.1. Puckered skin, patient with carcinoma of the breast.*

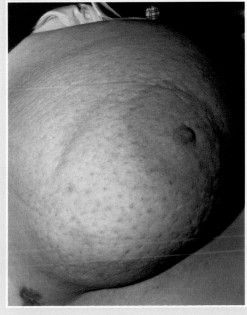

*Figure 6.2. Peau d'orange.*

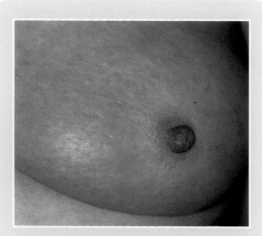

*Figure 6.3. Inflammatory breast cancer.*

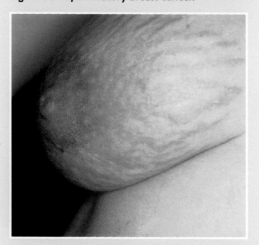

*Figure 6.4. Acute puerperal mastitis.*

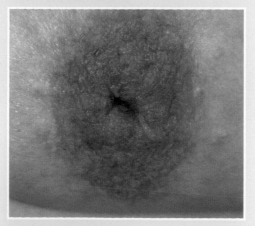

*Figure 6.5. Inverted nipple.*

developments in the skin. Palpation of the breasts should be done with the flat of the hand, pressing firmly over the whole of the breast area and up into the axilla (BreastCancer.org, 2008).

## Physical signs that may suggest breast cancer

### Dimpling, puckering or bulging of the skin

The most common presentation of breast cancer is a lump found by the patient. However, if this lump has become tethered to the skin there may be dimpling, puckering or bulging of the overlying skin (*Figure 6.1*). In this case, the patient had presented with a chest infection. During examination, puckering of the skin was noticed and a hard, irregular lump tethered to the skin, could be felt beneath it. This patient had chosen to ignore the symptom for 2 years. She was referred to the breast clinic and started on tamoxifen.

### Change in size, shape and colour of the breast

Inflammatory breast cancer (in which there has been invasion of the dermal lymphatics or small vessels of the skin) can cause a dimpled appearance like that of the peel of an orange (peau d'orange) (*Figure 6.2*).

If the cancer has invaded the lymphatics, presentation may also resemble that of inflammatory mastitis (*Figure 6.3*). This 68-year-old woman presented with a 3-week history of an inflamed area of the left breast. On examination she was afebrile, the skin felt warm and indurated, and there was an enlarged lymph node in the left axilla. She was referred urgently to the breast clinic where further investigation confirmed a poorly-differentiated carcinoma of the breast with blood vessel and lymph node involvement. A presentation such as this could be mistaken for infective mastitis but breast cancer is more common in the older age group (*Table 6.1*).

### Differential diagnosis

Acute mastitis would tend to have an acute onset, and most commonly occurs during the puerperal period. In *Figure 6.4*, the patient had been breastfeeding and developed cracked nipples. The inflammation had suddenly appeared and she was unwell and febrile. In her case, the condition quickly settled after a course of antibiotics. On subsequent examination, the breasts were found to be normal. Infection is usually due to *Staphylococcus aureus* or *Streptococcus*, and gains access through cracked nipples. Infection can result in abscess

| Table 6.1. Inflammatory breast cancer and infective mastitis | | |
|---|---|---|
| | **Inflammatory breast cancer** | **Infective mastitis** |
| **Aetiology** | Infiltration of cancer cells of the dermal lymphatics and small vessels<br>Rare under the age of 25 years | Infection - *Staphylococcus aureus* or *Streptococcus*<br>Usually associated with lactation and cracked nipples |
| **Presentation** | Afebrile - slower onset. Inflammation pain, swelling and induration. Peau d'orange effect, enlarged axillary lymph gland(s) | Acute onset - febrile and unwell<br>Inflammation of breast, red, tender<br>May progress to abscess formation |
| **Management** | Urgent referral to breast clinic | Antibiotics, analgesics, e.g. paracetamol, ice packs,<br>Continue breastfeeding unless abscess develops |

## Table 6.2. Paget disease or eczema of the nipple

|  | Paget disease of the nipple | Eczema of the nipple |
|---|---|---|
| **Aetiology** | Associated with intraduct carcinoma of the breast<br>Rare under age of 25 years | Personal or family history of atopy. Allergic response to contact allergen<br>May occur during lactation |
| **Presentation** | Erythema, rash, scaling, itching of nipple and areola<br>One nipple affected<br>Ulceration, destruction of the nipple<br>Lump under the nipple<br>Enlarged axillary glands | Inflammation, blisters, dry thickened areas, itching. Often both nipples involved the nipple |
| **Management** | Urgent referral to breast clinic<br>Oral antihistamine | Moisturizers, topical corticosteroid or ointment |

formation if not treated quickly with antibiotics. Ice packs and analgesics, such as paracetamol, should ease the pain. Breastfeeding may be continued unless the condition fails to subside and an abscess forms in the breast (with a fluctuant mass) (Encyclopædia Britannica, 2009).

### Nipple changes
#### Inversion of the nipple
Inversion of the nipple (*Figure 6.5*) is seen relatively frequently and may be a congenital problem resulting from short ducts restricting the nipple as the breast enlarges. It may also occur in inflammatory conditions that cause

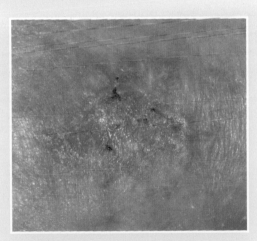

**Figure 6.6. Paget disease of the nipple with nipple destruction.**

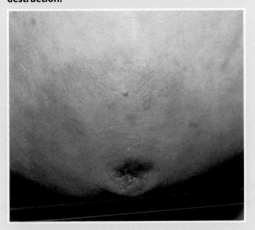

**Figure 6.7. Paget disease of the nipple with ulceration.**

scarring and shortening of the ducts (Breast Centre NZ, 2007). However, in some cases it may be more worrying, especially where there is recent change in one nipple and when it is not possible to evert the nipple in an older woman. In these cases, it may be associated with an underlying malignancy in which a lump is likely to be palpated below the nipple.

#### Inflammation, rash or scaling
Paget disease of the nipple is always associated with an underlying intraduct carcinoma of the breast. It presents with a unilateral, eczematous-type rash, with erythema, scaling and itching of the nipple and surrounding areola. The disease eventually destroys the nipple (*Figure 6.6*). In some cases, there may be discharge or bleeding from the nipple and the lesion may ulcerate (*Figure 6.7*).

Sometimes a lump may be palpated under the nipple, and in 50% of these cases, axillary metastases are found and the prognosis is less good. Cytology of a scrape from the nipple and mammogram should confirm the diagnosis (Kao, 2007). A presentation such as this must be distinguished from an eczematous change of the nipple (*Table 6.2*). *See Chapter 7 for more details on eczema of the nipple.*

### Ulceration of the skin
Metastatic spread from carcinoma of the breast may be to distant areas such as bones, liver, lungs or brain. Local spread may also occur with secondary deposits developing locally in the breast or the chest wall. These may present as nodules, as in the woman in *Figure 6.8*, who had undergone a mastectomy 14 years earlier. These may break down and ulcerate (*Figure 6.9*).

### Management
Any suspected case of carcinoma of the breast should be referred urgently to the breast clinic for full assessment by the team with a mammogram and/or ultrasound or MRI scan and needle biopsy. Depending on the findings, the choices are (Opatt, 2006):

* Surgery (lumpectomy, mastectomy and axillary clearance)
* Radiotherapy and chemotherapy.

For women with early stage breast cancer, which overexpresses human epidermal growth factor receptor-2 (HER2), follow-up treatment with trastuzumab may be considered (Joint Formulary Committee, 2008: 8.1.5).

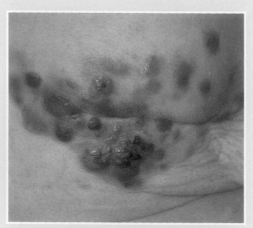

*Figure 6.8. Ulceration of skin secondaries from carcinoma of the breast.*

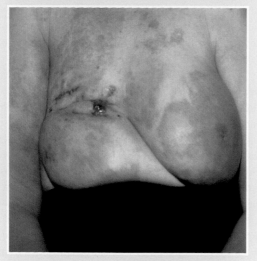

*Figure 6.9. Secondary nodular deposits develop 14 years after mastectomy (for carcinoma).*

However, trastuzumab is not recommended for those with certain heart problems or hypertension that is not well controlled (National Institute for Health and Clinical Excellence (NICE), 2006). The treatment is recommended to be taken at 3-week intervals for 12 months or until the cancer returns, and heart checks would need to be repeated every 3 months while on the treatment (NICE, 2006).

The clinic will take on much of the responsibility for managing a case of breast cancer, but the patient, family and/or friends will often need continuing support from the practice nurse and GP, to discuss his/her situation, treatment and any complications that may arise from it.

## References

BreastCancer.org (2008) Breast self-exam. www.breastcancer.org/symptoms/testing/types/self_exam/ (accessed on 17 February 2009)

Breast Centre New Zealand (2007) Nipple inversion. http://tinyurl.com/bxhm9h (accessed 17 February 2009)

Cancer Research UK (2005) Breast cancer survival statistics, 2003. http://tinyurl.com/ba2utq (accessed 17 February 2009)

Cancer Research UK (2008) UK breast cancer incidence statistics, 2005. http://tinyurl.com/b9snrq (accessed 17 February 2009)

Encyclopædia Britannica Online (2009) Mastitis. http://tinyurl.com/d3lbsw (accessed 17 February 2009)

Hoare C, Li Wan Po A, Williams H (2000) Systematic review of treatments for atopic eczema. *Health Technol Assess* **4**(37): 1-191

Joint Formulary Committee (2008), *British National Formulary* 56. September. BMJ and RPS Publishing, London

Kao GF (2007) Paget disease, mammary. *eMedicine* www.emedicine.com./derm/topic305.htm (accessed 17 February 2009)

National Cancer Institute (2005) Genetics of breast and ovarian cancer (PDQ). National Institutes of Health, USA. http://tinyurl.com/ch5fz9 (accessed 17 February 2009)

National Institute for Health and Clinical Excellence (2006) Trastuzumab for the adjuvant treatment of early-stage HER2-positive breast cancer. http://www.nice.org.uk/TA107 (accessed 17 February 2009)

Opatt DM (2006) Breast Cancer.*eMedicine* http://www.emedicine.com/plastic/topic521.htm (accessed 17 February 2009)

Vickers M (2005) HRT and breast cancer: Is there an association? *Practice Nursing* **16**(3): 128–32

## Test Your Knowledge

This elderly woman attended the surgery requesting treatment for a chesty cough. On examination of her chest, it was noticed that there were some changes in the breast that warranted further investigation. The nipple was being "pulled in" and there was adjacent puckering of the skin, beneath which was a hard lump, adherent to the skin above. The patient said that she had, in fact, noticed the changes in the last year, but had chosen to ignore them as she had no pain or other problems associated with it.

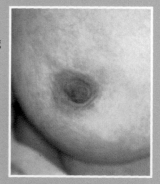

### Questions

1. What is the most likely diagnosis in this case and what further examination should you pursue at this first meeting?
2. What action would you take?
3. In this situation, how would you, as the Practice Nurse, follow up the patient?

# The nipple

Greater awareness of breast cancer and the benefits of early diagnosis and treatment has encouraged women to perform regular breast self-examination. Women should be encouraged to seek advice about any abnormal findings from health professionals.

This chapter will consider the nipple in particular and the kind of changes that raise concern and require advice. Changes that affect the nipple include discharge, ulceration, eczema, recent nipple retraction and skin distortion. Although women most commonly suffer these problems, men sometimes develop prolactinomas, eczema and malignancies too.

## Nipple discharge

If the nipple is squeezed, some discharge exudes from the nipple in about 29% of women. In many cases, this discharge is a physiological phenomenon that may occur in the neonatal period, during pregnancy and lactation or in association with hyper-prolactinaemia. However, in some cases a discharge may be associated with underlying pathology such as duct ectasia or papilloma or carcinoma of the breast.

To diagnose the problem it is important to observe whether the discharge is unilateral or bilateral, affects one or more ducts, its colour, whether it is blood stained and whether the discharge appears spontaneously or after expression (Surgical tutor, 2006) (*Table 7.1*).

## Galactorrhoea

Galactorrhoea is the spontaneous appearance of milk secretion from multiple ducts of both breasts. It may be of physiological origin and is usually associated with a raised level of prolactin. This occurs in pregnancy and lactation but it may also be found in association with certain drugs such as phenothiazines, haloperidol, methyldopa, oestrogens or opiates.

Pathological causes include hypothalamic or prolactin secreting pituitary tumours (prolactinomas), hypothyroidism or renal failure. Investigations include prolactin level, thyroid function, urea and electrolytes, a pregnancy test in women and a careful drug history.

In women, a prolactinoma leads to galactorrhoea (*Figure 7.1*), amenorrhoea or oligomenorrhoea. In men, problems tend to present later with loss of libido and the pressure effects of headache and visual disturbance.

If a prolactinoma is suspected the patient should be referred to an endocrinologist. Small micro-prolactinomas can usually be treated with drugs such as bromocriptine, that will control prolactin levels and symptoms. A prolactin level greater than 5000 mIU/litre, indicates a macroprolactinoma, which will require a magnetic resonance imaging scan and visual tests.

Bromocriptine may be sufficient but sometimes surgery or radiotherapy are needed (The Pituitary Foundation, 2006).

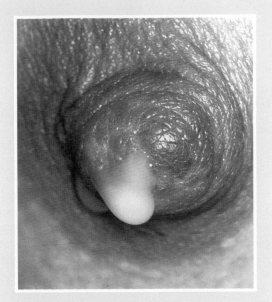

*Figure 7.1. Galactorrhoea.*

### Coloured discharge

Coloured discharge is usually bilateral, cream, green or white in colour and usually associated with duct ectasia, which occurs most frequently in women in their 40s and 50s. It occurs when fluid accumulates in the ducts, which become clogged and blocked with a thick, sticky substance. Patients with this problem may be reassured that no action is required. If the discharge is copious and troublesome, surgery may be indicated.

### Blood-stained discharge

Blood-stained discharge is of greater concern, particularly if the discharge is from a single duct and of recent onset, because it is more often associated with an underlying carcinoma of the breast or duct papilloma.

## Table 7.1. Differential diagnosis of nipple discharge

| | Galactorrhoea | Coloured discharge | Blood-stained discharge |
|---|---|---|---|
| *Cause* | • Physiological<br>• Drugs<br>• Prolactinoma | Blocked ducts | • Carcinoma of the breast<br>• Duct papilloma |
| *Investigations* | • Prolactin level<br>• Thyroid function<br>• Urea, electrolytes<br>• Pregnancy test<br>• Drug history | | • Haemostix to confirm blood |
| *Management* | • Bromocriptine may be sufficient<br>• Surgery<br>• Radiotherapy | • No further action unless troublesome<br>• Surgery if necessary | • Refer to breast clinic<br>• Mammography<br>• Cytology of discharge<br>• Exploration of duct system even if test negative<br>• Appropriate management if carcinoma found |

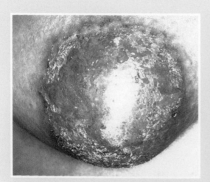

Figure 7.2. Acute eczema of the nipple.

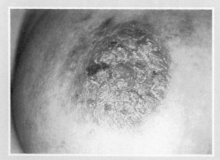

Figure 7.3. Chronic changes in eczema of the nipple.

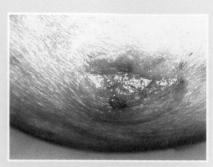

Figure 7.4. Paget's disease of the nipple with ulceration.

Haemostix may be used to confirm the presence of blood in the discharge. Such patients should be referred to a breast clinic for further investigation with mammography and cytological examination of the discharge. However, even if these prove negative, the duct system may still require exploration to finally exclude a ductal carcinoma *in situ* (Austoker et al, 1999).

## Eczema

Eczema is a common problem that affects about 20% of patients at some time in their lives. It is commonly seen on the areolae of the nipples. Eczema is often genetically determined. A patient or his/her family may have a history of eczema, hay fever or asthma. In others, allergies, irritant substances and stress may provoke eczema (DermNet NZ, 2005).

Eczema may present acutely with an erythematous rash that may be blistered, moist and swollen (*Figure 7.2*), or as a chronic, irritating condition with thickened, lichenified skin that the patient has probably scratched (*Figure 7.3*).

The edges of the changes are usually ill-defined. It is the areaola that is affected, tending to spare the nipple itself. Eczema usually affects both nipples and the patient often gives a history of intermittent recurrences.

### Management

Provided that there are no other abnormalities on breast examination, the problem may be treated with a mild topical steroid ointment. If there is no response to this treatment, referral should be made to a breast clinic for assessment with a mammogram and punch biopsy of the lesion to confirm the diagnosis.

## Paget's disease

Paget's disease of the nipple is not common. It usually occurs in women between the ages of 50 and 60 years and is less common in men. Mammary Paget's disease is associated with an underlying carcinoma *in situ* or more advanced malignancy.

Its presentation is very similar to that of a chronic eczema, with redness, scaling and swelling. Sometimes there is ulceration (*Figure 7.4*) of the nipple and/or an oozing of blood-stained discharge from the nipple. Because its presentation is similar to that of eczema, it is important to ensure an accurate diagnosis and take the appropriate action (*Table 7.2*).

Pointers to the diagnosis of Paget's disease are an itchy, unilateral lesion with a history of slow progression and an irregular but definite edge. The nipple itself is always involved and may be destroyed in advanced cases.

### Management

Confirmation of the diagnosis of Paget's disease is crucial and may be achieved by skin biopsy. However, this alone will not demonstrate an underlying problem and, therefore, a mammogram is also required. These checks are best done in a breast clinic. Urgent referral is required.

Treatment depends on the extent of the malignancy and varies from partial nipple excision, wedge excision, wide excision and/or radiotherapy and chemotherapy (DermNet NZ, 2006).

## Inverted nipple

In 10% of women nipple inversion (*Figure 7.5*) is a completely 'normal' congenital abnormality. However, in some cases it is related to an underlying problem such as duct ectasia or periductal mastitis. The abnormality is at the centre of the nipple and affects both breasts. It causes no problems when the woman wishes to breastfeed.

Concern is raised if there is recent development of inversion that may indicate an underlying malignancy. Sometimes a lump may be palpable on examination. In such cases, it is not possible to evert the nipple and the change normally affects one nipple only.

### Management

Urgent referral to a breast clinic is necessary for further investigation and management for those with a recent change and an associated breast lump (Kalbhen et al, 1998).

## Cracked nipples

Cracked nipples are a common problem in women who breastfeed their babies. They occur most commonly soon after delivery or when weaning the child, and the breasts are engorged. Severe pain may be associated with the cracked, bleeding nipples (*Figure 7.6*).

Cracked nipples provide a good portal of entry for infection, which may lead to mastitis, usually as a result of *Staphylococcus aureus* (GP Notebook, 2006). If this occurs, the woman will be unwell with fever and complaints of inflammation and tenderness of the breast

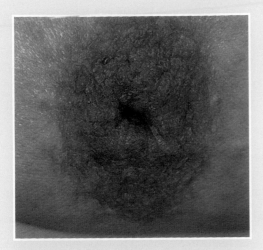

*Figure 7.5. Inverted nipple.*

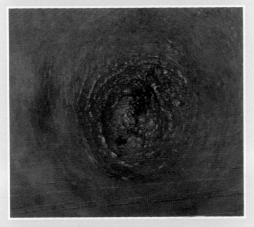

*Figure 7.6. Cracked nipple 5 days after delivery.*

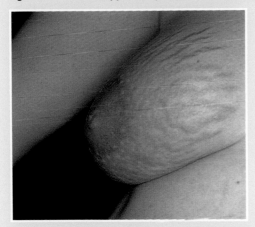

*Figure 7.7. Puerperal mastitis.*

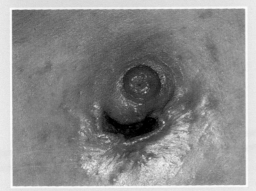

*Figure 7.8. Drained breast abscess.*

## Table 7.2. Differential diagnosis of eczema and Paget's disease

| | Eczema | Paget's disease |
|---|---|---|
| Symptoms | • Usually bilateral changes<br>• Areola affected<br>• Patient or family history of eczema, hay fever and/or asthma<br>• Erythematous, blistered, swollen, lichenified<br>• Itchy<br>• Acute onset, intermittent episodes<br>• Ill-defined edge | • Unilateral changes<br>• Nipple involved<br>• Erythema, scaling<br>• Dry or moist<br>• Itchy<br>• Slow progression<br>• Irregular but definite edge<br>• Lump under the nipple<br>• Lymphadenopathy in the axilla |
| Management | • If no response, refer to breast clinic for biopsy<br>• Moisturizers, topical corticosteroid or ointment | • Urgent referral to breast clinic<br>• Biopsy<br>• Mammogram<br>• If negative, explore the duct system |

(*Figure 7.7*). If left untreated, the infection may progress to abscess formation.

### Management

*Cracked nipples:* Feeding techniques should be discussed to ensure that the baby is well latched onto the breast, and positions changed so that a different area of the breast is exposed at each feed. Some of the milk rubbed on the nipples and allowed to dry will help them to heal. Bathing the nipples in plain water will help keep them clean. A simple analgesic such as paracetamol will ease the pain (Baby Centre USA, 2006).

*Mastitis* should settle with a course of systemic flucloxacillin or erythromycin. Breastfeeding may continue. Frequent feeds help maintain the supply of milk. If the breast is not completely emptied, a breast pump should be used to achieve emptying.

A *breast abscess* will need to be drained under local anaesthesia. Small abscesses can be drained with a needle but a larger abscess will require incision and drainage (NHS Direct, 2006) (*Figure 7.8*).

### Suppernumerary nipples

Supernumerary nipples (SN) are a relatively common congenital abnormality. Single SN may occur or they may number as many as eight, along the embryonic milk line on both sides. They may be seen in both men and women along a line that stretches from a point just beyond the axilla, down the chest and abdomen towards the groin. They may be associated with underlying breast tissue and the nipple itself may be present in part or whole.

Apart from embarrassment, SN are symptomless, but changes in pigmentation, swelling, tenderness and lactation may occur during menstruation and pregnancy.

No action is necessary unless the patient wishes to undergo cosmetic surgical removal. However, SN may undergo any of the same changes as a normal nipple or breast. It is important to notice any changes such as distortion, eczema or discharge and take the appropriate action. As in normal breast tissue, malignancies occur (Metzker, 2005).

## Test Your Knowledge

This patient is worried. For over 3 years she has had recurrent episodes of itching, soreness, inflammation and weeping of both nipples. She has tried a variety of creams and topical steroids but, although the symptoms ease for a while, they always come back. She is 7-months pregnant and is concerned that it may cause her problems with breastfeeding.

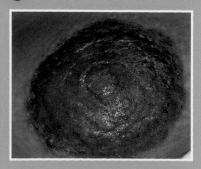

### Questions

1. What is the likely diagnosis?
2. What other information or findings might guide you to the true diagnosis?
3. How would you advise the patient?

### References

Austoker J, Mansel R, Baum M, Sainsbury R, Hobbs R (1999) Guidelines for referral of patients with breast problems. NHS Breast Screening Programme, Sheffield

Baby Centre USA (2006) Cracked or bleeding nipples. www.babycenter.com/refcap/baby/babybreastfeed/8493.html (accessed 23 August 2006)

DermNet NZ (2005) Dermatitis. www.dermnetnz.org/dermatitis/dermatitis.html (accessed 23 August 2006)

DermNet NZ (2006) Paget disease. www.dermnetnz.org/site-age-specific/paget.html (accessed 23 August 2006)

GP Notebook (2006) Puerperal mastitis. www.gpnotebook.co.uk/cache/1469710382.htm (accessed 23 August 2006)

Kalbhen C, Kezdi R, Rogus P, Dowling M, Flisak M (1998) Mammography in the evaluation of nipple inversion. *AJR Am J Roentgenol* **170**(1): 117–21

Metzker A (2005) Supernumerary nipple. *eMedicine*. www.emedicine.com/derm/topic735.htm (accessed 23 August 2006)

NHS Direct (2006) Breast abscess. www.nhsdirect.nhs.uk/articles/article.aspx?articleId=62&sectionId=4346 (accessed 23 August 2006)

Surgical Tutor (2006) Nipple discharge. www.surgical-tutor.org.uk/core/neoplasia/nipple.htm (accessed 23 August 2006)

The Pituitary Foundation (2006) Hyperprolactinaemia. www.pituitary.org.uk/gp-factfile/5-hyperprol.htm (accessed 23 August 2006)

# Brown pigmented lesions

Increased public awareness of sun damage and the risks of development of skin cancers can lead patients to be concerned about brown discolouration of the skin.

It is most important that any suspicion that a lesion could be malignant should be referred urgently for specialist care (Watkins, 2002). At other times, it may be obvious that the lesion is benign but the patient may require a more definitive diagnosis and advice on how to manage and reduce the discolouration.

This chapter considers the different diagnoses and advice that can be given on the management of lesions with a 'normal' skin surface that are brown, non-erythematous patches or plaques with poorly defined edges that do not normally present until after the age of ten according to Ashton and Leppard (2005: 262).

## Poikiloderma of Civatte
### Aetiology
Poikiloderma of Civatte is a relatively common problem that occurs in fair-skinned, middle aged and older women. The actual cause is unknown but exposure to Ultraviolet light (UVL) is a major factor in its development. Also it is thought to be related to a photosensitization to certain chemicals present in some cosmetics and perfumes. Research also suggests that the low oestrogen levels that occur at the menopause may play a part.

Genetic factors, in the form of autosomal dominance, may also be a factor and successive generations of families may be affected as Hawayek and Rubeiz (2006) have shown.

### Symptoms
The patient complains of symptomless, pigmentary changes on the sun exposed areas of the neck. Typically it does not affect the less exposed area under the chin (*Figure 8.1*). On examination, the affected skin is reddish brown with areas of telangiectasia and some atrophic changes.

### Management
The patient should avoid sun exposure and use sunscreens when outdoors. Also they should stop using perfumes and cosmetics as these products may have led to the development of the condition. If the patient is worried about the appearance of the lesions the New Zealand Dermatological Society (2005) recommends the use of pulsed dye laser (PDL) or intense pulsed light (IPL) as an effective way to improve the condition. However, the Society says topical treatments are not generally successful.

## Melasma
### Aetiology
Melasma (also known as chloasma) is unusual in men. Approximately 90% of cases occur in women after puberty. Melasma is related to, and becomes more obvious after, sun exposure. It is also more likely to occur in those with a darker skin type and there is thought to be a genetic predisposition to the problem.

Horminal influences do play a part in melasma in some instances but as yet it has not been established as to which hormones are involved. It is commonly seen in pregnant women and those on the contraceptive pill or hormone replace therapy and there is an increased incidence in those with thyroid disease.

### Symptoms
The patient is not always aware of the changes. However, a doctor or nurse in a family planning, HRT or pregnancy clinic will notice the development of a uniformly brown, blue or black colour over the cheeks, forehead, nose and/or upper lip. The discolouration is usually symmetrically distributed (*Figure 8.2*).

### Management
Many cases of melasma will gradually improve if the medication is discontinued or after the pregnancy is over. Of course, the patient should avoid aggravating the problem by further exposure to the sun and should be advised to wear a hat and use an effective sunscreen when outdoors. Topical depigmenting agents such as hydroquinone 2–4% can be used to lighten the darker areas of pigmentation. However, this topical treatment is not without its problems as hydroquinone can cause skin irritation, phototoxic reactions, secondary hyper-pigmentation and patchy discoloration.

Tretinoin cream may help but the response is slow and may take up to 6 months. It is important to observe that tretinoin must not be used during pregnancy.

Another alternative is azelaic acid cream (20%) This has the advantage of targeting only the hyperactive melanocytes and so will not lighten normal skin. The main side effect with this preparation is skin irritation. (Montemarano, 2006).

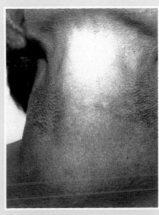

*Figure 8.1. Poikiloderma of Civatte. Notice the absence of the rash under the chin.*

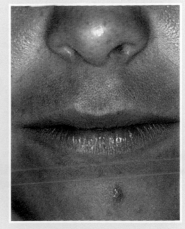

*Figure 8.2. Melasma affecting the upper lip.*

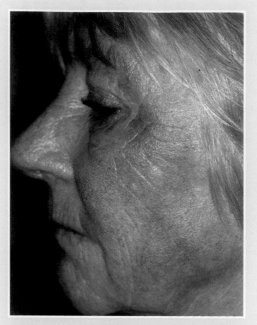

*Figure 8.3. Discolouration on the face of a patient taking long term minocycline.*

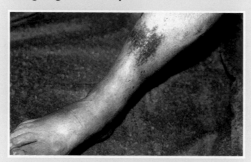

*Figure 8.4. Haemosiderin pigmentation in a patient with varicose veins.*

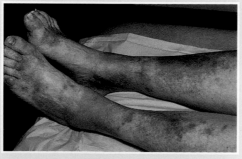

*Figure 8.5. Haemosiderein pigmentation in a man with varicose veins and a lifetime of standing at work.*

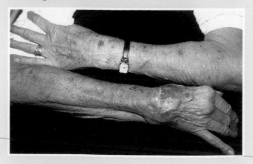

*Figure 8.6. Haemosiderin pigmentation in a patient who had developed purpura when on steroids.*

## Hyperpigmentation owing to drugs
### Aetiology
There are a number of drugs in common use today that may lead to problems of the development of patchy hyperpigmentation. The problem of melasma in relation to oestrogen and progesterone preparations has already been discussed but other drugs such as amiodarone, chloroquin and phenytoin may increase melanin in the skin. Chlorpromazine taken over long periods may also lead to a generalized hyperpigmentation (Ashton and Leppard, 2005).

### Symptoms
Patients on these drugs may become aware of colour changes. Not all these changes are related to melanin. For example, minocyline may cause a grey–blue or brown colour owing to the deposition of iron in the skin. The patient shown in *Figure 8.3* had been taking minocycline for many years for acne rosacea. The colour changes had developed and increased over the years (du Vivier, 2002).

### Management
The medication should be reviewed, stopped and an alternative found. Cosmetic camouflage may sometimes help to disguise the changes. The Red Cross run an excellent service to which patients can be refered by an NHS private Consultant or GP.

## Haemosiderin pigmentation
Haemosiderin staining is sometimes observed in the skin. It occurs as a result of breakdown of extravasated red blood cells that may occur in certain conditions. It may occur after episodes of purpura or as the result of venous hypertension that may occur in association with varicose veins (du Vivier, 2002).

### Symptoms
Discrete brown macules, which may merge into one another, occur in areas in where there has been leakage of blood cells into the tissues. The patient in *Figure 8.4* shows haemosiderin pigmentation in association with varicose veins.

Another patient had suffered with varicose veins for years (*Figure 8.5*). For 25 years he had worked in a job that required him to stand all the time. Over the previous 10 years he had noticed a gradual increase in the brown staining on his legs owing to stasis in the circulation in this area.

The patient in *Figure 8.6* developed a purpuric rash on her arms while on steroids (Ashton and Leppard, 2005: 354–55). Some of the patches are showing residual haemosiderin staining after the purpura has subsided.

There is no treatment for haemosiderin pigmentation other than attention to the underlying problem (du Vivier, 2005: 564).

## Schamberg's disease
### Aetiology
Schamberg's disease is a form of capillaritis that presents as pigmented purpuric lesions. It may occur at any age and is more common in men. The cause is unknown.

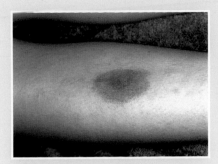

Figure 8.7. Schamberg's disease on the shin.

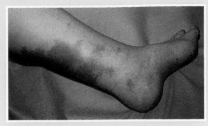

Figure 8.9. Post-inflammatory hyperpigmentation in a patient with recent cellulitis of that area.

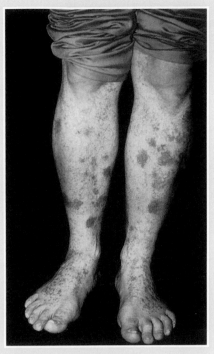

Figure 8.11. Post-inflammatory hyperpigmentation in resolved lichen planus.

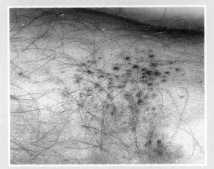

Figure 8.8. Schamberg's disease: cayenne pepper-like spots.

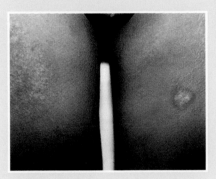

Figure 8.10. Post-inflammatory pigmentation years after severe burns.

## Symptoms

The patient develops an orange–brown bruise-like patch or patches (*Figure 8.7*) Within the area, small cayenne pepper-like spots are observed (*Figure 8.8*). They usually occur on the anterior surface of the lower limbs but do occasionally appear at other sites. The lesions may be symptomless but do sometimes itch (Jackson, 2005).

## Management

Schamberg's disease may settle spontaneously but more often runs a chronic course. It is a benign condition that does not pose any threat to health. Topical steroids are ineffective but oral steroids have cleared the condition. However, in view of the risks of side effects from this treatment, it is rarely used (Jackson, 2005).

## Post-inflammatory hyperpigmentation
### Aetiology

After any inflammatory condition affecting the epidermis, a discolouration caused by excess melanin pigmentation of the affected area may follow. It is therefore possible for it to occur in many situations such as skin infections, rashes, eczema, trauma and burns.

Changes in response to these inflammatory insults cause the release of substances that alter the activity of the immune cells and melanocytes. As a result the melanocytes produce more melanin causing the discolouration.

## Symptoms

The patient may complain of macular, brown patches, which may occur at any site. By the time the patient presents, all signs of the earlier problem may have disappeared. However, on careful questioning, it should be possible to ascertain that it has been preceded by some

rash, injury or other inflammatory condition prior to its development. (Ngan, 2005).

For example, the woman shown in *Figure 8.9* was worried about the large, brown area on her leg. It transpired that a few weeks before she had developed a cellulitis of the leg following an insect bite. The infection had cleared but the staining followed.

Often it is more marked in those with dark skin. Another woman was severely burned at the age of seven when her clothes were set alight when she was standing too close to the fire. She spent 3 months in hospital at the time. Now in adult life there is still evidence of hyperpigmentation in the scars on her thighs (*Figure 8.10*).

Another patient had a florid itchy rash that was diagnosed as lichen planus. Although the itching had settled, there remained a marked brown staining where the rash had been (*Figure 8.11*). This is a common problem with lichen planus but the patient can be reassured that, once there is improvement in the rash and the itching has settled, the active disease is over and no more treatment will be required.

## Management

There is no treatment for post-inflammatory hyperpigmentation. The discolouration tends to decrease over the ensuing months or years.

## Conclusions

It is evident from current research that there are several conditions which can present as brown-pigmented lesions on the skin. Some patients may fear that these lesions are malignant melanomas. Careful examination, knowledge of patient history and awareness of the symptoms related to different dermatalogical conditions are crucial to correctly diagnose and manage such cases (*Table 8.1*).

**Table 8.1. Differential diagnoses of brown, pigmented lesions of the skin**

| Disease | Cause | Age/sex | Symptoms | Management |
|---|---|---|---|---|
| Poikiloderma of Civatte | Unknown, possibly:<br>• Chemical photosensitivity<br>• Hormonal factors<br>• Genetics | • Middle age<br>• Women | Pigmentary changes Telangiectasia Sun exposed areas neck | • Stop perfume cosmetics and sun exposure<br>• Occasionally PDL or IPL |
| Melasma | • Hormonal factors<br>• Genetics<br>• Darkens on sun exposure | • After puberty<br>• Usually women | Symmetrical brown/black stain on cheeks, forehead, nose, upper lip | • Stop contraceptive pill or HRT<br>• Avoid sun<br>• Topical depigmentation agents |
| Drug-induced pigmentation | Induced by drugs, e.g:<br>• Chlorpromazine<br>• Amiodarone<br>• Chloroquin<br>• Phenytoin<br>• Minocycline | Any age | • Brown discolouration<br>• Blue/grey/brown with minocycline | • Stop the offending drug<br>• Cosmetic camouflage as needed |
| Haemosiderin pigmentation | Breakdown of extravasated red blood cells as with varicose veins or purpura | Any age | Discrete brown macules - may merge | No treatment Investigate any underlying problem |
| Schamberg's disease | Unknown | • Teens/young adults<br>• More common in men | • Orange/brown 'bruise'<br>• Cayenne pepper spots<br>• Usually lower limbs | • No treatment<br>• Very occasionally oral steroids, but beware side effects |
| Post-inflammatory hyperpigmentation | Melanocytic response to inflammation of the epidermis | Any age | • Macular brown areas<br>• History of recent inflammatory skin disease | • No treatment<br>• Gradually improves |

HRT = hormone replacement therapy; IPL = intense pulsed light; PDL = pulsed dye laser

# Test Your Knowledge

This woman attended the surgery with concerns about this mark on her leg. At first she thought that it was just a bruise, although she could not actually remember any recent injury. The mark was painless and had persisted for several weeks without change. She was anxious and needed some explanation.

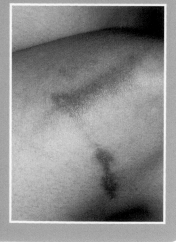

### Questions

1. What is the likely diagnosis?
2. How could you elucidate the cause?
3. What advise would you give to the patient?

## References

Ashton R, Leppard B (2005) *Differential Diagnosis in Dermatology.* 3rd edn. Radcliffe, Oxon

du Vivier A (2002) *Atlas of Clinical Dermatology.* 3rd edn. Churchill Livingstone, Edinburgh

Hawayek L, Rubeiz N (2006) Poikiloderma of Civatte. www.emedicine.com/DERM/topic603.htm (accessed 23 June 2006)

Jackson C (2005) Pigmented purpuric dermatoses. www.patient.co.uk/showdoc/40024698 (accessed 23 June 2006)

Montemarano A (2006) Melasma. www.emedicine.com/DERM/topic260.htm (accessed 23 June)

New Zealand Dermatalogical Society Incorporated (2005) Poikiloderma of Civatte. DermNet. http://dermnetnz.org/colour/poikiloderma-civatte.html (accessed 23 June 2006)

Ngan V (2005) Post inflammatory hyperpigmentation. www.dermnetnz.org/colour/postinflammatory-pigmentation.html (accessed 23 June 2006)

Watkins J (2002) Dermatology clinic. *Practice Nursing* **13**(3): 126–8

Red Cross (2005) Red Cross Beauty Care and Cosmetic Camouflage Service. www.timewarp.demon.co.uk/redcross.html (accessed 23 June 2006)

# Telangiectasia

Telangiectases are common. They are described as 'visible small blood vessels in the upper dermis, which blanch on pressure' (Lawrence and Cox, 2002: 306). They may be seen on the skin, nailfolds and mucous membranes. In many cases there is no obvious cause. In others there may be an inherited factor, while in some, telangiectasia may be an indication of an associated disease process, related to the effect of a medication or an insult to the skin such as sun exposure or radiotherapy (Lawrence and Cox, 2002). Telangiectasia need not suggest specific diagnosis, but may be a sign that will sometimes add weight to the possibility of an underlying disease or aggravating cause.

## Hereditary disease

A few, uncommon, hereditary problems may be associated with telangiectasia, such as ataxia telangiectasia, a rare, progressive condition that presents in childhood with poor balance, slurred speech and delayed development. Telangiectases occur on the cheeks, ears and around the eyes. The prognosis in these cases is poor with the likelihood of death in the teens or early 20s. Only symptomatic treatment is available (National Institutes of Health, 2007).

### Hereditary haemorrhagic telangiectasia

Hereditary haemorrhagic telangiectasia, or Osler-Weber-Rendu syndrome, is an inherited autosomal dominant condition (du Vivier, 2002: 479). The diagnosis may be easily recognized if a patient presents with problems of nose bleeds, telangiectasia and a family history of the condition. However, the presentation is not always so clear. It is suggested that, if only two of these factors are present, the diagnosis is unlikely (Shovlin et al, 1999).

Usually, symptoms first occur after puberty with nose bleeds and/or bleeding from the gut, genito-urinary tract or lungs. Visible telangiectases often appear only later in life. When they do, they may be widespread and have a tendency to bleed. The patient sometimes develops an iron deficiency anaemia resulting from occult intestinal bleeding. Telangiectases are often seen on the tongue, palate, on the nasal septum and the lips (*Figure 9.1*).

They may also be found on other parts of the body, particularly the hands (*Figure 9.2*), feet, ear and chest.

### Management

Hereditary haemorrhagic telangiectasia is a potentially serious condition. The outcome can be improved if it is recognized early, and the appropriate treatment implemented. Initially, any bleeding should be controlled, as well as possible, with icepacks, pressure and rest. If further treatment is required, cautery or laser treatment of individual lesions is available. In severe cases and where anaemia from blood loss is a problem, iron or blood transfusion may be necessary (University of Michigan Health System, 2003). Where gastrointestinal bleeding is a problem, endoscopy may allow a bleeding point(s) to be identified and treated by laser. Oestrogen therapy can also be effective in hereditary telangiectasia, but may cause problematic side effects in men (Porteus, 2007).

## Idiopathic disease

Patients may seek advice about a number of vascular lesions related to the dilation of cutaneous venules, which in most cases do not cause major problems. Such lesions include generalized essential telangiectasia, Campbell de Morgan spots and spider naevus.

### Generalized essential telangiectasia

Generalized essential telangiectasia tends to present in middle age with widespread, persistent dilation of small vessels in the skin, for no apparent reason. They are of no particular significance unless patients are embarrassed by them. If they are concerned about appearance, cover-up make-up may be beneficial. Advice regarding this can be obtained if the patient is referred to the Red Cross Service (Red Cross, 2007). If absolutely necessary, laser treatment may be helpful (DermNet NZ, 2007a).

### Campbell de Morgan spots

Campbell de Morgan spots, or cherry angiomas, are small haemangiomas which tend to occur in adults and increase in number during middle age, usually around the mid-trunk (*Figure 9.3*). Sometimes where multiple angiomas develop

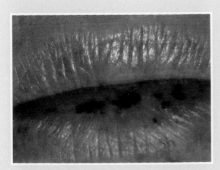
*Figure 9.1. Hereditary telangiectasia— lesion on the lip.*

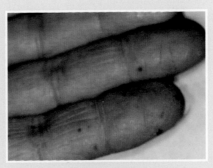
*Figure 9.2. Hereditary telangiectasia— lesions on the fingers.*

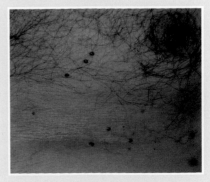
*Figure 9.3. Campbell de Morgan spots.*

*Figure 9.4. Spider naevus.*

*Figure 9.5. Spider naevus blanched by pressure from microscope slide.*

over a short time, it may be an indication of an underlying malignancy.

### Management

No treatment or investigation is required unless there is doubt about the diagnosis, or the angiomas are causing problems such as haemorrhage. If there is concern about the possibility of an underlying problem, further investigations will be required (DermNet NZ, 2007b). If treatment is considered necessary, the choices rest between shave excision, curettage and electrocautery, laser treatment or cryotherapy (Brown, 2006).

### Spider naevus

Spider naevus consists of a central arteriole with small radiating vessels (*Figure 9.4*) which blanch when the central vessel is compressed (*Figure 9.5*). Spider naevi are common, particularly on the face, upper trunk and arms. Usually there is no obvious cause but they appear most commonly in pregnancy or in those taking oral contraceptives. Some patients with cirrhosis of the liver or other liver problems may suddenly develop a number of spider naevi.

### Management

If the spider naevi are thought to have been stimulated by hormones, as in pregnancy or users of hormonal contraception, the patient can be reassured that spontaneous resolution usually occurs within 9 months of delivery or stopping the pill. The question of continuation of a hormonal contraceptive pill should be discussed. If this is considered to be a factor, alternative contraception can be offered. In patients with numerous lesions, liver function should be assessed. Treatment is unnecessary unless the

patient is unhappy about his/her appearance but cold point cautery under local anaesthetic can be applied to the central vessel. The patient should be warned that he/she may be left with a scar.

## Secondary disease

A number of factors and conditions that lead to the development of telangiectasia.

### Chronic vasodilation

Chronic vasodilation may occur in association with excess sun exposure, varicose veins and rosacea.

### Rosacea

The cause of rosacea is unknown. It is most common in people aged 30–60 years and presents with a red facial flush

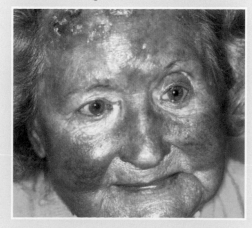

*Figure 9.6. Acne rosacea with multiple telangiectasia on the cheeks.*

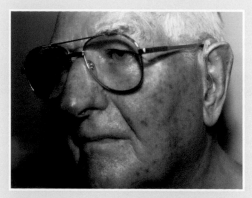

*Figure 9.7. Early rhinophyma with thickening, redness and telangiectasia on the nose.*

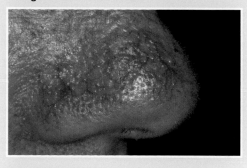

*Figure 9.8. Severe flare of rosacea in a woman who had been applying a potent topical steroid to her face.*

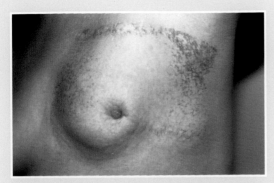

Figure 9.9. Multiple telangiectasia following lumpectomy and radiotherapy for carcinoma of the breast.

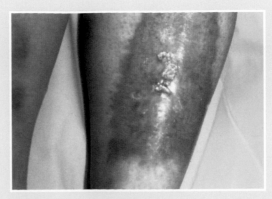

Figure 9.10. Necrobiosis lipoidica.

and/or telangiectasia, papules and sometimes pustules, mainly on the cheeks, forehead, nose and chin (*Figure 9.6*). Unlike acne vulgaris, there are no comedones. The eyes may also feel gritty, with conjunctival hyperaemia. In some there is thickening and sebaceous hyperplasia of the nose, which looks unsightly and is known as rhinophyma (*Figure 9.7*). Aggravating factors include anything that leads to flushing such as heat or sun exposure, hot spicy foods or alcohol. Similar rosacea-like signs, including perioral dermatitis may also follow the use of potent steroids on the face (Kupiec-Banasikowska and Ogholikhan, 2007).

## Management

It is usually possible to make a clinical diagnosis of this condition but, if necessary, a biopsy will exclude problems such as lupus or sarcoidosis. It is important never to treat rosacea with steroids as, although they may subdue symptoms temporarily, they recur with renewed energy when the steroids are discontinued (*Figure 9.8*). The approach should be to avoid trigger factors and to recommend sunscreen when out of doors.

A tetracycline oral antibiotic 500 mg twice daily for 6–12 weeks helps control the inflammation. It may need to be repeated intermittently. Alternatives are erythromycin, doxycycline or minocycline. Topical metronidazole may be sufficient for mild cases. In persistent cases and those resistant to treatment, oral isotretinoin is often effective, but requires hospital advice and prescription. It may need to be continued at low levels for a number of years.

Vascular laser treatment may improve the appearance of telangiectasia. Carbon dioxide laser or surgical reshaping of the nose may be required for rhinophyma (DermNet NZ, 2007d).

## Atrophic disorders

Atrophic changes in the skin cause it to lose its elasticity and become thin, translucent and wrinkly with telangiectasia. Owing to a diminution of the dermis and epidermis, it occurs as a normal part of ageing. Such changes may also be caused by outside influences that damage the skin or be part of the presentation of disease in which there are atrophic changes in the skin. Once the changes have occurred, the skin should be protected from further damage, and emollients applied if the skin is dry.

There are many causes of atrophic skin changes.

### Physical damage

Telangiectasia may develop in areas that have been exposed to a variety of insults such as physical damage from heat, as in erythema ab igne, excess sun exposure over the years, or radiation. As in the patient in *Figure 9.9*, multiple telangiectasia occurred in the area in which she had received a course of radiotherapy, following a lumpectomy for carcinoma of the breast (Huang et al, 2002). In the same way, telangiectases are often seen in scars following radiation of lesions such as basal cell carcinoma. Patients should be warned of this possible complication before treatment.

### Disease

A number of conditions lead to atrophic skin changes, and with it the likelihood of the development of telangiectases. Problems that may result in these changes include necrobiosis lipoidica, poikiloderma, lichen sclerosis et atrophica, discoid lupus eryrthematosus, morphea, scleroderma and dermatomyositis.

Necrobiosis lipoidica is seen most often in people with type 1 diabetes. Yellow patches on the shins, that become shiny and pale may display telangiectases in the lesion (*Figure 9.10*). The cause of necrobiosis lipoidica is unknown. It is usually painless, but ulceration may easily occur following a minor injury (DermNet NZ, 2006).

In lichen sclerosus et atrophicus, sharply demarcated, smooth, ivory white, atrophic patches develop, particularly around the vulva and anus in women, or the foreskin and glans of the penis in men. Similar 'cigarette paper-like patches' may be found on other parts of the body. In a small percentage of cases, vulval or penile carcinoma may develop. It is therefore necessary to continue to observe patients (DermNet NZ, 2007c).

### Discoid lupus erythematosus

Discoid lupus erythematosus is most common in women between the ages of 20–50 years. Red scaly patches appear on the cheeks, nose, and ears, which settle, leaving post-inflammatory pigmentation and atrophic white scars. The scalp is also often involved, causing scarring alopecia (DermNet NZ, 2007).

### Dermatomyositis

Dermatomyositis is most common between the ages of 50–70 years. The initial signs are often reddish or purple

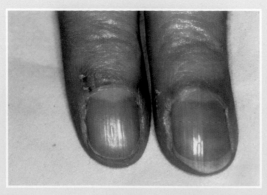

Figure 9.11. Periungual erythema and telangiectasia in a patient with dermatomyositis.

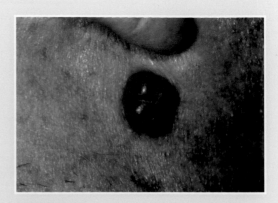

Figure 9.12. Cystic basal cell carcinoma with telangiectasia.

## Table 9.1. Types, causes and management of telangiectasia

| Types | | Characteristics | Action |
|---|---|---|---|
| **Hereditary disease** | Ataxia telangiectasia, haemorrhagic telangiectasia | • Poor balance, slurred speech, developmental delay<br>• Nose bleeds, family history | • Supportive, symptomatic<br>• Control bleeding, cautery or laser treatment of lesions<br>• Oestrogens<br>• Blood transfusion if necessary |
| **Idiopathic disease** | Generalized essential telangiectasia | • Generalized dilated small vessels<br>• Middle age<br>• No apparent reason | • Cosmetic camouflage<br>• Laser treatment |
| | Campbell de Morgan spots | • Multiple angiomas<br>• Middle age—mid trunk electrocautery, laser, cryotherapy<br>• Investigate possible malignanc, if indicated | • Treat only if necessary<br>• Shave excision, curettage, |
| | Spider naevi | • Occasionally underlying malignancy<br>• Central arteriole with radiating vessels<br>• Cause unknown—may develop in pregnancy or from oral contraceptives or liver disease | • If hormone induced—clears within 9 months of delivery or stopping contraception<br>• Liver function tests if indicated<br>• Cold point cautery, local anaesthetic |
| **Secondary disease (chronic vaso-dilatation)** | Rosacea | • Cause unknown, age 30–60 year<br>• Facial flush, telangiectasia, papules<br>• Eye involvement<br><br>• Rhinophyma | • Tetracycline 6–12 weeks, repeat if necessary<br>• Mild cases—topical metronidazole<br>• Biopsy if diagnosis in doubt<br>• Laser for telangiectasia<br>• Surgical reshaping<br>• Carbon dioxide laser |
| **Secondary disease (atrophy)** | Physical damage: sun, radiotherapy, heat, potent topical steroids | Thin, translucent, wrinkly with telangiectasia | Prevent further damage, e.g. sun proctection emollients |
| | Necrobiosis lipoidica | Often insulin dependent diabetics | Check blood glucose |
| | Lichen sclerosus et atrophicus | • Yellow patches, shiny, pale, telangiectases on shins<br>• Women 20–50 years<br>• May occur in children | Watch for malignant change |
| | Discoid lupus erythematosus | • Red, scaly patches cheeks, nose, ears<br>• Atrophic scars. Scalp involvement<br>• Age 50–70 years | Refer for investigation and management |
| | Dermatomyositis | • Red/purple patches sun exposed area<br>• Nailfold telangiectasia<br>• Triggers—infection, drugs, malignancy | Refer for investigation and management |
| **Localized lesions** | Nodular basal cell carcinoma | • Small translucent growth—usually head or neck<br>• Central area may ulcerate<br>• Cystic lesions with telangiectasia | • Biopsy if necessary<br>• Excision, shave, curettage and cautery, radiotherapy<br>• Further observation for other Suspicious lesions |

patches on the skin in sun-exposed areas. A further feature may be nailfold telangiectasia with ragged cuticles (DermNet NZ, 2006a) (*Figure 9.11*). The cause of dermatomyositis is unknown, but is thought to be an autoimmune defect and it is sometimes triggered by infection, drugs or an underlying malignancy.

## Management

A factor in these atrophic disorders may be the presence of telangiectasia in the skin lesions. Once an associated disease is suspected, the patient will require referral to a doctor for further investigation, treatment and follow-up.

## Localized lesions

Telangiectasia may be a feature of localized lesions such as kerato acanthoma or basal cell carcinoma.

Nodular basal cell carcinomas are most commonly seen on the face. They present with a small translucent growth which, if the contents are soft, is called cystic. The central area may break down leaving an open sore, often called a rodent ulcer. Frequently, telangiectasia can be seen on the surface of the lesion (*Figure 9.12*).

The treatment of choice for a nodular basal cell carcinoma is probably excision, providing the patient is agreeable and the size and positioning of the lesions do not make this a difficult procedure. Alternative approaches are shave, curettage and cautery, or radiotherapy. Providing the lesion is completely removed, there should be no recurrence, but the patient must be aware that further lesions may develop, and that sun protection should be used in the future.

## Test Your Knowledge

This 26-year-old woman attended the surgery with concern about the crop of 'red spots' that had recently appeared on the neck and upper chest. They caused her no discomfort but she was unhappy about her appearance and concerned that friends had recently remarked on them. Her general health was good. On examination, the lesions were found to be telangiectasia.

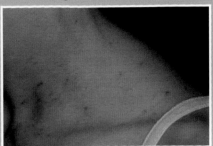

### Questions

1. How would you confirm that these were actually telangiectasia?
2. What further history would you require in order to ascertain the cause of her problem?
3. What advice and/or treatment would you offer?

## References

Brown C (2006) Cherry hemangioma. www.emedicine.com/DERM/topic73.htm (accessed 7 August 2007)

du Vivier A (2002) *Atlas of Clinical Dermatology*. 3rd edn. Churchill Livingstone: 479

DermNet NZ (2006) Necrobiosis lipoidica. http://dermnetz.org/dermal-infiltrative/necrobiosis-lipoidica.html (accessed 4 July 2007)

DermNet NZ (2006a) Dermato-myositis. http://dermnetnz.org/immune/dermatomyositis.html (accessed 4July 2007)

DermNet NZ (2007) Cutaneous lupus erythematosus. http://dermnetnz.org/immune/cutaneous-lupus.html (accessed 4 July 2007)

DermNet NZ (2007a) Generalized essential telangiectasia. http://dermnetnz.org/vascular/essential-telangiectasia.html (accessed 4 July 2007)

DermNet NZ (2007b) Haemangioma. http://dermnetnz.org/vascular/haemangioma.html (accessed 4 July 2007)

DermNet NZ (2007c) Lichen sclerosus. http://dermnetnz.org/immune/lichen-sclerosus.html (accessed 4 July 2007)

DermNet NZ (2007d) Rosacea. http://dermnetnz.org/acne/rosacea.html (accessed 4 July 2007)

Duffy B (2006) Undifferentiated connective-tissue disease. www.emedicine.com/med/topic2937.htm (accessed 4July 2007)

Huang E, Chen H, Wang G et al (2002) Predictive factors for skin telangiectasia following post-mastecstomy electron beam irradiation. *Br J Radiol* **75**(893): 444–7

Kupiec-Banasikowska A, Ogholikhan M (2007) Rosacea. www.emedicine.com/derm/topic377.htm (accessed 4July 2007)

Lab Tests Online (2007) Autoimmune disorders. www.labtestsonline.org/understanding/conditions/autoimmune.html (accessed 4 July 2007)

Lawrence C, Cox N (2002) *Physical Signs in Dermatology*. 2nd edn. Elsevier Science Ltd: 306–9

National Institutes of Health (2007) Ataxia telangiectasia information page. www.ninds.nih.gov/disorders/a_t/a-t.htm

# Viral warts

Viral warts are common presentations in general practice. Prevalence rates are 3.9–4.9% in children and adolescents (Williams et al, 1993). Adults may also be affected—the adult prevalence rate is 3.5% (Williams et al, 1993). Patients usually ask nurses and doctors to 'get rid of them', but treatment is not always the best option; 60–70% of warts resolve spontaneously in 3 months and no single treatment of warts is 100% effective (Sterling et al, 2000). The following chapter considers the types of warts that may present in general practice and highlights causes for concern and the options available to deal with them.

## Causes

The human papilloma virus (HPV) is responsible for most warts. There are many genotypes of HPV, each of which prefers different settings in which to thrive. For example, some may prefer the cornified, stratified, or squamous epithelium (i.e. any area of the skin) while others prefer the mucous membranes.

Wart virus infection may be transmitted from person to person by direct contact or by contact with fomites on surfaces such as the floor. Macerated skin or skin damaged by local trauma encourages such spread. Swimming pools and bathrooms are areas where patients may be at risk of acquiring warts (Johnson, 1995). Genital warts may be transmitted sexually (Wright, 1998) and have an infectivity rate of 60%, with an incubation period of 2–8 months (Adler, 1995).

Warts are particularly common in immunosuppressed patients. In such cases patients will often be troubled by numerous lesions (*Figure 10.1*). For example 50% of patients who have had a renal transplant will develop warts within 5 years of the procedure (Rudlinger et al, 1986).

## Presentation of warts

Depending on the genotype of the HPV, warts of different type and in different situations may display different features. Common warts (HPV types 1, 2, 4 and 57) (*Figure 10.2*) may be single or multiple, discrete, flesh-coloured papules or nodules with a firm, roughened, keratotic surface. They may be seen on any skin surface but are particularly common on the hands and feet.

Plane warts (HPV types 3 and 10) present as slightly raised, pigmented or flesh-coloured, flat-topped papules (*Figure 10.3*). They may occur anywhere but are particularly common on the face, hands and limbs. If they are treated with a topical steroid, by mistake, they will spread.

Plantar warts (verrucae) (HPV types 1, 2, 4 and 57) present as discrete 'sago grain-like' papules that develop a keratotic, roughened surface. Small haemorrhages can be seen because involution occurs as a result of thrombosed capillaries (*Figure 10.4*).

Verrucae usually occur on the sole of the foot and may cause considerable pain on walking. However, they are occasionally found on the palm of the hand. When pared with a scalpel, small bleeding points appear. This will distinguish the lesion from a corn, in which the skin appears more normal as it is pared.

Mosaic warts (HPV type 2) occur when numbers of verrucae coalesce together to form plaques of roughened skin. They may be found on the feet (*Figure 10.5*) or present in clusters around the nails (periungual warts) (*Figure 10.6*). They tend to be persistent and difficult to treat but generally are not painful.

## Complications and concerns

Malignant change is almost unknown in immunocompetent patients with simple warts on the skin. However, there could occasionally be a problem with periungual warts in patients who also have genital HPV infection (Sterling et al, 2000).

Some genital warts are associated with one of the 13 types of HPV that have a moderate risk for neoplastic

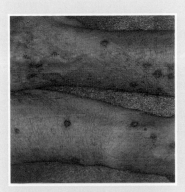

Figure 10.1. Multiple warts in a patient with a renal transplant. (These warts have been treated by cryotherapy.)

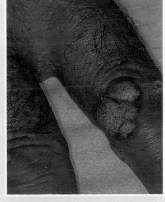

Figure 10.2. Common wart on the finger.

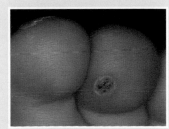

Figure 10.4 Verruca

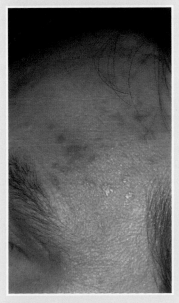

Figure 10.3. Plane warts on the forehead.

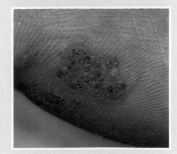

Figure 10.5. Mosaic wart on the ball of the foot.

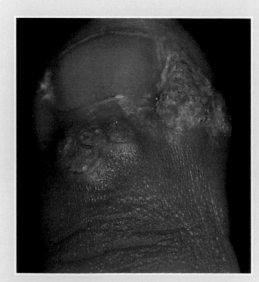

*Figure 10.6. Periungual warts.*

conversion and two (HPV tyoes 16 and 18) that are considered high risk. Areas most likely to be affected are the penis, vagina, cervix, perineum and perianal area and these changes may occur after a latent period of months or many years (Sterling et al, 2000). It has been found that 25% of those with genital warts also carry another sexually transmitted disease (Wright, 1998). *See Chapter 11 on Genital Warts for more infomation.*

### Psychosocial problems

When dealing with patients with warts it is important to be aware that a number of problems may be causing them anxieties. The health professional must give patients the opportunity to air their particular fears and concerns and discuss them. Health professionals should help patients make decisions about how to resolve or adapt to their difficulties. A number of points should be considered in such a discussion.

*Social contacts and employment* may be important factors. For example, friends may have remarked on the warts or employers may have expressed concern that an unsightly lesion could upset colleagues or customers. Patients may fear that their job is under threat or that their social life will be curtailed if they do not get rid of the warts.

*Swimming pools, schools, gymnasiums* must also be considered because the patient may fear that he/she will be excluded from swimming or some sports. The patient may not realize that this problem can be overcome by wearing plastic verruca socks or waterproof plasters (Health Protection Agency, 2003).

*Genital warts* can affect or break up relationships with the realization that the warts are sexually transmitted. Partners may be blamed and the patient may feel guilt and shame. Embarrassment may cause the patient to avoid sex. Further transmission of the virus may occur through failure to use condoms in a new relationship.

The present partner may be blamed and discussion must acknowledge that the incubation period can be long and date from an earlier liaison. Any new partner may need to be checked in case he/she has more recently acquired the infection.

*Pregnant women* should be informed that vaginal delivery may lead to transmission of the virus to the child. The patient should discuss this problem with the obstetrician who may sometimes offer the patient a Caesarean section (Kazzi and Ghadishah, 2002).

## Treatment

A number of treatment options are available (including no treatment) (*Table 10.1*). Each case must be considered on its own presentation. Often the correct approach is to await spontaneous resolution which should occur in 60–70% of patients within 3 months. The main reasons for treatment are for those with pain, where function is interfered with, or where the patient finds the wart(s) a cosmetic problem, for example, when working in a food shop. A number of treatments are available in general practice.

Salicylic acid clears 67% of hand warts and 84% of plantar warts in 12 weeks and it has been found that the results of this treatment are as good as any of the other readily available treatments. (Bunney et al, 1976; Veien et al, 1991; Gibbs et al, 2002).

A number of preparations can be used. Before application of the preparation, excess keratin should be pared away or sanded down with an emery board and the area softened by soaking in warm water. Gels, ointments, flexible collodion or liquid should be applied daily to the warts, taking care to protect the surrounding skin with Vaseline (Joint Formulary Committee, 2004: 560–1).

Facial warts should not be treated with wart paints, which could result in irritation and scarring. In addition, plane warts may Koebnerize and the problem may be exacerbated (Sterling et al, 2000). The Koebner phenomena occurs when an eruption of the underlying condition is induced along the line of any trauma such as a scratch or burn. It may occur in three conditions including plane warts, lichen planus and psoriasis.

Formaldehyde may be used daily as a 0.7% gel or in a 3% solution as a short soak. Or glutaraldehyde 10–20% solution can be applied daily for common, plantar or mosaic warts (Joint Formulary Committee, 2004: 560–1).

Cryotherapy can be used to treat a single or double freeze of warts every 3–4 weeks. A number of attendances may be required (Sterling et al, 2000).

Cryotherapy causes the equivalent of a burn on the skin and may be painful and cause blistering. Particular care should be taken when treating warts over tendons and patients with poor circulation. The lower leg, particularly in older people, may fail to heal well after treatment. In addition, the area may be affected by hypo- or hyperpigmentation after treatment, particularly in those with black skin (Larsen and Laurberg, 1996).

Warts may be excised surgically but the patient should be informed of the risk of scarring (Sterling et al, 2000).

Laser therapy has been used to treat viral warts and may be helpful in periungual and subungual warts that can be difficult to eradicate by other methods. Pain and scarring may be problems afterwards, but appear to be less with pulsed laser dye (Kenton-Smith and Tan, 1999) than with CO laser (Street and Rÿnigk, 1990).

### Periungual warts

Periungual warts are particularly difficult to clear. One option is to provide encouragement to await spontaneous resolution, which will occur in two thirds of patients within 2 years. Where this is not possible cryotherapy or chemical agents such as salicylic acid may achieve results.

For really stubborn problems the dermatologist may find other approaches helpful. These might include laser, intralesional bleomycin interferon or 5-fluorouracil. Decisions to treat in this way are the responsibility of the specialist and therefore referral would be required if the GP believed it was necessary.

### Table 10.1. Treatment choices for specific types of warts

| | No treatment | Salicylic acid | Glutaldehyde or formaldehyde | Cryotherapy | Surgery | Other |
|---|---|---|---|---|---|---|
| Common warts | ✓ | ✓ Not face | ✓ Not face | ✓ | Curettage and cautery under local anaesthetic occasionally | |
| Plantar warts | ✓ | ✓ | ✓ | ✓ | Curettage and cautery under local anaesthetic occasionally | |
| Plane warts | ✓ | Not face | Not face | With care if really necessary | | |
| Mosaic warts | ✓ | ✓ | ✓ | ✓ | Contra-indicated | |
| Periungual warts | ✓ | ✓ | ✓ | ✓ | | CO laser Dermatologist advice |

### References

Adler M (1995) *ABC of Sexually Transmitted Diseases*. 3rd edn. BMJ Books, London: 42–4

Bunney M, Nolan M, Williams D (1976) An assessment of methods of treating viral warts by comparative treatment trials based on a standard design. *Br J Dermatol* **94**(6): 667–9

du Vivier A (2002) Viral disorders of the skin: Warts. In: *Atlas of Clinical Dermatology*. 3rd edn. Churchill Livingstone, London: 300

Gibbs S, Harvey I, Stirling J et al (2002) Localised treatments for cutaneous warts. *Cochrane Database Syst Rev* 2002(3). Update Software, Oxford

Johnson L (1995) Communal showers and the risk of plantar warts. *J Fam Pract* **40**(2): 667–9

Joint Formulary Committee (2004) *British National Formulary*. 47. March. British Medical Association and Royal Pharmaceutical Society of Great Britain, London

Kazzi A, Ghadishah D (2002) Warts, genital. www.emedicine.com/emerg/topic640.htm (accessed 9August 2004)

Kenton-Smith J, Tan ST (1999) Pulsed Dye Laser Therapy for viral warts. *Br J Plast Surg* **52**(7): 554–8

Larsen P, Laurberg G (1996) Cryotherapy of viral warts. J Dermatolog Treat **7**: 29–31

Health Protection Agency (2003) Guidelines on the management of communicable diseases in schools and nurseries. Warts and verrucas. www.hpa.org.uk/infections/topics_az/schools/guideline_info/warts.htm (accessed 9 August 2004)

Rudlinger R, Smith I, Bunney M (1986) Human papilloma virus in a group of renal transplant recipients. *Br J Dermatol* **115**: 681–92

Sterling J, Handfield-Jones, Hudson P (2000) Guidelines for the management of cutaneous warts. British Association of Dermatologists, London. www.bad.org.uk/doctors/guidelines/cw.asp (accessed 9August 2004)

Street M, Rÿnigk R (1990) Recalcitrant periungual verrucae: The role of carbon dioxide laser vaporization. *J Am Acad Dermatol* **23**(1): 115–20

Veien NK, Madsen SM, Avrach W et al (1991) The treatment of plantar warts with a keratolytic agent and occlusion. *J Dermatolog Treat* **2**: 59–61

Williams H, Potter A, Strachan D (1993) The descriptive epidemiology of warts in British schoolchildren. *Br J Dermatol* **128**(5): 504–11

Wright T (1998) Genital warts: Their etiology and treatment. *Nursing Times* **94**(7): 52–4

## Test Your Knowledge

This teenage girl was worried about the scaly lesion on the ball of her foot. It had been present for some time but since starting at college, to which she had to walk quite a distance: it was so painful that she had had difficulty reaching there. Her friend had told her that it was a verruca and apart from the pain, that she would not be able to go to the swimming baths until it was better. She bought a wart paint (containing salicylic acid) from the chemist, and had been applying it for several weeks without any signs of improvement. Now, with college access being a problem and summer and swimming soon to be enjoyed, she wanted a more instant cure.

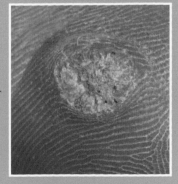

### Questions

1. What is the diagnosis and what particular findings would lead you to the conclusion?
2. What treatment would you suggest for this patient?
3. What advice could you give her about attendance at a swimming pool?

# Genital warts

Genital warts are the most common of the sexually transmitted infections (STIs). Over the past 20 years there has been a dramatic increase in the incidence of this problem (Health Protection Agency (HPA), 2007). In 2006 there were 83 745 new diagnoses of genital warts (a 3% increase from 2005), in addition to 44 655 recurrent episodes and 17 821 re-registered cases (HPA, 2007). The incidence is highest among women aged 17–19 years (767 per 100 000) (HPA, 2007).

Lesions are most likely to develop within 3 months of contact with an infected partner, but sometimes there may be a latency period of years (Kazzi and Hindiyeh, 2007). Infidelity should not therefore be assumed if warts develop during a long-term relationship where there have been risks of acquiring the problem previously.

Risk factors include smoking, oral contraceptives, multiple sexual partners and early involvement in sexual activities. We see many patients, both male and female, in the surgeries and clinics with genital warts. Primary health professionals must be in a position to recognize genital warts and advise patients as to the treatment and future management. Also, with the knowledge that the wart virus infection is usually acquired sexually, any patient with this problem should be checked or referred to a genitourinary (GU) department, so that other STIs may be recognized and dealt with.

## Aetiology

About 75 different types of the double-stranded HPV papoviruses have been isolated and many of them are associated with malignant change. About 90% of genital warts are of the HPV types 6 and 11 (Reisinger et al, 2007). These are the strains that cause the most visible warts, but which tend not to lead to neoplastic change. HPV types 16 and 18 have the greatest potential to precipitate such change (Kazzi and Hindiyeh, 2007). It is therefore important to be aware of the risks and follow patients up, so that pointers to the possibility of malignant change may be spotted early.

## Vaccination

From September 2008, HPV vaccine will be offered to all females at the age of 12–13 years, as well as a catch-up programme for those aged 16–18 years from autumn 2009 (NHS Cervical Screening Programme, 2007). Past this age is considered likely that many girls will already have been exposed to the virus but if, after discussion with the patient, the risks of having contracted the disease are seen to be small, it may be considered up to the age of 26 years.

The Department of Health has decided to restrict the vaccination programme to the prevention of cervical cancer. A bivalent vaccine has been chosen for the programme which protects against HPV types 16 and 18, despite the availability of a quadrivalent vaccine which would also have protected against HPV types 6 and 11, the cause of 90% of genital warts.

## Clinical presentation

In many cases the patient may remain symptomless and the wart virus infection detected only by a routine cervical smear. Some may complain of Pruritus and discharge. Others, particularly those affected by HPV 6 and 11, will develop small, pearly, filiform or smooth eruptions in the genital area. Commonly these are on the penis in a male (*Figure 11.1*) or the cervix, vagina, vulva or perineum in the female (*Figure 11.2*). Sometimes they may occur in the perianal area (*Figure 11.3*), particularly in those who have practised anal intercourse or where there are problems of immuno-suppression. In some cases the lesions may be florid and cauliflower-like (*Figure 11.4*).

Children with genital warts are of particular concern as they may raise fears about sexual abuse. However, it is important not to jump to the wrong conclusion, as it is possible for the infection to be acquired through manual contact or, as in the case of this baby (*Figure 11.5*) following a vaginal delivery in a mother with genital warts (Kazzi and Hindeiyeh, 2007).

### Bowenoid papulosis

Bowenoid papulosis is an uncommon precancerous condition caused by HPV. Men develop small, red or

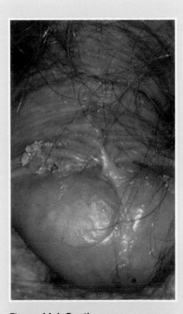

*Figure 11.1. Penile warts.*

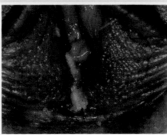

*Figure 11.2. Vulval warts.*

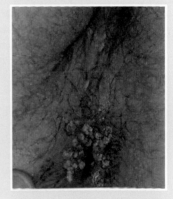

*Figure 11.3. Perianal warts.*

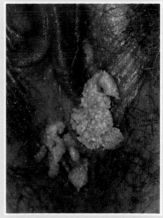

*Figure 11.4. Cauliflower type of genital warts.*

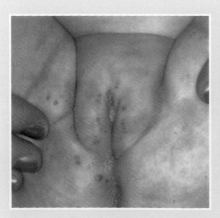

Figure 11.5. Genital warts in a young child.

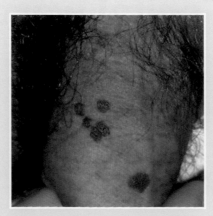

Figure 11.6. Bowenoid papulosis (Penile intraepithelial neoplasia) of the penis.

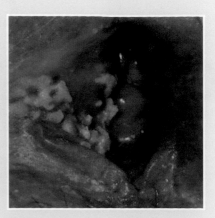

Figure 11.7. Vulval intraepithelial neoplasia.

brown, warty lesions caused by penile intraepithelial neoplasia, on the shaft of the penis (*Figure 11. 6*). Usually these lesions are symptomless, but occasionally they may become inflamed, painful and itchy. Spontaneous resolution may occur, but there should be regular follow-up of patients to note changes that could indicate early progression to a squamous cell carcinoma (SCC).

In women, Bowenoid papulosis is a type of vulvar intraepithelial neoplasia (VIN) (*Figure 11.7*). The diagnosis may be confirmed by biopsy of a lesion (DermNet NZ, 2008).

## Complications
### Transmission to others
Unprotected sexual contact with a partner, and close contact with actual warts, are likely to lead to transmission of the virus to that partner (*Table 11.1*).

### Pregnancy
Viral warts in pregnancy may cause problems with bleeding and occasionally obstruction to a vaginal delivery. Although neonatal infection may occur during passage through the birth canal, Caesarean section is not usually recommended unless obstruction is likely to be a problem.

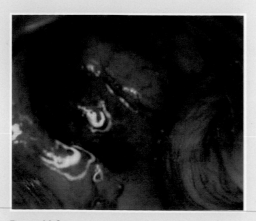

Figure 11.8.
Carcinoma of the cervix.

### Malignant change
The more visible manifestation of HPV is usually associated with types 6 and 11, the types that are least likely to progress to malignant change. The more worrying types, 16 and 18, may remain symptomless and be picked up only when a cervical smear is taken or, as in one case, where a woman complained of intermenstrual bleeding. She was found to have a stage B1 squamous cell carcinoma of the cervix (*Figure 11.8*) and underwent a Wertheim's hysterectomy.

Such problems may not be restricted to the genital region. Some patients will develop warts on the hands and fingers that may have resulted from direct contact with the genital area. Occasionally such areas may raise concerns that malignant change is occurring in these warts, as in this patient with a florid collection of periungual warts (*Figure 11.9*). However, a biopsy excluded malignancy.

### Psychological effects
Little research has been done into the psychological effects on patients with genital warts. A small study of the reactions of patients to such a diagnosis exposed fear, not only of the diagnosis, but also the subsequent treatment and possible outcomes of embarrassment, shame, guilt, sexual and relationship problems (Shepherd et al, 1995). This suggests that attention should be paid to these matters when dealing with patients with genital warts.

### Diagnosis
When obvious warts are present in the genital area, the diagnosis is usually clear. In cases of doubt, a biopsy may be taken. Wart virus infection is also

| Table 11.1. Complications of HPV and genital warts |
| --- |
| Transmission to others |
| Malignant change |
| Pregnancy - obstruction in labour |
| Psychological |

most frequently picked up in patients, with or without symptoms, when abnormalities are seen in a cervical smear. Although typing of the virus is possible, it is not yet done routinely in the surgeries and clinics of the UK; it may sometimes be done at colposcopy or when a lesion is biopsied. For those at greater risk of anal HPV, such as those practising receptive anal sex or those with HIV, an anal smear should also be taken (Cancerbackup, 2007).

## Management

Any patient with a HPV infection should have a full check to exclude other STIs. If this cannot be done in the surgery, the patient should be referred to the GU clinic.

In principle, it is normally recommended in the NHS that cervical smears are taken every 3 years from the age of 25–49 years and every 5 years from 50–64 years (Cancerbackup, 2008). For those with suspicious symptoms or abnormal results, extra smears or more frequent follow-up may be recommended by the laboratory.

If left untreated, warts may remain unchanged, increase or resolve spontaneously. In some cases, treatment is offered. However, the underlying infection may persist even after the warts are cleared. Treatment may be required for symptoms such as itching, bleeding, pain, anxiety or embarrassment. The following approaches are the ones most usually considered:

- Podophyllotoxin—applied twice daily for 3 days to the warts and, if necessary, repeated at weekly intervals up to four times. This causes them to shrink or disappear. Patients may apply this themselves at home, unless lesions are bigger than 4 cm or if they are pregnant (Joint National Formulary, 2008)
- Imiquimod—applied three times a week at night until the lesion resolves, or for up to 16 weeks. This enhances the patient's immune responses and recurrence of the warts is less likely to follow.

## Table 11.2. Differential diagnosis of genital warts

| | Cause | Presentation | Diagnosis | Management |
|---|---|---|---|---|
| Genital warts | Warts: HPV type 6, 11 Few symptoms: HPV types 16, 18 | Warts – small, pearly, filiform or smooth eruptions in genital area Sometimes florid cauliflower like lesions Abnormal cervical smear | Clinical Cervical smear Colposcopy Biopsy | Check for other STIs Await spontaneous resolution or: Podophyllotoxin Imiquimod Cryotherapy Electrocautery Excision or cautery Laser ablation |
| Pearly penile papules | Uncertain – may be more common in uncircumcised men | Asymptomattic early, flesh-like, dome-topped or filiform papules round corona or sulcus of glans penis | Clinical | Reassurance No treatment necessary Laser ablation, electrocautery, curettage or excision |
| Milia | Epidermoid cyst Underdevelopment or disruption of sweat gland | Single or multiple Cream or white papules | Clinical | Spontaneous resolution No need to treat Prick with sterile needle to express contents |
| Molluscum contagiosum | Poxvirus | Small, pearly, umbilicated papules | Clinical Biopsy | Check for other STIs if sexual transmission is suspected Spontaneous resolution usual in a few months Curettage, cryotherapy or needle electrocautery |
| Seborrhoeic wart | Benign abnormality of basal cell maturation More common in elderly | Well-defined, rough surfaced papule or plaque. | Clinical Biopsy | None necessary Cryotherapy, curettage and cautery or excision |

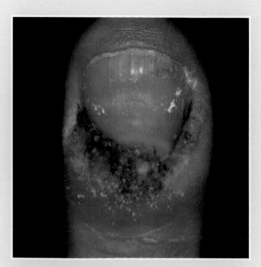

*Figure 11.9. Periungual warts.*

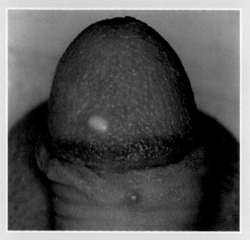

*Figure 11.10. Milium of the penis.*

Imiquimod can be used by the patient, but not in pregnancy. (Joint National Formulary, 2008)

- Cryotherapy—may be painful and cause blistering but can be used for both internal and external warts and is, perhaps, preferable in pregnancy
- Electrocautery—can be used to burn the warts under local or general anaesthetic
- Excision or curettage—to remove the warts
- Laser ablation—in cases of an abnormal smear the laboratory may recommend referral to a gynaecologist for colposcopic examination and/or biopsy (Cancer research, 2007).

## Prevention

The adoption of the quadrivalent HPV vaccine would have offered great hope for the future that this common virus, with all its suffering and implications, would be controlled. Until a vaccine is offered to the UK population, however, sexual abstinence and monogamy will remain the best protective measures available. Condoms may help, but they do not protect against transmission from uncovered lesions.

## Differential diagnosis

There are certain lesions in the genital area which may be mistaken for warts. Therefore a careful differential diagnosis is required (*Table 11.2*).

### Pearly penile papules

These asymptomatic, pearly, flesh-like, dome-topped or filiform papules tend to form around the corona or sulcus of the glans penis. These lesions are extremely common and likely to persist through life.

Pearly penile papules are harmless. No treatment is required, but patients are sometimes concerned and will need reassurance that they have not acquired an STI. If a patient insists on treatment, laser ablation, electrocautery and curettage or excision can be offered (Large Penis Support Group, 2006).

### Milia

A milium is an epidermoid cyst that is thought to form as the result of underdevelopment or disruption of a sweat gland.Milia are symptomless, single or multiple cream or white papules which commonly occur on the face, but may also appear elsewhere in the body, including the penis (*Figure 11.10*).

Frequently, no treatment is required and they will resolve spontaneously. If it is necessary, the lesion may be pricked with a sterile needle and the contents expressed or it may be excised (du Vivier, 2002).

### Molluscum contagiosum

Molluscum contagiosum is a viral-infection of the skin caused by a poxvirus. It is transmitted by direct contact with a lesion or through contaminated items such as towels. It is most common in children and more likely to be a problem in the immunosupressed. Direct transmission may also occur during sexual contact.

At first the lesions develop as small papules that form raised, pearly nodules with an umbilicated centre, 2–5 mm in diameter (*Figure 11.11*). The lesions are painless. A spontaneous resolution of the lesions can usually be expected within a few months, and no treatment is normally necessary. The diagnosis can usually be made from the clinical appearance but if necessary a biopsy can be taken. Lesions may be surgically removed by scraping, freezing or needle electrocautery.

### Genital naevi

A variety of pigmented lesions may be found on the genitalia of both men and women. The majority of them will be benign and include seborrhoeic keratoses, which develops in later life (*Figure 11.12*). Naevi in these areas are no different to those found on other parts of the body, but occasionally they may be mistaken for genital warts (Selim, 2008).

Although most naevi in the genital area are benign, in a few cases there may be a possibility of malignant change or malignant melanoma. In cases where this may be suspected, a biopsy should be taken and action carried out according to the results. Benign naevi do not normally require treatment, unless the patient is embarrassed by them or they are causing problems with chafing and soreness. The options then available are cryotherapy, curettage and cautery or excision.

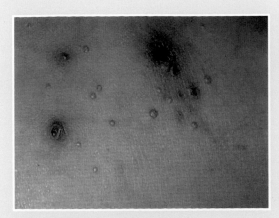

*Figure 11.11. Molluscum contagiosum.*

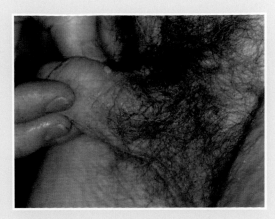

*Figure 11.12. Seborrhoeic wart on the penis.*

## References

Cancerbackup (2007) Human papilloma virus (HPV) www.cancerbackup.org.uk/Aboutcancer/Causes/Viruses/HumanpapillomavirusHPV (accessed 24 June 2008)

Cancerbackup (2008) Cervical screening. www.cancerbackup.org.uk/Aboutcancer/Screening/Cervicalscreening (accessed 24 June 2008)

Cancer Research UK (2007) Cervical cancer tests. www.cancerhelp.org.uk/help/default.asp?page=2760 (accessed 24 June 2008)

DermNet NZ (2008) Bowenoid papulosis. http://dermnetnz.org/site-age-specific/bowenoid-papulosis.html (accessed 24 June 2008)

du Vivier A (2002) Benign tumours of the Skin. In: *Atlas of Clinical Dermatology.* 3rd edn. Churchill Livingstone: 126–7

Health Protection Agency (2007) Trends in genital warts and herpes diagnoses in the United Kingdom. *Health Protection Report* **1**(35). http://tinyurl.com/6qja9m (accessed 27 June 2008)

Joint Formulary Committee (2008) *British National Formulary* 55. March. BMJ Publishing Group Ltd and RPS Publishing, London

Kazzi A, Hindiyeh R (2007) Warts, Genital. www.emedicine.com/emerg/topic640.htm (accessed 24 June 2008)

Large Penis Support Group (2006) Pearly penile papules (PPP) www.lpsg.org/29213-pearly-penile-papules-ppp.html (accessed 24 June 2008)

NHS Cervical Screening Programme (2007) Possible future developments. www.cancerscreening.nhs.uk/cervical/#future (accessed 23 June 2008)

Reisinger KS, Block SL, Lazcano-Ponce E et al (2007) Safety and persistent immunogenicity of a quadrivalent human papillomavirus types 6, 11, 16, 18 L1 virus-like particle vaccine in preadolescents and adolescents: a randomized controlled trial. *Pediatr Infect Dis J* **26**(3):201 9(accessed 24 June 2008)

Selim A (2008) Atypical Genital Naevi. *Journal Watch Dermatology* http://dermatology.jwatch.org/cgi/content/full/2008/314/1 (accessed 24 June 2008)

Shepherd S, White M, Waltzman M (1995) Genital warts: just a nuisance? *Genitourin Med* **71**: 194–5

UK Health Care (2007) HPV vaccine use guidelines http://ukhealthcare.uky.edu/press/releases/hpv_providers.htm (accessed 24 June 2008)

## Test Your Knowledge

This 40-year-old man had been troubled by a sore area in his left groin for 6 months. It caused him problems, particularly when he was hot and sweating as it became rubbed and inflamed. On examination there was some inflammation around clusters of small warty areas that were clearly genital warts. He was concerned that he might have 'caught something' from his girlfriend of 3 years' standing and their relationship was suffering as he was accusing her of having 'played away'.

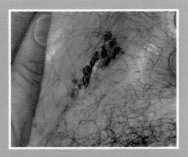

### Questions

1. Which type of HPV is likely to be associated with these warts and what advice would you give the patient about follow-up and the risks of malignant change?
2. What advice would you give to the patient about treatment of the warts and his condition?
3. How could you discuss his question of his girlfriend's suspected infidelity and what advice would you offer for her?

# Diagnosing spots and vesicles

Immunization has resulted in the reduction or near eradication of many infectious illnesses. The Department of Health (DH) has now commissioned the Joint Committee on Vaccination and Immunisation (JCVI) to consider the evidence for the introduction of a chickenpox vaccines. This vaccine is already in use for nonimmune (seronegative) health workers in primary care and hospitals who have direct contact with patients (Chief Medical Officer et al, 2003) but as yet there are no plans to start routine immunisation of children (Rull, 2009).

Chickenpox appears in general practice, but other 'spotty' conditions also occur. Therefore, it is important to recognize these conditions and offer the appropriate advice when they present.

## Chickenpox (varicella)

### Aetiology

Chickenpox is caused by the varicella (herpes) zoster virus, which is spread by respiratory droplets and/or direct contact with the vesicles (Papadopoulos, 2007). It is common in children, but adults who have not had chickenpox are also at risk of infection.

Initial infection should provide lifelong immunity. Occasionally, previously immunized children may develop a mild, modified form of the disease, without a fully developed rash. The incubation period for varicella is 11–21 days. School exclusion with chickenpox is recommended for 5 days after the onset of the rash not, as previously recommended, until all the lesions have dried and crusted (Health Protection Agency (HPA), 2007).

### Clinical presentation

The patient usually presents with a rash, without any prodromal symptoms. The patient will develop crops of itchy papules that blister over the trunk, abdomen and face, before spreading to other parts of the body (*Figure 12.1*), including the mouth and urogenital area. The early spots have the typical 'tear-drop' appearance (*Figure 12.2*).

Initially, the patient will complain of much itching. The vesicles become crusted and dried before finally clearing. Scars may follow.

### Diagnosis

The diagnosis can usually be made on clinical grounds alone but, if necessary, examination of the vesicular fluid may culture the virus.

Immunofluorescence is likely to produce more reliable results (Papadopoulous, 2007) as it has greater sensitivity. Culture of the fluid from the vesicle will not always show a positive result.

### Complications

Chickenpox in children usually settles without problems, but there is a risk of a secondary bacterial infection of the lesions. Scarring is then more likely.

The immunocompromised and adults are more likely to suffer complications, some of which may be serious, e.g. pneumonia, haemorrhagic lesions or bullous chickenpox, hepatitis or encephalitis (Papadopoulous, 2007).

Serious complications are more likely in women who develop chickenpox during pregnancy. Before the introduction of antiviral therapy, mortality rates of 25–40% were reported. Pneumonia occurs in 10% of pregnant women with chickenpox and is likely to be more severe in late pregnancy (Royal College of Obstetricians and Gynaecologists, 2007).

Chickenpox in the first 3 months of pregnancy does not seem to increase the rate of miscarriage, but there is a possibility of fetal varicella syndrome if the woman suffers chickenpox in the first 20 weeks of pregnancy. This risk is small but the child may have a number of developmental abnormalities including eye defects, neurological problems or limb hypoplasia. If chickenpox occurs in the mother at term, the child is at risk of developing the disease, with severe consequences for the child, such as disseminated varicella and possible fatal results (Royal College of Obstetricians and Gynaecologists, 2007).

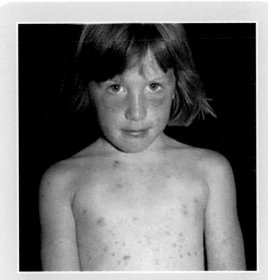

*Figure 12.1. Chickenpox rash.*

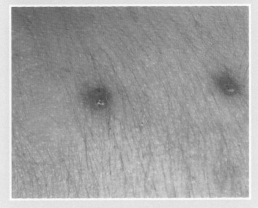

*Figure 12.2. Chickenpox: 'tear-drop' spots.*

## Management

Symptomatic treatment is all that is usually required in the treatment of chickenpox, with paracetamol and topical calamine lotion to ease the itching (*Figure 12.3*). An antiviral agent such as aciclovir may be considered in adults or the immunocompromised, as they are more likely to have a severe infection. In the immunocompromised, aciclovir should be administered intravenously.

Secondary infection of the lesions may require topical or oral antibiotics, depending on the extent of the problem.

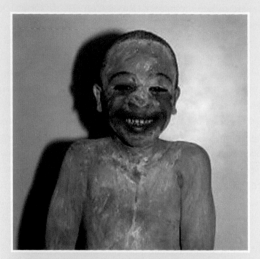

*Figure 12.3. Child with chickenpox, covered in calamine lotion to reduce the itching.*

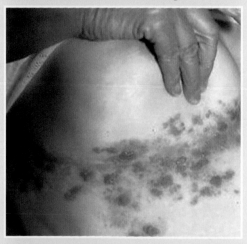

*Figure 12.4. Shingles rash on chest.*

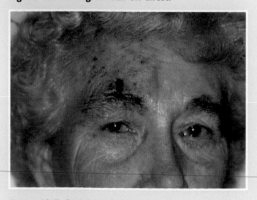

*Figure 12.5. Ophthalmic herpes zoster.*

Those in contact with chickenpox who are at greater risk of severe problems, particularly nonimmune pregnant women, can be helped by varicella-zoster immunoglobulin, if given within 96 hours of contact. Although it may not prevent chickenpox, it can modify the course of the disease (Dermnet NZ, 2007).

To reduce the risk to a fetus, aciclovir should be given within 24 hours of the onset of the rash, providing the pregnancy is more advanced than 20 weeks. Although there appears to be no risk of fetal abnormalities if given earlier, there is a risk of teratogenesis if used in the first trimester; and it is, therefore better avoided (Royal College of Obstetricians and Gynaecologists, 2007).

# Shingles
## Aetiology

After chickenpox, the varicella-zoster virus remains dormant in the dorsal root ganglia of the spinal cord. Sometimes, for reasons that are not fully understood, the virus is reactivated and shingles occurs. The risk of shingles is greater in those with reduced immunity and the elderly (Melton, 2006). Although it may occur in young people it is more common in the elderly. It is possible to transmit chickenpox to susceptible contacts if there is direct contact with the rash. Providing the rash is covered, crusted or dried, there should be no risk of transmission.

## Clinical presentation

Initially, the patient may complain of unilateral pain along the area supplied by the involved nerve. The patient may feel unwell and complain of headache and fever. After several days the rash appears, which may be erythematous, and vesicular before becoming pustular and crusting over (*Figure 12.4*). Secondary bacterial infection of the area is possible.

Healing is gradual, but the patient may be left with post-herpetic pain, which may be severe, along the distribution of the rash. This pain may persist for many weeks or months or even years. Particular problems can arise if shingles affects the ophthalmic division of the trigeminal nerve. This is associated with visual complications that may be serious including conjunctivitis, keratitis, ulceration cornea, uveitis, glaucoma and blindness. In these cases the rash presents over the forehead and extends to the tip of the nose (Hutchinson's sign) (Melton, 2006) (*Figure 12.5*).

## Diagnosis

A clinical diagnosis can usually be made but, if necessary, biopsy for direct immunofluorescence assay will identify varicella zoster and distinguish it from herpes simplex (Melton, 2006).

## Management

Antiviral agents such as aciclovir, if given early, help modify the course of disease and reduce the incidence of post-herpetic neuralgia. They are recommended for all immunocompromised patients, those over 60 years of age and those with zoster affecting the neck, limbs and perineum. In severe cases add additional corticosteroids have been tried. Analgesics are required for pain. NICE recommends amitryptilline or pregabalin for post herpeic neuralgia and referral to a specialist pain unit. If this is not sufficient, using tramadol or topical lindocaine while awaiting appointment. Using and topical calamine lotion or wet dressings with 5% aluminium acetate several times a day may help reduce the discomfort of the rash. If secondary infection occurs, antibiotics are needed, Any indication of eye involvement requires urgent referral to an ophthalmic unit.

## Molluscum contagiosum
### Aetiology
Molluscum contagiosum is a skin infection caused by a DNA poxvirus (Kauffman and Beatty, 2007). It is spread by direct contact with the lesions. The incubation period is 14–50 days, although no period of isolation is recommended for this mild condition (HPA, 2007). It is more common in the immunosuppressed or those with atopic eczema and may occur at any age; however, it is most common in children and young adults.

### Clinical presentation
Small, firm, smooth, umbilicated, flesh-coloured or white papules may be seen, often in clusters (*Figure 12.6*). Some patients will complain of itching, but many are symptomless. Those with eczema are likely to have more widespread lesions. Spontaneous resolution can be expected, but it may take many months or even years. Secondary infection of the lesions is possible and lesions on the eyelid may lead to conjunctivitis (Kauffmann andBeatty, 2007).

### Diagnosis
The diagnosis can usually be made on clinical grounds but a biopsy is possible if necessary.

## Table 12.1. Diagnosis and management of spots and vesicles

| | Chickenpox | Shingles | Molluscum contagiosum | Hand-foot-and-mouth disease |
|---|---|---|---|---|
| **Cause** | Varicella-zoster virus | Reactivation of dormant varicella-zoster virus | DNA poxvirus | Coxsackievirus A16 Enterovirus 71 |
| **Incubation** | 11–21 days | | 14–50 days | 3–5 days |
| **School exclusion** | 5 days after onset of rash | No risk of transmission if rash covered or crusted and dried  Risk of chickenpox only to individual who has not had chickenpox | None | None |
| **Symptoms** | • Itchy papules, blisters on the trunk, abdomen and face, then limbs and oral or urogenital ulcers | • Unilateral pain along distribution of affected nerve<br>• Unwell, headache<br>• Erythema, vesicular rash after several days along line of affected nerve<br>• Rash crusts and dries | • Small, smooth, flesh coloured or white, umbilicated papules<br>• Often in clusters | • 1–2 days: Slightly unwell, sore mouth, cough<br>• Then erythematous, macula rash and small oval blisters mainly on hands, feet and buttocks<br>• Painful mouth ulcers |
| **Diagnosis** | • Clinical<br>• Immunofluorescence<br>• viral swab for culture | • Clinical<br>• Immunofluorescence | • Clinical<br>• Biopsy if necessary | • Clinical<br>• Swab from vesicle for virus culture |
| **Complications** | • Rare in children— secondary infection<br>• Greater risk in adults, immunocompromised – pneumonia, haemorrhagic lesions, hepatitis, encephalitis<br>• In pregnancy—small risk in the first 20 weeks of fetal varicella syndrome. At term—varicella in newborn may be serious | • Secondary infection<br>• Post-herpetic pain<br>• Ophthalmic herpes – conjunctivitis, keratitis, ulceration cornea.<br>• Uveitis, glaucoma and blindness | • Secondary infection | • Occasionally dehydration if fluids refused because of sore mouth |
| **Management** | • Symptomatic - paracetamol, calamine lotion<br>• Antibiotic if secondary infection<br>• Antiviral, e.g. aciclovir for at risk patients—VZIG within 96 hours of contact | • Antiviral, e.g. aciclovir<br>• Topical calamine or aluminium acetate dressings<br>• Analgesics<br>• Amitryptilline<br>• Pregabalin<br>• Tramadol<br>• Topical lindocaine | • Preferably nil<br>• Can prick lesions, or apply podophyllin (not in pregnancy) or trichloracetic acid<br>• Retinoin, imiquimod<br>• Cryoytherapy or curettage | • Symptomatic<br>• Analgesics<br>• Antiseptic mouth wash |

VZIG=varicella-zoster immunoglobulin

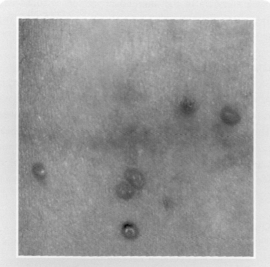

*Figure 12.6. Molluscum contagiosum.*

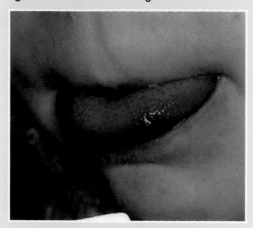

*Figure 12.7. Hand, foot and mouth disease—mouth ulcer.*

### Management

Masterly inactivity is the best approach. Scratching should be discouraged as this may lead to autoinoculation. Direct contact with others and the sharing of towels or razors should be avoided.

Treatment is often more upsetting to a child than the condition. Sometimes, if the spots are pierced with an orange stick, inflammation occurs and the spots may then clear. If a local anaesthetic is applied to the area first, the discomfort of the procedure is lessened. If it is felt necessary to treat, as may be the case in the immunocompromised, preparations such as topical podophyllin or trichloracetic acid, retinoin, imiquimod,

cryotherapy or curettage can be used. Podophyllin and imiquimod should not be used in pregnancy (British Association of Dermatologists, 2004). Molluscum on the eyelid should be referred to an ophthalmologist.

## Hand-foot-and-mouth disease

Hand-foot-and-mouth disease is a highly infectious viral infection caused by Cox-sackievirus A16 or enterovirus 71. It tends to occur in late summer and early autumn. It is unrelated to the foot and mouth disease of animals.

The incubation period is 3–5 days and school exclusion for this mild disease is unnecessary (HPA, 2007). Spread is thought to be through droplets or direct contact with secretions from the respiratory tract or faeces. Hand-foot-and-mouth disease is most common in children, but may also be seen in adults (Graham, 2007).

### Clinical presentation

The patient may feel unwell, with a low-grade fever, sore mouth and cough for 1–2 days before the rash develops. A few painful mouth vesicles on an erythematous base develop (*Figure 12.7*), which may hinder eating. On the body, an erythematous, macular rash, with a central vesicle, appears mainly on the hands, feet and buttocks (*Figure12.8*). Typically, the lesions are oval in shape (*Figure 12.9*). Spontaneous resolution follows in 1 week.

Hand-foot-and-mouth disease is generally mild, but occasionally complications of dehydration occur if children fail to take sufficient fluids because of the painful mouth ulcers. If a woman acquires the disease in the first 3 months of pregnancy, there is a risk of spontaneous abortion (Graham, 2007)

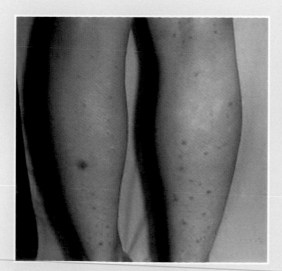

*Figure 12.8. Hand, foot and mouth disease—rash on the legs.*

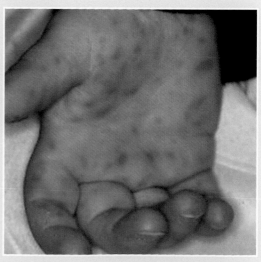

*Figure 12.9. Hand-foot-and-mouth disease:oval lesions on palm.*

Diagnosis of hand-foot-and-mouth disease is normally be made on clinical grounds, but the virus can be cultured by a swab from the vesicles or a stool specimen, if necessary.

Symptomatic treatment is usually all that is required with plenty of cold fluids and soft foods. Analgesics may be required for pain, and antiseptic mouth washes may help any oral discomfort (DermnetNZ, 2006).

## References

British Association of Dermatologists (2004) Molluscum contagiosum. Patient information leaflet. www.bad.org.uk/public/leaflets/molluscum.asp (accessed 5 February 2008)

Dermnet NZ (2007) Chickenpox (Varicella) www.dermnetnz.org/viral/varicella.html (accessed 5February 2008)

Chief Medical, Nursing, Dental and Pharmaceutical Officers (2003) Chickenpox (varicella) immunisation for health care workers. Letter, 4 December. http://tinyurl.com/2slpuh (accessed 13 February 2008)

Dermnet NZ (2006) Hand foot and mouth disease. http://dermnetnz.org/viral/hand-foot-mouth.html (accessed 5 February 2008)

Graham B (2007) Hand-foot-and-mouth disease. *eMedicine*. www.emedicine.com/derm/topic175.htm (accessed 5 February 2008)

Health Protection Agency (2007) Guidelines on the management of communicable diseases in schools and nurseries. www.hpa.org.uk/infections/topics_az/schools/schools.pdf (accessed 5February 2008)

Kauffman C, Beatty C (2007) Molluscum contagiosum. *eMedicine*. www.emedicine.com/derm/topic270.htm (accessed 5February 2008)

Melton C (2006) Herpes zoster eMedicine. www.emedicine.com/emerg/topic823.htm (accessed 5 February 2008)

Papadopoulos AJ (2007) Chickenpox. *eMedicine*. www.emedicine.com/derm/topic74.htm (accessed 5 February 2008)

Royal College of Obstetricians and Gynaecologists (2007) Chickenpox in pregnancy. Green-top Guideline 13. www.rcog.org.uk/index.asp?PageID=514 (accessed 5 February 2008)

Rull G (2009) Chickenpox (variella). Patient Plus www.patient.co.uk/chickenpox.patientplus (accessed 30.07.2010)

# Test Your Knowledge

This patient was 27 years of age. She presented in the surgery with a 3-day history of an itchy rash that had started on her face and back, and was now rapidly spreading to the rest of her body. She complained of feeling unwell, hot and feverish and with a headache. She was particularly worried as she was 3 months pregnant. The rash of erythematous papules and blisters was extensive and there were ulcers in her mouth that made it difficult to eat.

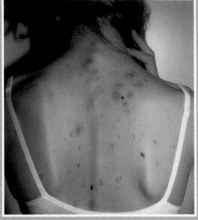

## Questions
1. What is the likely diagnosis?
2. What particular concerns might you have about the pregnancy?
3. How would you advise the patient?

# Plaque psoriasis

Psoriasis is a common condition of the skin that affects 1–2% of the UK population (British Association of Dermatologists (BAD), 2006). The effect on those who have psoriasis can be profound, not only in symptoms, but also in the effect on their social lives, both at home and at work.

Psoriasis may present in a number of different ways, but when considering the problem of plaque psoriasis, it is important to make the correct diagnosis, assess the severity of the problem as seen by the practice nurse and the patient, and then to advise and institute the best programme of treatment to fit the circumstances. There are a number of other conditions which may present with rashes that mimic plaque psoriasis and it is therefore necessary to consider alternative possibilities before embarking on management.

This chapter will discuss the presentations of plaque psoriasis, possible confirmatory signs to look for, some of the other conditions with which it may be confused and ways in which they may be distinguished.

## Plaque psoriasis
### Aetiology
The exact cause of psoriasis in which there is hyper-proliferation of epiermal cells is unknown, but a number of different factors have been implicated. These include:

- Evidence suggests it to be an autoimmune disease
- Related to excess T-cell activity (Gordon 2010)
- Genetic factors—frequently patients with psoriasis will know of other members of the family with the condition. HLA-B13, B17 and CW6 have all been found to be associated with plaque psoriasis (Lui and Mamelak, 2007)
- Environmental—trauma, strepotococcal infection, HIV, stress, smoking and alcohol
- Drugs—psoriasis may be exacerbated by lithium, beta-blockers, nonsteroidal anti-inflammatory drugs (NSAID), some antimalarials and withdrawal of systemic steroids
- Sunlight—may occasionally aggravate psoriasis, but usually improves it (Lui and Mamelak, 2007)
- Age—psoriasis may present in children, but most often first appears in the late-teens, early-20s or in the late-50s.

### Presentation
The patient typically complains of well-defined, red, scaly patches that may be covered in a silvery scale, and some may be itchy. They may be isolated lesions or widespread, and tend to be symmetrically distributed (*Figure 13.1*). These may appear anywhere on the body, but sites commonly affected are the extensor surfaces of the elbows and knees (*Figure 13.2*), or the scalp (*Figure 13.3*).

Some of the lesions may coalesce to form large plaques (*Figure 13.4*). In some more acute cases, the plaques may be inflamed, red and sore without the scale and silvery

appearance (*Figure 13.5*). Where precipitated by injury such as burns, cuts, grazes or surgical wounds, the psoriatic rash may appear at the site of the trauma. This is known as the Koebner phenomenon (Lui and Mamelak, 2007) (*Figure 13.6*).

### Diagnosis
Psoriasis can usually be diagnosed on clinical grounds and, although skin biopsy will confirm the diagnosis, further investigations are rarely necessary.

When faced with a rash that might be plaque psoriasis, it is worth looking for other signs that will support this diagnosis. Lesions on the elbows and/or knees are commonly present, even in patients with minimal symptoms, or there may be scalp involvement. Also, it is always important to check the nails because these

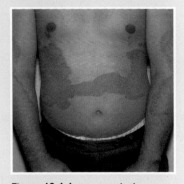
Figure13.2. Psoriatic lesions on the extensor surface of the knees.

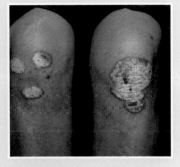
Figure 13.4. Large psoriatic plaque on the abdomen.

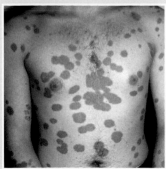
Figure 13.5. Acute phase of plaque psoriasis with red inflamed lesions.

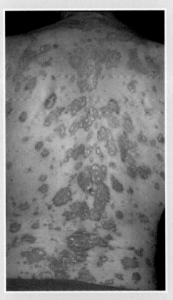
Figure 13.1. Widespread plaque psoriasis.

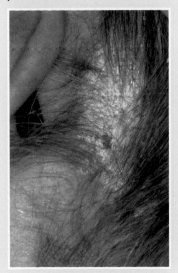
Figure 13.3. Scalp psoriasis.

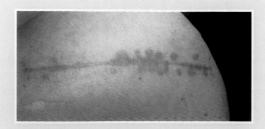

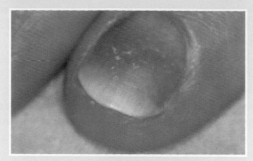

*Figure 13.6. Koebner phenomenon following total hip replacement.*

*Figure 13.7. Nail psoriasis with pitting and onycholysis.*

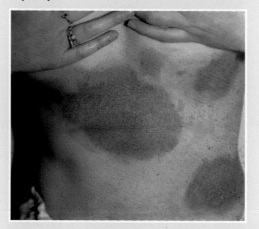

*Figure 13.8. Burnt areas following the application of dithranol.*

frequently show signs such as pitting, onycholysis (*Figure 13.7*), subungual keratosis or dystrophy (Lui and Mamelak, 2007).

## Management

Psoriasis cannot be cured. The patient is likely to suffer exacerbations and remissions. Treatment is aimed at inducing remissions so that the patient can feel more comfortable and lead as normal a life as possible, bearing in mind that even relatively minor lesions may interfere with acceptability among friends or in the workplace.

As certain drugs may precipitate or worsen the condition, the need to continue with such drugs should be reviewed and alternatives substituted if possible. The adverse effects of alcohol and smoking should be discussed and the patient encouraged to change his/her habits.

If the patient is in a stressful situation, discussion or counselling could be recommended. If at the end of this further treatment seems necessary, alternatives and their likely effects and side effects should be considered when deciding which path to follow. The patient should discuss the management plan and have specific instruction on how to apply or seek any treatment.

There are a number of treatment options (Joint Formulary Committee, 2008: 13.5.2) (*Table 13.1*).

## Emollients

Emollients soften the scale and may be especially helpful in inflammatory psoriasis.

## Topical coal tar

Topical coal tar 1–5% is often effective in inducing remission but patients are often deterred from its use by the smell and the fact that it is messier to use. Although, recent research has raised concerns of carcinogenicity of coal tar products, these concerns remain unproven and topical tar preparations remain available (BAD, 2006).

Topical tar combined with a (mostly mild) corticosteroid may help avoid the stronger tar preparations that tend to be so messy.

## Table 13.1. Treatments for plaque psoriasis

| Product | Ingredient/trade name | Preparation | Adult dose |
|---|---|---|---|
| Topical coal tar | Coal tar 10% (Carbo-Dome)<br>Coal tar 12% (Cocois)<br>Coal tar 1% (Exorex)<br>Coal tar 6% (Psoriderm)<br>Coal tar 12% (Sebco) | Cream<br>Scalp lotion<br>Lotion<br>Cream<br>Scalp lotion | 1–3 times daily |
| Topical coal tar/corticosteroid | Coal tar extract 5%, hydrocortisone 0.5%, allantoin 2% (Alphosyl HC) | Cream | Thinly twice daily |
| Topical dithranol | Dithranol 0.1–2% (Dithrocream)<br>Dithranol 1–3% (Micanol)<br>Dithranol 0.11–1.6% (Psorin) | Cream<br>Cream<br>Ointment | Once or twice a day depending on the preparation (see British National Formulary section 13.5.2) |
| Vitamin D analogues | Calcipotriol (Dovonex)<br>Calcitriol (Silkis)<br>Tacalcitol (Curatoderm) | Cream, ointment<br>Ointment<br>Ointment | 1–2 times daily (maximum 100 g/week)<br>Twice daily (maximum 30 g/day)<br>Once daily (maximum 10 g/day) |
| Vitamin D analogue/corticosteroid | Calcipotriol and betamethasone (Dovobet) | Ointment | Once daily (maximum 15 g/day or 100 g/week) to no more than 30% of body surface |

From: Joint Formulary Committee, 2008.

## Topical corticosteroids

Cosmetically, patients like corticosteroids but it must be remembered that psoriasis may rebound on ceasing the steroid. It is recommended that 'no topical steroid should be used for more than a month without careful review' (BAD, 2006). Tolerance may develop. Moving on to the more potent topical steroids may lead to thinning of the skin and permanent striae. Occasionally overuse leads to toxicity and pituitary adrenal suppression. The rule is that no more than 100 g of a moderately potent or potent topical steroid should be used in 1 month and for no longer than 7 days (BAD, 2006). Stronger steroids may be used on the palms, soles and scalp.

## Topical dithranol

Topical dithranol is a cheap and effective way of treating stable plaque psoriasis but correct application by the patient may be difficult and a trained nurse who can teach the patient may be required. Application of gradually increasing strengths of the cream must be to the plaques alone, as the surrounding normal skin may be burned. (BAD, 2006) (*Figure 13.8*).

## Vitamin D analogues

Calcipotriol and tacalcitol are often more acceptable to the patient as they neither stain nor smell. They work well in mild-to-moderate chronic plaque psoriasis. They should not be used in children under 6 years nor in pregnancy. If calcipotriol is combined with betamethasone, good results are sometimes achieved, although long-term

---

### Table 13.2. Resources

**The Psoriasis Association**
www.psoriasis-association.org.uk
2 Queensbridge, Northampton NN4 7BF
*Tel* 0845 676 0076
(Mon. to Thurs. 09.15 to 16.45, Fri. 09.15 to 16.15)
*Email* mail@psoriasis-association.org.uk

---

data on relapse rates are incomplete. It may be useful in stable plaque psoriasis when calcipotriol alone has failed (BAD, 2006).

## Ultraviolet light

Ultraviolet light (UVL) may be helpful and may also help topical preparations to work better.

## Scalp psoriasis

Intially a tar-based shampoo should be used. A 2.5% salicylic acid preparation, coconut oil combined with the above, calcipotriol or potent topical steroid may also be tried (BAD, 2006).

## Advice and support

Further advice may be required for patients with severe problems or those that have not sufficiently responded to one of the above. The dermatologist may offer UVL, photochemo-therapy (PUVA), methotrexate, acetretin, ciclosporin and hydroxycarbamide.

Support groups may be of great help to patients (see Psorisis Association) (*Table 13.2*).

---

### Table 13.3. Differential diagnoses of plaque psoriasis

| Diagnosis | Aetiology | Presentation | Investigations |
|---|---|---|---|
| Plaque psoriasis | Cause- unknown. Factors - excess T-cell activity, genetic, trauma, infection (HIV) Drugs, sunlight (usually beneficial) First episode usually late teens to early 20's or late 50's | Well-defined, red, scaly patches, silvery scale Symmetrical. Some may be itchy Acute case - red, sore no silvery scale Koebner phenomenon along lines of injury | Usually clinical diagnosis Confirmatory signs - plaques elbows, knees scalp Nails—pitting, onycholysis, subungual keratosis, dystrophy Skin biopsy if necessary |
| Bowen's disease | Pre-invasive intradermal carcinoma Affects sun damaged skin or arsenic exposure or HPV16 | Sharply demarcated erythematous or scaly plaque. Usually isolated lesion | Biopsy Check rest of possible areas of sun damage |
| Discoid eczema | Cause unknown May follow trauma or in children with atopic eczema | Single or multiple, coin shaped plaques Dry, rough, red, scale Most common on lower leg Often secondary infection | Clinical diagnosis If necessary bacterial swab, mycology to exclude fungal infection, and patch testing if allergy suspected |
| Discoid lupus erythematosus | Cause unknown Occasionally genetic link Most often women 20-50 Precipitated by sun exposure | Affects sun exposed areas Erythematous plaques, scale Separate lesions, merge Localized or widespread Post-inflammatory hypopigmentation, scars | Skin biopsy |
| Pityriasis rosea | Cause unknown, possibly viral | Herald patch—initial isolated patch, round or oval, up to 5cm diameter, salmon colour, wrinkled centre, red surround and colarette of scale Within 10 days - more generalized rash trunk, thighs and upper arms | Look for herald patch Clinical diagnosis Mycology if fungal infection suspected Skin biopsy to exclude other conditions |
| Mycosis fungoides | Cutaneous T-cell lymphoma Cause unknown Usually develops about the age of 50 years | Patches, plaques and later tumors. Well-defined, irregular outline Single or multiple, flat erythematous macules Later plaques Asymmetrical distribution | Biopsy |

---

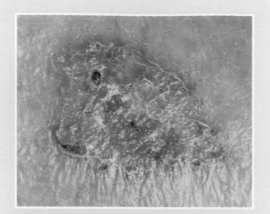

Figure 13.9. Bowen's disease on the lower leg.

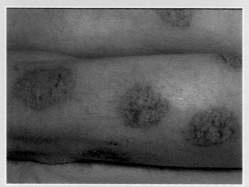

Figure 13.10. Discoid eczema.

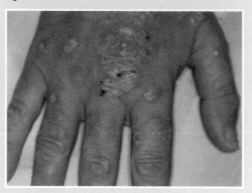

Figure 13.11. Discoid lupus erythematosus.

## Differential diagnosis

When faced with a new presentation of a plaque-like lesion or lesions, particularly in patients with no previous history of psoriasis, it is important to consider any possible conditions with which it might be confused. In all these cases, the history, clinical findings and sometimes further investigations will be needed to determine the problem (*Table 13.3*). Having confirmed the diagnosis, future management and treatment can be agreed.

## Bowen's disease
### Aetiology

Bowen disease is a form of pre-invasive intradermal carcinoma that may, in time, progress to a squamous cell carcinoma (SCC). It occurs more commonly in the elderly, especially in those who have suffered sun damage to the skin, following exposure to arsenic or in association with the human papillomavirus (HPV) type 16 (Welch, 2008).

### Presentation

Lesions usually present on sun-exposed areas of the skin with a history of a sharply demarcated, erythematous or scaly plaque that gradually increases in size (*Figure 13.9*). In the majority of cases the lesion may be an isolated one.

### Investigations

• A full examination of the patient to ensure that no other suspicious lesions are present, particularly on sun exposed areas, should be carried out
• A skin biopsy should be conducted to confirm the diagnosis.

## Discoid eczema
### Aetiology

The cause of discoid eczema is unknown and may occur at any age (DermnetNZ, 2008). On occasions it may follow minor trauma or occur in children with atopic dermatitis.

### Presentation

Single or multiple, well-defined, itchy, coin-shaped lesions appear, which may be dry, rough, red and covered in scales. They may occur anywhere on the body but are most common on the lower leg. Secondary infection often follows, leading to weeping and crusting (*Figure 13.10*). The patches may last for months.

### Investigations

• The diagnosis is normally made on clinical grounds, but it is worth checking for other signs of psoriasis
• A bacterial swab should be taken in case of secondary infection
• Skin scraping for mycology is needed if tinea corporis suspected
• Patch testing should be used if allergy is suspected.

Response to topical potent steroids for 2 weeks is usually good, but the patient may need an antibiotic if there is a secondary infection.

## Discoid lupus erythematosus
### Aetiology

The cause of discoid lupus erythematosus (DLE) is unknown, but it is likely that some patients have a genetic predisposition. It is more common in women between the ages of 20–50 years, and in those with dark skin. It is precipitated by sun exposure. Sunscreens do not always prevent it.

### Presentation

Sun exposed areas, particularly the face, the 'v' of the neck and the backs of the hands are most commonly affected. The patient usually presents with erythematous plaques that may scale (*Figure 13.11*). Separate lesions may merge and lesions may be localized or widespread. On resolution the patient is left with post-inflammatory hypopigmentation and permanent scars.

### Investigations

• The diagnosis may be confirmed by skin biopsy
• Further advice will be required to manage the case.

## Pityriasis rosea

### Aetiology

The cause of pityriasis rosea is unknown, but the fact that it tends to occur in groups of patients with contact, in the spring and autumn suggests that it may be viral in origin (Lichenstein, 2008).

### Presentation

A single 'herald patch' may appear for up to 3 weeks before the development of a more generalized rash on the trunk and spreading to the limbs, but not the face. The herald patch usually occurs on the trunk. It is round or oval, up to 5 cm in diameter, with a salmon-coloured, wrinkled central area and surrounding darker red area and colarette of scale (*Figure 13.12*). This is sometimes mistaken for ringworm or psoriasis. The herald patch will help confirm a diagnosis of pityriasis rosea when the main rash appears within the next 10 days. The main rash comprises smaller replicas of the herald patch and may spread in a Christmas-tree fashion, like the ribs of a fir tree. Usually the rash is symptomless, but can occasionally be very itchy. The condition usually resolves spontaneously in about 2–3 months.

### Investigations

- There is no specific test that will diagnose pityriasis rosea, which is usually a clinical diagnosis
- A herald patch should help confirm the diagnosis
- Skin scrapings for fungal infections would rule out tinea
- Blood test should exclude secondary syphilis
- A skin biopsy is not diagnostic, but might exclude other conditions (Lichenstein, 2008).

## Mycosis fungoides

### Aetiology

Mycosis fungoides is the most common form of cutaneous T-cell lymphoma. Its cause is unknown (Pinter-Brown, 2006). It most commonly develops around the age of 50 years.

### Presentation

Patches, plaques and tumours develop on the skin over many years. Single or multiple patches of flat, erythematous macules occur which may later develop into palpable plaques, with asymmetrically distributed, well-defined but irregular outline and central clearing (*Figure 13.13*). Later, mushroom-like tumours occur. In the earlier stages of the disease the diagnosis may be confused with psoriasis.

### Investigations

A skin biopsy should confirm the diagnosis.

### Management

Further advice will be required to decide on any further investigations and the management of the case.

## References

Callen J (2007) Lupus erythematosus, discoid. *eMedicine*. www.emedicine.com/DERM/topic247.htm (accessed 29 October 2008)

DermnetNZ (2008) Discoid eczema. http://dermnetnz.org/dermatitis/nummular-dermatitis.html (accessed 29 October 2008)

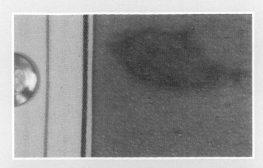

*Figure 13.12. Herald spot of pityriasis rosea.*

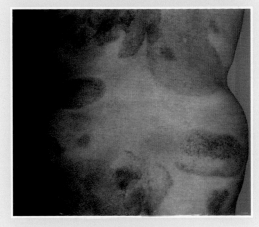

*Figure 13.13. Mycosis fungoides.*

Gordon R (2010) Psoriasis *eMedicine*. www.emedicine.medscape.com.dermatology (accessed 30.07.2010)

Joint Formulary Committee (2008) *British National Formulary* 56. September. BMA and RPS Publishing, London

Lichenstein R (2008) Pityriasis Rosea. *eMedicine*. www.emedicine.com/emerg/topic426.htm (accessed 29 October 2008)

Lui H, Mamelak AJ (2007) Psoriasis, plaque. *eMedicine*. www.emedicine.com/derm/topic365.htm (accessed 29 October 2008)

Pinter-Brown LC (2006) Mycosis fungoides. *eMedicine*. www.emedicine.com/med/topic1541.htm (accessed 29 October 2008)

Smith CH, Anstey AV, Barker JNWN et al (2006) British Association of Dermatologists guidelines for use of biological interventions in psoriasis 2005. *Br J Dermatol* 153: 486–97. http://tinyurl.com/5vm3xw (accessed 29 October 2008)

Welch M (2008) Bowen disease. *eMedicine*. www.emedicine.com/DERM/topic59.htm (accessed 29 October 2008)

# Test Your Knowledge

James was 22 years old. In the past few months he had been bothered by this plaque on his right shin. It caused him no particular problems but he was worried that it would cause comment when he went swimming on a holiday to Spain in a few weeks time. He had never suffered with any skin problems in the past and wanted to know what the problem might be.

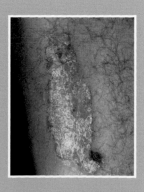

### Questions

1. What is the most likely diagnosis in this case?
2. What further findings would help you to feel that you had made the right decision?
3. How would you discuss the matter with him and what sort of advice would you give about future management?

# Lichen planus

Patients often present in the surgery complaining of a rash. Their particular concerns tend to be 'What is it?', 'Is it contagious?' or 'Could it be meningitis?' If the rash is in an exposed area, the patient often wants a rapid cure, because the symptoms may be distressing, or the patient is embarrassed to be seen in public.

For the professional, a careful history of the presentation and development of the rash, itching, previous medical history, the patient's job, any medications that may have been used recently, and the family history should be taken. On examination, the type of rash and its distribution should be noted. As the results are put together, a fair idea of possible diagnosis may be assumed and decisions made as to whether further investigations would be required to confirm the diagnosis and what treatment, if any, may be appropriate (Collins, 2007).

This chapter will consider the condition of lichen planus, looking at specific features that help clarify the diagnosis, and help practice nurses recognize and learn how to distinguish some of the other conditions with which it may be confused.

## Lichen planus
### Aetiology

Lichen planus may occur at any age, but more often affects adults aged between 30 and 60 years. It is not infectious and the cause remains unknown, but it is thought to be related to an abnormal immune response to a virus (possibly hepatitis C) or a drug.

Occasionally there may be a family history of others who have been affected. These may show an increase in frequency of human leucocytic antigen B7 (HLA-B7) that would suggest a genetic predisposition to the problem in some patients (Chuang and Stitle, 2008).

### Presentation

The initial complaint is usually a sudden appearance of an itchy rash, commonly on the flexor surfaces of the limbs, especially the wrists, or legs, genital area or trunk. Lesions tend to be distributed symmetrically. Scratching or other injury may lead to the spread of the rash along the line of the insult. This is known as the Koebner phenomenon (*Figure 14.1*). This also occurs in cases of psoriasis and plane warts.

Typically the rash consists of sharply demarcated, flat-topped papules, 2–5 mm in diameter, that may form clusters or plaques. They are usually very itchy. Lesions tend to be purple in colour, and on the legs in particular lesions may be hypertrophic and thickened (*Figure 14.2*).

As the condition resolves, residual brown lesions may remain for some time. This is a sign that the condition is

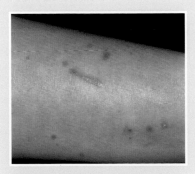

*Figure 14.1. Initial presentation of lichen planus with rash and Koebner phenomenon.*

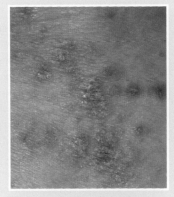

*Figure 14.3. Wickham's striae*

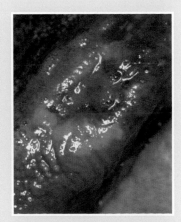

*Figure 14.5. Ulceration of the tongue in lichen planus*

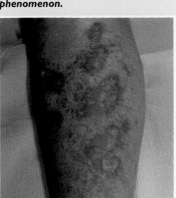

*Figure 14.2. Hypertrophic lesions on the leg.*

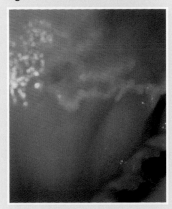

*Figure 14.4. Oral lichen planus*

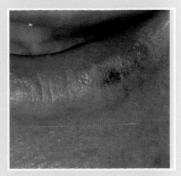

*Figure 14.6. Lip erosions in lichen planus.*

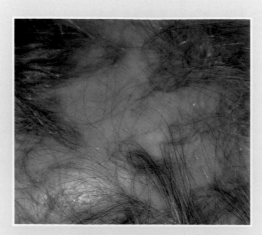

*Figure 14.7. Scarring alopecia of the scalp in lichen planus.*

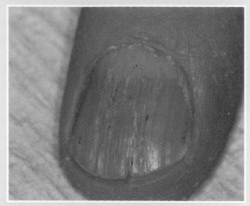

*Figure 14.8. Longitudinal ridging of the nail lichen planus.*

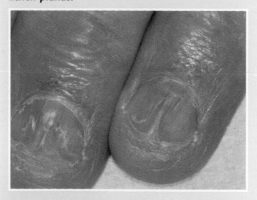

*Figure 14.9. Pterygium of the nail in lichen planus.*

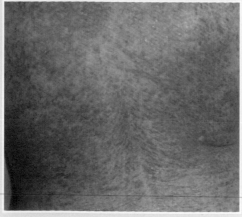

*Figure 14.10. Lichenoid drug-induced rash.*

quiescent and no further treatment is required. Another distinguishing feature of the rash is Wickham's striae: fine white lines running across the lesions (*Figure 14.3*). The initial localized rash may become more generalized in the ensuing weeks.

Confirmation of lichen planus is often found in the mouth. Linear, lacy or reticulate white or grey streaks may be seen on the buccal mucous membrane (*Figure 14.4*). These may be symptomless or slightly sore or tender. Painful ulcers may also develop on the tongue (*Figure 14.5*). These should be followed up with care as they may sometimes undergo malignant change. Erosions are sometimes seen on the lips (*Figure 14.6*). Genital lesions may also occur.

Involvement of the scalp (lichen planopilaris) is also common in lichen planus. Itchy, scaly papules may be found and progression may lead to a permanent scarring alopecia in the area (*Figure 14.7*). It is important to find such lesions, because early intervention with treatment may avoid permanent bald patches developing.

Further evidence may be found in nail changes that will be present in 10% of cases of lichen planus, with longitudinal ridging (onychorrhexis) (*Figure 14.8*). These changes may occur in other conditions such as old age, rheumatoid arthritis, Darrier's or peripheral vascular disease; however, taken in conjunction with other changes they may be helpful in making the diagnosis (Thornton and Tomecki, 2005). Occasionally more severe, permanent damage to the matrix may lead to pterygium formation which tends to occur only in lichen planus (*Figure 14.9*). In some cases there may be complete loss of the nail (Chuang and Stitle, 2008).

### Investigations

The diagnosis of lichen planus can normally be made on clinical grounds, but if in doubt, biopsy of the rash should give confirmation. However, where mouth ulcers are persistent, biopsy may be necessary to exclude malignancy. Malignant changes may take years to develop and, therefore, biopsies of ulcerated oral lesions may need to be repeated so that later changes are not missed.

### Management

The usual course of lichen planus is for spontaneous resolution after a period of about a year to 18 months. If the rash is symptomless, there is no need to treat, other than to advise the patient that the condition is neither serious nor infectious. For those with troublesome itching, an oral antihistamine and/or a mild or moderate topical steroid should be able to control symptoms. Ultraviolet light (UVL) therapy may be helpful in cases of widespread lichen planus. Systemic steroids would be recommended only in severe cases.

Oral lesions may be helped by steroid pastes, inhalant powders. Beclometasone spray is another option (unlicensed indication) (Joint Formulary Committee, 2008: 12.3.1).

In lichen planus of the scalp early intervention is important because, if it is allowed to progress, the patient is likely to be left with permanent areas of alopecia. Choices are a potent topical steroid, intralesional triamcinolone for large, itchy areas, or systemic cortico-steroids in severe cases. The hope is that the condition resolves, but there is a possibility of recurrence years later (Dermatology Channel, 2008).

If nail changes are noticed, early treatment may reduce the risks of permanent deformity or loss of the nail. Choices include intralesional triamcinolone into the nail fold, or antimalarials such as chloroquine. Unfortunately, recurrences are common after ceasing the treatment (Prevost and English, 2007).

## Differential diagnoses
### Lichenoid drug eruption
Part of the history of any skin rash must include a list of medication, either prescribed or bought over the counter. In some cases presenting with a rash resembling lichen planus, it may be suspected that the drug could be responsible for the skin reaction. Of many drugs that may

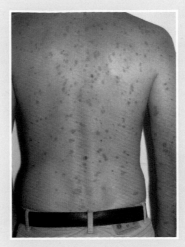
Figure 14.11. Guttate psoriasis.

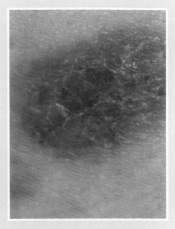
Figure 14.12. Pityriasis rosea: herald patch.

## Table 14.1. Differential diagnoses of lichen planus and management

| Condition | Aetiology | Rash | Confirmatory signs | Management |
|---|---|---|---|---|
| Lichen planus | Unknown Possibly abnormal immune response to virus Affects adults aged 30–60 years Not infectious Possible genetic predisposition | Sudden onset of itchy rash Flexor surfaces limbs, especially wrists. Trunk or genital area Symmetrical, flat topped papules, plaques. Purplish colour Hypertrophic lesions especially on legs Become brown as resolving | Koebner phenomenon Wickham's striae Oral lesions: lacy or streaks of white on buccal mucous membrane. Ulcers Lip erosions Scalp itchy, scaly papules Permanent scarring alopecia Nails—longitudinal ridging Pterygium, nail loss | Clinical diagnosis or biopsy if necessary Biopsy persistent mouth ulcers Expect spontaneous resolution in 12–18 months No treatment unless symptoms Topical steroids Antihistamines for itching UVL therapy Occasionally systemic steroids Potent topical steroids for scalp Intralesional steroids—scalp and nails Chloroquine—nails |
| Lichenoid reaction | Reaction to drug, most commonly gold, ACE inhibitors, antimalarials | Lichenoid type of rash as of lichen planus | History of drug intake | Stop the offending drug |
| Guttate psoriasis | Follows 2–3 weeks after streptococcal infection Adolescents, young adults | Crops of discrete red, drop-like spots with silvery scaly over a few days Trunk, upper arms, thighs | Recent history of sore throat | No treatment necessary unless symptoms Topical steroids, tar-based cream, calcipotriol UVL Antibiotic if evidence of persisting infection |
| Pityriasis rosea | May be related to herpes virus 6 and 7 and some drugs Children, young adults | Oval, pink papules with scaling at edges. Not usually itchy Fir-tree look Mainly on the trunk | Herald patch—appears up to 3 weeks before the main rash | No treatment required unless symptoms Emollients, topical steroids, UVL |
| Lichen simplex | Repeated scratching Usually adults | Thickened, itchy patch of skin Occurs within reach of fingers, often on one shin | Usually unilateral No purplish colour | Topical steroids—may need potent steroids under occlusion Stop scratching |
| Tinea corporis | Dermatophyte fungal infection | Itchy, round or oval, inflammatory patches with central clearing Mainly affects trunk and limbs Tinea of the scalp—patchy hair loss with scaling and erythema of the scalp | Skin scrapings for microscopy and culture | Antifungal agent, e.g. terbinafine Topical agent for localized lesions Systemic agent for scalp and more widespread infection |
| Syphilis | Infectious sexually transmitted disease Gram-negative spirochaete bacterium Treponema pallidum | Widespread red or brownish macules Papules on soles of feet Patchy hair loss Raw areas on mucous membranes, mouth and genitalia Fever and malaise | History of primary chancre | Refer to genitourinary department Investigate contacts Treated with intramuscular penicillin |

lead to this reaction, the most common are gold, antimalarial drugs and captopril (DermNet NZ, 2007).

This patient (*Figure 14.10*) presented with a widespread lichenoid-type rash that had been a problem to him for 3 years. It transpired that the rash had first appeared after he had been prescribed the ACE inhibitor, perindopril, for his hypertension. After the drug was discontinued and an alternative hypotensive agent substituted, the rash quickly cleared.

### Guttate psoriasis

Guttate psoriasis occurs most commonly in adolescents and young adults. It presents with the sudden appearance, over a period of 2 or 3 days, of a crop of discrete, red, drop-like spots (*Figure 14.11*), which may be covered in a silvery scale. It may be slightly itchy and tends to be mainly on the trunk, upper arms and thighs. On inquiry, one can usually obtain a history of a sore throat a 2–3 weeks before. Often the rash will subside and clear spontaneously without treatment. However, in troublesome cases, topical steroids, tar-based creams, calcipotriol or UVL may be helpful. The rash follows a recent streptococcal infection. If there is any evidence of persistent infection, an antibiotic may be indicated. Once clear some patients will have no further problems. Others may have problems of psoriasis later, especially if there is a family or previous history of the condition (DermNetNZ, 2008).

### Pityriasis rosea

Pityriasis rosea occurs most commonly in children and young adults. The first sign is a single, scaly patch that usually occurs somewhere in the 'T-shirt-trunks' area. The plaque is oval, 2–5 mm in diameter and has a collarette of scale around its margin (*Figure 14.12*). It may develop up to 3 weeks before subsequent eruption of smaller oval, pink papules, with the scaly edging appearing (*Figure 14.13*). Itching is not usually a feature. This rash is mainly on the trunk, but may spread to the neck, upper limbs and thighs. Sometimes these may follow the line of the ribs giving a fir tree-like look. The rash usually fades and clears spontaneously within about 3 months. Treatment is not normally required, but the application of emollients may be helpful and topical steroid creams or ointments may ease itching, if it occurs. If the rash is persistent, UVL may help.

Pityriasis rosea occurs most often in children and young adults and may be related to human herpes virus 6 and 7 (HHV6 and 7). It may also be stimulated by certain drugs, including barbiturates, captopril, metronidazole, isotretinoin and D penicillamine (Lichenstein, 2008).

Other conditions presenting with rashes that might be confused with lichen planus include the following.

### *Lichen simplex*

Lichen simplex usually occurs in adults who present with an itchy patch of skin that becomes thickened and may display scratch marks. It is common on the shin, or other places within reach of fingers that scratch. It lacks the purplish colour of lichen planus and should respond to topical steroids, providing the patient is persuaded to stop

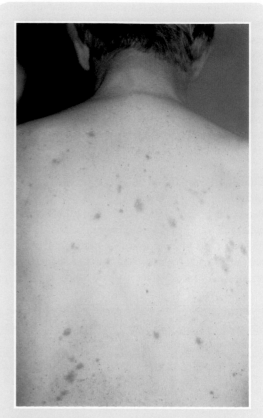

*Figure 14.13. Pityriasis rosea rash.*

scratching. Often potent topical steroids, sometimes under occlusion, are required (DermNet NZ, 2007).

### *Tinea corporis*

This may present with the sudden appearance of itchy, round or oval, inflamed patches, that may appear to be healing centrally, mainly on the trunk and limbs. Scaly, inflammatory areas of alopecia may occur if the scalp is affected (tinea capitis).

It is caused by a dermatophyte fungus and the diagnosis can be confirmed if skin scrapings are taken for microscopy and culture. The infection may be acquired from dogs (microsporum canis) or the feet (tinea pedis or athlete's foot), or nails. Treatment is with an antifungal agent such as terbinafine. Depending on the extent of the rash this may be used topical or systemically (DermNet NZ, 2008).

### *Secondary syphilis*

This is a sexually transmitted disease. The primary chancre, of syphilis, a single, painless, small, red papule on the genitalia may pass unnoticed but may be followed, up to 3 months later, by a rash of red or brownish spots that may appear anywhere on the body. This may be accompanied by fever, malaise, headache and lymphadenopathy. Knowledge of the patient or the partner's lifestyle may lead the physician to be more likely to consider this diagnosis.

An initial nonspecific treponemal blood test (TPHA and TTPPA) is generally used for screening. If fluorescent treponemal antibody absorption (FTA-ABS) test is positive, in a high proportion of patients syphilis can be used as a confirmatory test for postive VDRL and RPR test findings (Tidy, 2010). The patient should be referred to a genitourinary specialist for further tests and treatment for the patient and any contacts (DermNet NZ, 2007).

All these conditions may need to be considered and investigations undergone if one is unsure of the diagnosis of lichen planus.

## References

Chuang T-Y, Stitle L (2008) Lichen Planus. *eMedicine*. www. emedicine.com/DERM/topic233.htm (accessed 5 January 2009)

Collins R (2007) Rash, general. In: *Differential Diagnosis in Primary Care*. Lippincott Williams and Wilkins

Dermatology Channel (2008) Baldness (alopecia). http://www. dermatologychannel.net/alopecia/lichen_planopilaris.shtml (accessed 5 January 2009)

DermNet NZ (2008) Guttate psoriasis. http://dermnetnz.org/scaly/ guttate-psoriasis.html (accessed 5 January 2009)

DermNet NZ (2007) Lichen simplex. www.dermnetnz.org/ dermatitis/lichen-simplex.html (accessed 5 January 2009)

DermNet NZ (2007) Syphilis. www.dermnetnz.org/bacterial/ syphilis.html (accessed 5 January 2009)

DermNet NZ (2008) Tinea corporis. www.dermnetnz.org/fungal/ tinea-corporis.html (accessed 5 January 2009)

Joint Formulary Committee (2008) *British National Formulary* 56. September. BMA and RPS Publishing, London

Lichenstein R (2008) Pityriasis rosea. *eMedicine*. www.emedicine. com/emerg/topic426.htm (accessed 5 January 2009)

Prevost NM, English JC (2007) Palliative treatment of fingernails in lichen planus. *Journal of Drugs in Dermatology* February: findarticles.com/p/articles/mi_m0PDG/is_2_6/ai_n19171467 (accessed 5 January 2009)

Thornton S, Tomecki K (2005) Nail disease: Signs for the internist. www.clevelandclinicmeded.com/diseasemanagement/ dermatology/naildisease/naildisease.htm (accessed 5 January 2009)

Tidy C (2010) Syphilis. Patient Plus www.patient.co.uk (accessed 30 July 2010)

## Test Your Knowledge

This 50 year old woman had been attending the surgery for nearly a year. She had first noticed a few itchy spots on the front of her wrists but since that time the rash had spread and become more widespread. In particular the rash on her legs had worsened and become thickened. She had been using a moderately potent topical steroid on the rash. Initially this had seemed to help but at this stage it provided little or no relief. Her general health was good and she had never before suffered with any skin problems.

### Questions

1. What is the likely diagnosis in this case and what particular features of the rash would help you to come to this conclusion?
2. What other features would you look for to confirm your suspicions of the diagnosis?
3. What treatment would you suggest?

# Intertrigo

Intertrigo is a common problem that affects the site of contact of two skin surfaces. Such contact creates a warm, sweaty enclosed space. Friction between the surfaces may lead to the development of soreness and erythema that may itch, sting or burn.

An opportunity for the proliferation of microbes and for the growth of yeasts or fungi is created in the warm sweaty enclosed space between the two skin surfaces. If untreated, the area becomes more inflamed and swollen. It may progress to develop vesicles, pustules and crusts that break down leaving raw, weeping areas that frequently become secondarily infected and may lead to constitutional symptoms of malaise or fever. The most common sites to be affected are under the breasts, the groins, axillae or between the toes (Marks, 1987).

Intertrigo in its broad sense, i.e. referring to skin problems within the flexures, is easily recognized. Secondary infection may require different management, depending on the organism involved.

In addition, there are other conditions that may simulate a simple intertrigo but require specific treatment. These conditions will be discussed, together with the investigations necessary to ascertain and offer the correct care.

## Aetiology

The development of intertrigo in a patient may be encouraged by a variety of causes (Anon, 2003). Patients living in a humid climate where excessive sweating is a problem are more likely to suffer this condition, especially if they are obese or hygiene is poor (*Figure 15.1*). Intertrigo from any cause may be associated with a secondary infection that may be either bacterial and/or fungal.

## Recognizing infections that complicate intertrigo

*Candida albicans* usually presents with pustules and surrounding, itchy erythema. As the pustules become confluent and break, the skin becomes red, raw, thickened and macerated, and develops a white appearance (*Figure 15.2*). Candida commonly complicates intertrigo from any cause and is particularly likely to occur in patients with diabetes mellitus (Zuber and Baddam, 2001: 9).

## Dermatophyte infections (ringworm)

**Tinea cruris** (Dhobi itch) is most common in young men and must be distinguished from candida or a simple intertrigo. It is usually caused by *Trichophyton rubrum* or *Epidermophyton floccosum*. The rash presents as a red, scaly rash with a margin that is slightly raised. The central area tends to be clear. It occurs in the groin area and often spreads onto the buttocks and medial thighs (*Figure 15.3*) (du Vivier, 2002: 235–7). Often it is associated with ringworm in other parts of the body, e.g. athlete's foot. Skin scrapings should confirm the diagnosis.

**Interdigital tinea pedis** (athlete's foot) (*Figure 15.4*) usually starts in the toe web and presents with an asymmetrical, itchy erythema and peeling between the toes. It may spread to the under surface of the foot and is open to develop secondary bacterial infection. It is usually caused by *T. rubrum* or *E. floccosum* (Brooks and Bender, 1996).

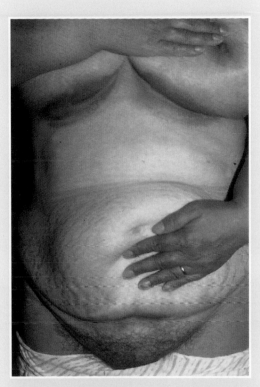

Figure 15.1. Intertrigo under the breasts and between the abdominal folds in an obese woman.

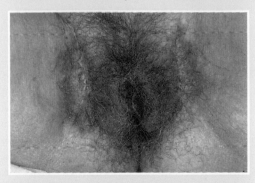

Figure 15.2. Candida in a vulval intertrigo.

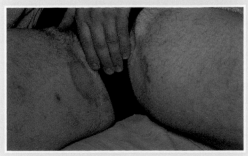

Figure 15.3. Tinea cruris.

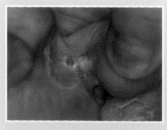

Figure 15.4. Interdigital tinea
pedis.

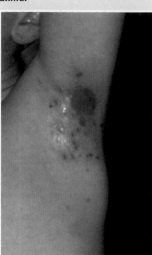

Figure 15.5. Erythrasma in the
axilla.

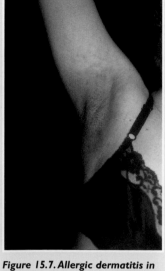

Figure 15.7. Allergic dermatitis in
the axilla caused by deodorant.

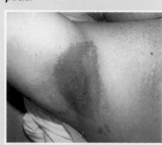

Figure 15.6. Impetigo in the axilla.

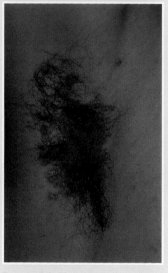

Figure 15.8. Seborrhoeic eczema
in the axilla.

**Erythrasma** is caused by *Corynebacterium minutissium* and usually affects the flexures, presenting with a well-defined brown discolouration which has a scaly, wrinkly surface (*Figure 15.5*). It can remain symptomless but the patient may sometimes complain of irritation. Lesions tend to be less inflamed than those of ringworm or seborrhoeic dermatitis. Diagnosis can be made by using Wood's lamp, which produces an ultraviolet light (ADAM, 2003b). When the light is shone on the affected area a coral pink fluorescence appears. Skin scrapings should be taken to confirm the diagnosis.

### Bacterial infections
Bacterial infections, e.g. impetigo (*Figure 15.6*), may present with the rapid spread of blisters and purulent exudate that dries and forms a 'golden' crust. They are usually caused by *Staphylococcus aureus* or *beta haemolytic streptococci*. The diagnosis may be confirmed by taking a swab from the area for culture and sensitivities.

## Differential diagnosis
An accurate diagnosis of intertrigo is important. There are a number of conditions that are difficult to distinguish from intertrigo (*Table 15.1*).

### Allergic reactions
The occluded areas of the axillae allow for enhanced penetration for the constituents of cosmetics, perfumes and perfumed deodorants. Many of these contain formaldehyde, which can cause problems. Colophony and balsam of Peru (natural resinous substances derived from trees) are often present in fragrances. Sensitization to these substances is therefore common and patients present with irritating, erythematous areas (*Figure 15.7*) or blisters that break down and weep.

The distribution of the rash gives a clue to its cause. For example, where both axillae are affected, it is likely to be related to the use of a deodorant. Patch testing at a later stage should identify the causative substance (du Vivier, 2002: 62).

### Seborrhoeic dermatitis
Seborrhoeic dermatitis is commonly seen in adults. It affects the face, scalp and chest and occasionally presents in the flexures with a symmetrical, pink or bright red and sore rash (*Figure 15.8*). It is associated with an overgrowth of the yeast *Pityrosporum ovale* and is most often seen in obese, middle-aged patients and the immunosuppressed. It is important to exclude erythrasma as well as ringworm, candida and other secondary infections, by taking a swab and skin scrapings.

### Psoriasis
Psoriasis commonly occurs in the flexures, under the breasts, axillae and in the genital region. The skin may be red, but scaling may be absent in these areas (*Figure 15.9*). In this case, the well-defined scaly lesions around the edge of the 'intertrigo' suggested the diagnosis. The patient will usually have a family history, personal history or actual signs of psoriasis elsewhere on the body. A swab should be taken as well as skin scrapings because secondary infection of the area may also be present (du Vivier, 2002: 69–84).

## Investigations
Taking a swab from the affected area for culture and sensitivity will help confirm *C. albicans* or bacterial infection, e.g. *S. aureus* or beta haemolytic streptococci.

Skin scrapings will help identify fungal elements and culture, including tinea cruris or tinea pedis (usually *T. rubrum* or *E. floccosum*), erythrasma (from which *C. minutissium* may be cultured) and seborrhoeic dermatitis (the skin scrapings may demonstrate *P. ovale*).

Wood's lamp will show the presence of erythrasma if a coral pink fluorescenece appears.

If allergy problems are suspected, patch testing should be able to suggest the causal allergen (du Vivier, 2002: 64–5).

A urine test should always be taken to check for glucose and to exclude diabetes in a patient with candida because it may be the presenting symptom of diabetes mellitus in some patients (Forbes and Jackson, 1993).

## Treatment

It is most important to gain relief for the moist, compressed areas, but this is difficult to achieve. As well as encouraging the patient to lose weight, he/she should be advised to carefully dry the affected areas after bathing. Attempts to 'prop open' the skin folds should be made, and non-restrictive clothing should be worn. Mild cases without secondary infection may be helped temporarily by topical hydrocortisone 1% cream (ADAM, 2003a).

### Candida albicans

The following medication options can be used to help treat *C. albicans*:

- Topical antifungal agents—imidazole or nystatin cream should be applied two to three times a day
- Systemic antifungal agents, e.g. fluconazole, for more severe, wide-spread or persistent cases
- Imidazole cream with mild corticosteroid, which may better alleviate symptoms in the first few days
- Antifungal vaginal pessaries, e.g. clotrimazole,

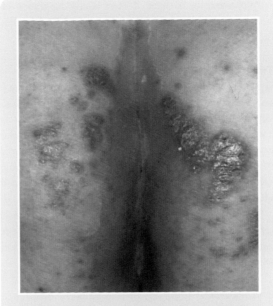

*Figure 15.9. Flexural psoriasis in the natal cleft.*

## Table 15.1. Differential diagnosis of intertrigo and other conditions

| Condition | Signs and symptom | Investigations | Treatment |
|---|---|---|---|
| Intertrigo | Pink and brown inflammation in flexures | • Swab for culture and sensitivities | • Dry carefully, aerate,<br>• Lose weight<br>• Hydrocortisone 1% |
| *Candida albicans* | Itchy erythema, pustules<br>Thickening, maceration<br>White appearance | • Swab for *Candida albicans*<br>• Urine check for glucose | • Topical imidazole or nystatin cream and or pessaries<br>• Severe—systemic fluconazole |
| Dermatophyte infections | Groin: red scaly rash, raised margin and central clearing<br>Often associated with interdigital: itchy, asymmetrical erythema, peeling between toes | • Skin scrapings for *Trichophyton rubrum* or *Epidermophyton floccosum* | • Topical terbinafine or imidazole cream<br>• Severe—systemic terbinafine, itraconazole or ketoconazole |
| Erythrasma | Well-defined brown discolouration, wrinkly surface | • Wood's lamp - Coral fluorescence<br>• Skin scrapings for *Corynebacterium* | • Erythromycin—oral |
| Bacterial infections | Rapidly spreading blisters<br>Purulent exudates, Golden crusts | • Swab for *Staphylococcus aureus* or *beta-haemolytic streptococci* | • Cleanse, soak crusts<br>• Topical fusidic acid or mupirocin<br>• Oral antibiotic— penicillin V, erythromycin, flucloxacillin |
| Allergic reactions | Itchy, erythema, blisters that break down usually related to areas of contact with allergen | • Patch testing (later) to check possible allergens | • Stop all possible contact with allergens<br>• Mild—moderately potent topical steroid<br>• Severe—systemic steroids |
| Seborrhoeic dermatitis | Symmetrical, pink or red raw, sore rash | • Swab or skin scrapings to exclude secondary infection | • Topical—weak or moderate steroid<br>• Combined steroid and antifungal/ bacteria creams<br>• Saline, pot permanganate soaks<br>• Severe—systemic antibiotics and/ or hospital admission |
| Psoriasis | Red rash. No scaling<br>Patient history, family history or other evidence of psoriasis | • Swab or skin scrapings to exclude secondary infection | • Topical—moderately potent steroid cream or ointment |

miconazole or nystatin, if there is any suggestion of vaginal involvement (Joint Formulary Committee, 2003: 386).

### Tinea cruris or tinea pedis

Topical antifungal agents, such as econazole, miconazole, ketoconazole creams (twice daily until better and for a further 2 weeks) or terbinafine cream (once daily for 2 weeks) will usually clear this problem (Joint Formulary Committee, 2003: 569–71). However, topical steroids should not be used, and the combined use of an antifungal agent with a corticosteroid preparation is not normally advised (Zuber and Baddam, 2001: 13).

Systemic antifungal agents, e.g. terbinafine for 4 weeks, is very effective in combatting severe or widespread problems. Itraconazole or ketoconazole may also be used (Joint Formulary Committee, 2003: 293–4).

### Erythrasma

To treat erythrasma, erythromycin 250 mg should be taken four times daily by mouth for 2 weeks. No topical application is required.

### Bacterial infections

Cleanse the area and soak off the crusts with arachis oil. A topical fusidic acid or mupirocin ointment may be sufficient in localized problems, but for more widespread problems an appropriate oral antibiotic, such as penicillin V, erythromycin or flucloxacillin, may be required (Joint Formulary Committee, 2003: 259–64, 276).

### Allergic reactions

If an allergic reaction is suspected, the patient should stop the use of all suspect preparations and a patch test should be taken to elucidate the allergen(s). A moderately potent topical steroid ointment (e.g. clobetasone 0.05% or betamethasone 0.025%) should control the problem but it will recur if there is contact with the allergen again (Leppard, Ashton, 1998: 64). Severe cases may require systemic steroids, e.g. prednisolone, as a short, sharp course (du Vivier, 2002: 65).

### Seborrhoeic dermatitis

Mild cases of *seborrhoeic dermatitis* should respond well to a weak topical steroid, e.g. hydrocortisone 1%. Combined preparations of antibacterial, antifungal and hydrocortisone 1% are often used as there is frequently infection with candida or bacteria. In severe cases saline, aluminium acetate or potassium permanganate soaks, or systemic antibiotics (e.g. erythromycin or flucloxacillin) should be prescribed. If extremely severe, hospital admission may be necessary (du Vivier 2002: 49).

Moderately potent topical steroids, e.g. clobetasol 0.05% or betamethasone 0.025%, or combined preparations of an antifungal (nystatin), antibiotic (oxytetracycline) and a steroid, may also be required to control the problem.

### Psoriasis

The skin in the flexural areas and genitalia tends to become sore if preparations of dithranol or tar are used. Moderately potent topical steroids (clobetasone 0.05% or hydrocortisone 0.1% 17-butyrate cream or ointment twice-daily) may be helpful (Leppard and Ashton, 1999: 177).

## References

ADAM (2003a) Intertrigo. Medline Plus Medical Enclyopedia. www.nlm.nih.gov/medlineplus/ency/article/003223.htm (accessed 6February 2004)

ADAM (2003b) Wood's Lamp. Medline Plus Medical Encyclopedia. www.nlm.nih.gov/medlineplus/ency/article/003386.htm (accessed 6February 2004)

Anonymous (2003) Intertrigo. GP Notebook. Oxbridge Solutions Ltd. www.gpnotebook.co.uk/cache/-1442447332.htm (accessed 6February 2004)

Brooks KE, Bender JF (1996) Tinea pedis: diagnosis and treatment. *Clin Podiatr Med Surg* **13**(1): 31–46

du Vivier A (2002) *Contact Dermatitis: Atlas of Clinical Dermatology* 3rd edn. Churchill Livingstone

Forbes C, Jackson W (1993) *A Colour Atlas and Text of Clinical medicine: Diabetes Mellitus.* Wolfe, England: 327

Joint Formulary Committee (2003) *British National Formulary* 46. Sept. British Medical Association and Royal Pharmaceutical Society of Great Britain, London

Leppard B, Ashton R (1998) *Treatment in Dermatology* Book E-H. Radcliffe Medical Press: 64

Marks R (1987) *Skin Disease in Old Age.* Dunitz, London: 40–2

Zuber T, Baddam K (2001) Superficial fungal infection of the skin. *Postgraduate Medicine online* **109**(1): 117–32 www.postgradmed.com/issues/2001/01_01/zuber.htm (accessed 6February 2004)

# Test Your Knowledge

This man had noticed a slight itching in the axilla for a few days. When he looked, he was surprised to find this brownish rash in both armpits. He made an appointment to see the nurse.

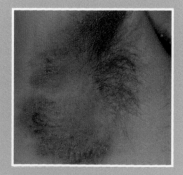

### Questions

1. What is the most likely diagnosis and which particular features of the rash would make you consider this?
2. What is the cause of this condition and how would you confirm the diagnosis?
3. What treatment would you recommend?

# Scaly feet/Keratoderma

A scale is defined as a flaking of the skin owing to increased loss from the stratum corneum. This may be caused by the production of abnormal keratin or keratin that is produced at an increased rate, as occurs, for example, in psoriasis. Damage to the stratum corneum also leads to scaling, and scaling may be associated with eczema and infections. In keratoderma, the horny keratin layer of the skin is formed normally but is not shed at the normal rate. As a consequence, there is a build-up of a thickened keratin layer of the skin that does not scale, but may create a similar effect of dry flaking skin. This problem may result from an underlying congenital abnormality affecting the skin or as the result of persistent pressure and trauma (du Vivier, 2002: 11).

When faced with a 'scaly foot' in the surgery it is important to decide if any investigation is necessary to make an accurate diagnosis of the problem, and suggest the appropriate management depending on the cause. The following chapter considers some of the conditions that may cause confusion.

## Keratoderma

Palmar-plantar keratoderma occurs in a variety of forms. It affects both the palms of the hands and the soles of the feet. In general, it is inherited as an autosomal, dominant problem. Patients are usually aware of other members of their family suffering with the same problem. Specific gene mutations are associated with the different types of keratoderma (Ratnavel and Griffiths, 1997). Patients present with a symmetrical, thick, diffuse hyperkeratosis over the palms and soles. The thickened skin often has a yellowish appearance (*Figure 16.1*). The hands feel rough, tend to crack and are painful at times. The problem may be first noticed in infancy and persists throughout life. In some types of the condition there may be associated meta-bolic problems or carcinoma of the oesophagus, but this is rare (Lucker et al, 1994).

In general, treatment is unsatisfactory but some symptomatic relief can be gained from salt water soaks, paring the hard skin, topical keratolytics such as salicylic acid 5–10%, lactic acid 10% or urea in a suitable base, topical or (sometimes) oral retinoids. A potent topical steroid ointment may be appropriate if there is inflammation.

Supervision by a chiropodist is important and shoes should be chosen with care. There is always the risk of secondary fungal infection and this should be checked for (Gruber and Ratnavel, 2003).

### Keratoderma climactericum

Keratoderma climactericum (KC) usually develops in women after the age of 40 years, often in those who are obese. Initially sides of the feet and the pressure areas of the soles and heels are affected by erythema, hyperkeratosis and painful fissures (*Figure 16.2*). Sometimes the central part of the palm is also affected.

The cause of KC is unknown. Although it tends to begin at the menopause, no hormonal connection has been proven. Emollients play a large part in the treatment, but topical calcipotriol and occasionally oral retinoids may be used (Gruber and Ratnavel, 2003).

## Inflammatory and reactive dermatoses
### Pompholyx eczema

Acute attacks of pompholyx eczema (or vesicular palmoplantar eczema) may occur at any age but are most common in young adults aged between 20 and 30 years (Gramvussakis and Wilkinson, 2002). Pompholyx eczema presents with erythema, vesiculation and blisters on the palms and the soles (*Figure 16.3*). It may occur in atopic people as a sensitivity reaction to contact with a variety of allergens, or it may be related to stress. (Gramvussakis and Wilkinson, 2002). Often it is a recurrent problem and it is more common in the spring and summer. The patient complains of a pricking, burning or itching sensation. Within 2–3 weeks the blisters usually dry out and the area desquamates. Some patients suffer further attacks but these tend to lessen with age (Gramvussakis and Wilkinson, 2002).

In subacute episodes there may be some erythema, dryness and/or scaling. Patients often develop painful fissures (Gramvussakis and Wilkinson, 2002) (*Figure 16.4*).

In cases of chronic hyperkerototic eczema thick keratotic plaques and fissuring develop (*Figure 16.5*).

The cause all these problems may remain a mystery but the contribution of atopy, stress, increased sweating or sensitivity to allergens such as rubber should be considered.

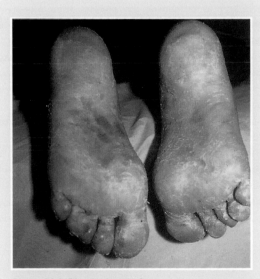

*Figure 16.1. Plantar keratoderma.*

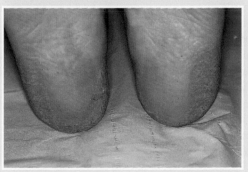

*Figure 16.2. Keratoderma climactericum.*

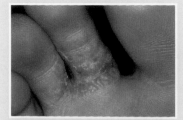

Figure 16.3. Acute pompholyx eczema.

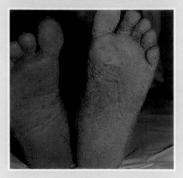

Figure 16.4. Sub-acute pompholyx eczema.

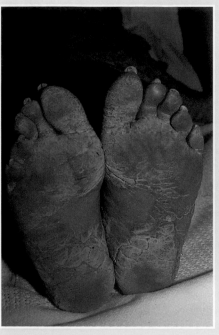

Figure 16.5. Chronic hyperkeratotic eczema.

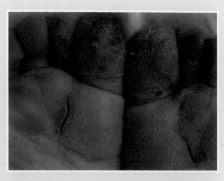

Figure 16.6. Juvenile plantar dermatosis.

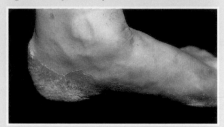

Figure 16.7. Psoriasis: Plaques are sharply demarcated with silvery scale.

Subacute and hypertophic problems often persist for years and are difficult to clear (Gramvussakis and Wilkinson, 2002).

Investigations include skin scrapings to exclude fungal infection, patch testing for an offending allergen, biopsy (if necessary) to distinguish the problem from psoriasis or keratoderma, and swabs, if infection is suspected (Gramvussakis and Wilkinson, 2002).

Management of the acute phase comprises rest, wet soaks or soaks in potassium permanganate solution. Potent topical steroids are useful in mild and moderate cases. Systemic antibiotics are necessary to treat secondary infections.

In the subacute phase potent topical corticosteroids are used.

The hyperkeratotic phase is very difficult to treat and specialist advice may be required. Relief is sometimes obtained using a number of options, including retinoids (etretinate or acitretin), potent topical glucocorticosteroids (sometimes under occlusion), low-dose oral steroids, (psoralen and ultraviolet light (PUVA) therapy, azathioprine, cyclosporin or methotrexate (Gramvussakis and Wilkinson, 2002).

### Juvenile plantar dermatosis

Juvenile plantar dermatosis occurs in children and adolescents. It is probably related to the fashion for trainers and the wearing of synthetic materials in shoes and socks, which are less porous and more occlusive (du Vivier, 2002: 53). It occurs most often in atopics who may have related problems of asthma, eczema or hay fever.

Patch testing is unhelpful because there does not seem to be an allergic element to this problem (du Vivier, 2002: 53). The skin of the forefoot becomes shiny, scaly and painful. Cracks develop under the toes and the ball of the foot (*Figure 16.6*).

The patient should be advised to reduce the pressure of any footwear with padding such as extra cotton socks and open or leather shoes, so that the feet can 'breathe'. The fissures should be kept covered and clean and emollients applied liberally. Topical steroids do not provide much benefit.

### Psoriasis

Patients with psoriasis affecting the feet may, or may not, have signs of the condition elsewhere on the body, e.g. on the scalp or nails, with pitting, onycholysis and subungual hyperkeratosis. Slightly raised, red plaques covered in a silvery white scale and a clearly demarcated margin are observed (*Figure 16.7*). On the soles the scaling may be thicker and more waxy. Some patients will also have associated problems of arthritis in the distal interphalangeal joints of the fingers and toes (Neale and Adams, 1989).

In *plantar pustular psoriasis* the patient develops plaques and yellow, sterile pustules that turn brown on the soles of one or both feet. Sometimes they occur on the palms. Psoriatic scaling is observed occasionally.

It is questioned whether this is a true psoriatic condition. Some patients will recall a family history of psoriasis or display other signs of the psoriasis. It is more common in older women and smokers, and may be associated with diabetes mellitus and thyroid disease (du Vivier, 2002: 73).

Plantar pustular psoriasis is particularly difficult to treat. In the case shown in *Figure 16.8* there was no response to PUVA but some improvement was achieved with acitretin.

Some patients will improve spontaneously. For others, a number of management options are available. Smoking cessation is important in those who smoke. Coal tar preparations or dithranol can be useful. Salicylic acid is a keratolytic and may be helpful to remove scale and allow better penetration of other medicaments.

Potent topical steroids may appear to help psoriasis but relapse is likely once they are stopped. Topical or systemic retinoids, ultraviolet light or PUVA therapy, methotrexate, ciclosporin or tacrolimus may help problem cases. These decisions should be taken by an experienced doctor.

## Lichen planus

Patients with lichen planus may develop lesions on the feet (*Figure 16.9*). Diagnosis of this patient was difficult. At first it was thought that this man had pompholyx eczema. When the problem persisted and he was found to have other signs of lichen planus at the wrist and white lacy patterns on the mucous membranes of the mouth, it was realized that this was a hypertrophic form of the disease.

Hypertrophic lesions are very itchy and may affect both the dorsum and soles of the feet. Discrete, itchy, flat violaceous papules may occur. These may fuse to form larger plaques that may scale. The lesions tend to persist and leave residual pigmentation when they resolve.

Lichen planus may occur at any age but is most common between 30 and 60 years of age. The cause is unknown but thought to be a cell-mediated immune response (Chuang and Stitle, 2003). A diagnosis of lichen planus is usually made on clinical grounds but, if necessary, it can be confirmed by biopsy.

Lichen planus normally resolves within 8–12 months without treatment. Topical steroids may be used if the rash is very itchy. Potent topical steroids may be used on the soles of the feet. Systemic steroids are rarely required unless the disease is widespread or, in the case of the feet, the problem is very troublesome and mobility is compromised. Sometimes referral to a dermatologist is necessary (Chuang and Stitle, 2003).

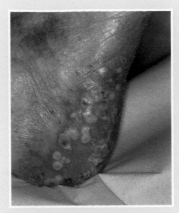 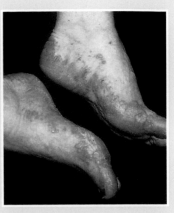

*Figure 16.8. Plantar pustular psoriasis.*

*Figure 16.9. Hypertrophic lichen planus.*

## Callosities and corns

Callosities and corns are common in locations where constant friction of the skin occurs (*Figure 16.10*). Owing to clubbed feet, this man walked on the balls of his feet. The skin became thickened and tender, and hyperkeratotic corns arose over bony prominences (du Vivier, 2002: 304).

The diagnosis must distinguish between corns and verrucas. Verrucas are identified if small bleeding points appear when a lesion is pared. Corns become more normal in appearance when the skin is pared.

### Table 16.1. Differential diagnosis for scaly feet

| Condition | Age | Cause | Symptoms |
|---|---|---|---|
| Palmar plantar keratoderma | Infancy onwards | Genetic-autosomal dominant | Hyperkeratosis (soles and palms) |
| Keratoderma climactericum | Women over 40 | Associated with obesity | Hyperkeratosis, erythema, fissures over soles and palms |
| Pompholyx eczema | Usually 20–30 years but may be any age | Sometimes associated with atopics, stress and sensitivity reactions | Erythema, vesiculation, blisters (soles and palms) Acute, sometimes recurrent |
| Sub-acute pompholyx eczema | | | Erythema, dryness, scaling, fissures |
| Chronic hypertrophic pompholyx eczema | | | Thick keratotic plaques, fissures |
| Juvenile plantar dermatosis | Children and adolescents | Most common in atopics | Scaly, shiny forefoot Painful fissures under toes |
| Psoriasis | Infancy onwards | Genetic | Raised, demarcated, red plaques with silvery scale Often other signs psoriasis elsewhere |
| Pustular psoriasis | Later in life | Associated with smoking | Plaques, yellow, sterile pustules that turn brown |
| Lichen planus | Usually 30–60 years | Unknown | Itchy, violaceous papules, plaques |
| Callosities | Children and adults | Ill-fitting footwear | Hyperkeratosis with central, painful core over bony prominences |
| Tinea pedis | Children and adults | *Trichophyton rubrum* *T. mentagrophytes* *Epidermophyton floccosum* | Maceration, fissures between toes. Itchy, scaly soles of feet |
| Pitted keratolysis | | Associated with hyperhidrosis and occlusive footwear | Smelly feet Maceration, small pits and erosions |

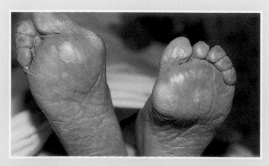

Figure 16.10. Callosities in a man with clubbed foot.

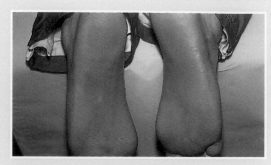

Figure 16.11. Pitted keratolysis.

Callosities and corns are best managed by a chiropodist. Advice will include suggestions about footwear, a variety of foot supports and splints, padding, salicylic acid plasters, paring and sometimes excision and curettage (Neale and Adams, 1989: 196–203).

## Infections

### Fungal infections

Tinea pedis is a very common infection of the foot and is therefore not discussed in full detail here. The key considerations for its diagnosis are outlined in *Table 16.1*. The infection may be transmitted by contact with infected scales. Protective footwear is advised (Elewski, 1999).

Investigation is made using skin scrapings, which may be taken from the affected area, mixed with potassium hydroxide and examined under the microscope. This should reveal fungal elements. Alternatively, skin scrapings can be sent to a laboratory (Martin and Elewski, 2004).

Topical imidazoles applied twice daily work well in localized infections. Terbinafine cream once or twice daily for 1 week is more effective but more expensive (Joint Formulary Committee, 2004: 569). For persistent problems or more widespread infection, terbinafine 250 mg tablets are prescribed daily for 2–6 weeks (Joint Formulary Committee, 2004: 292–4).

### Pitted keratolysis

Pitted keratolysis is the result of an infection that affects the soles of the feet and the toes. It is usually caused by a *Corynebacterium, Micrococcus sedentarius* (English, 2003).

The patient can usually be diagnosed as he/she enters the room because of the unpleasant problem of 'smelly feet' (Gardner and Elston, 1998). On examination of the soles and toes of the feet, symmetrical, small pits and irregular erosions can be seen in the stratum corneum, which becomes macerated from sweating (*Figure 16.11*). Occlusive footwear aggravates this problem.

Investigation is usually unnecessary because the odour betrays the diagnosis, but organisms can be demonstrated in gram-stained scrapings (du Vivier, 2002: 596). Examination under a Wood's lamp in the dark reveals a coral pink fluorescence (du Vivier, 2002: 10).

Management entails the avoidance of occlusive footwear and the use of absorbent cotton socks. Sweating may be reduced by applying an antiperspirant (e.g. aluminium hydroxide 20%). Topical erythromycin or clindamycin, or oral erythromycin, should clear the condition and the smell in 3–4 weeks (English, 2003).

## References

Chuang T-Y, Stitle L (2003) Lichen planus. www.emedicine.com/derm/topic233.htm (accessed 13October 2004)

du Vivier A (2002) *Atlas of Clinical Dermatology*. 3rd edn. Churchill Livingstone, London

Elewski BE (1999) Tinea pedis and tinea manuum. In: Demis DJ, ed. *Clinical Dermatology* vol 3, unit 17–19: 1–11

English JC III (2003) Pitted keratolysis. www.emedicine.com/derm/topic332.htm (accessed 13October 2004)

Gardner T, Elston D (1998) A rash with a foul odour. *Phys Sport Med* **26**: 104–6

Gramvussakis S, Wilkinson JD (2002) Vesicular plantopalmar eczema. www.emedicine.com/derm/topic608.htm (accessed 13 October 2004)

Gruber PC, Ratnavel R (2003) Keratosis palmaris et plantaris. www.emedicine.com/derm/topic589.htm (accessed 13 October 2004)

Joint Formulary Committee (2004) *British National Formulary 48*. September BMA and Royal Pharmaceutical Society of Great Britain, London

Lucker G, Van de Kerkhof P, Steijlen P (1994) The hereditary palmoplantar keratoses: An updated review and classification. *Br J Dermatol* **131**(1): 1–14

Martin ES, Elewski BE (2004) Tinea pedis. www.emedicine.com/derm/topic470.htm (accessed 13October 2004)

Neale D, Adams I (1989) *Common Foot Disorders*. 3rd edn. Churchill Livingstone, London: 113

Ratnavel RC, Griffiths WA (1997) The inherited palmoplantar keratodermas. *Br J Dermatol* **134**(4): 485–90

## Test Your Knowledge

This 80-year old woman presented with a 6-week history of an ery-thematous, pustular, scaly rash on both feet. Initially the pustules were yellow but some were becoming brown. She complained it was starting to cause her slight discomfort but mentioned that it was not particularly itchy. She said that she had never had any skin problems previously.

### Questions

1. What is the likely diagnosis?
2. What further questions, examination or investigations would you pursue?
3. What advice and treatment would you suggest?

# Hand dermatitis/ Tinea manuum

Patients often present with eczematous eruptions on the hands. It is easy to give a quick diagnosis of 'eczema', advise on protecting the hands from aggravating factors and prescribe moisturizing creams and topical corticosteroids. However, without taking a history and understanding why the patient may be reacting to any aggravating substances, the real problem may never be identified and the condition will remain poorly controlled. Problems such as tinea on the hands may be confused with dermatitis. If the wrong treatment is applied, the hands will fail to heal.

## Hand eczema

Primary contact irritant dermatitis of the hands may occur in association with any occupation in which the hands are exposed often to water and/or other irritants such as detergents, shampoos, polishes, cement dust, oils and greases (du Vivier, 1993; Rook et al, 1979: 4.3–4.4). Hairdressers, nurses, cooks, housewives, building labourers and engineering workers are at the greatest risk of this problem. It is also more common in those who had atopic eczema in childhood. Once it has developed, even minor re-exposure to the irritant substance will keep it active.

Eczematous changes often begin under a ring and spread from there (*Figure 17.1*). They tend to affect the backs of the hands more than the palms. In more severe cases the area may blister and/or weep. In milder or earlier cases, examination will reveal ill-defined, pink, rough, fissured patches and the patient will complain of itching. If the skin around the posterior nail fold is involved, horizontal linear ridges may appear across the nail plate (*Figure 17.2*). The palms of the hands are normally spared but may show changes in severe cases (*Figure 17.3*).

Diagnosis is usually made by taking a full history including any occupational hazards or exposure to irritant substances. Sometimes the problem is the result of an allergic reaction to something the patient has been handling. It is always worth considering a patch test to identify any allergies (*Figure 17.4*). In a patch test small patches containing dilutions of suspect substances are applied to the hairless skin of the back. The patient returns after 2–4 days so that the patches may be removed and any inflammatory reaction to the substances recorded. Patch testing is usually done in a hospital (English, 2000).

## Treatment

Treatment depends on the severity of the condition and the stage at which it presents (Leppard and Ashton, 1999: 63–4). If the allergen is known, it should be removed. Blisters can be dried up with soaks in a 1:10 000 solution of potassium permanganate for 10 minutes twice a day (Leppard and Ashton, 1999: 61).

For dry eczema a dilute potent topical corticosteroid applied to the area 2–3 times daily should help to control the condition. Betamethasone valerate 0.025% or beclometasone dipropionate diluted 1:4 are suitable choices (British Medical Association and Royal Pharmaceutical Society of

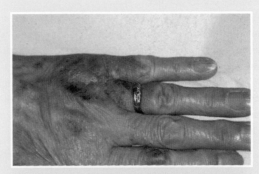

*Figure 17.1. Eczema often spreads from under a ring.*

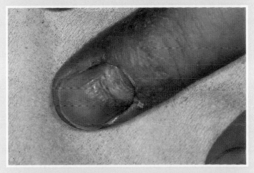

*Figure 17.2. Horizontal ridges across the nail plate.*

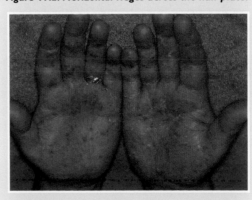

*Figure 17.3. Eczema on the palms.*

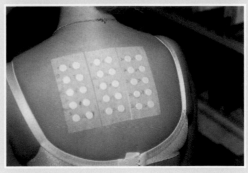

*Figure 17.4. Patch testing.*

Great Britain, 2002: 543–4). Ointments containing white soft paraffin are preferable to creams. Creams that contain preservatives and lanolin may be allergenic.

Rubber gloves can protect the hands during contact with water or detergents. If contact with rubber causes a problem, the patient should use cotton-lined PVC gloves instead.

Once the eczema is under control the patient should be referred for patch testing, which may suggest a cause. If a cause is established, the patient should be advised which products to avoid. This may involve serious changes in life style or a change of employment if contact with the substance occurs at work.

Engineers working with oils or those with problems on contact with cement dust may have difficulty working with gloves. They may either have to find alternative work or find another way of doing it.

Contact irritant eczema is an industrial disease. Patients may be eligible for industrial benefit, but a dermatologist's opinion may be required to substantiate this (Leppard and Ashton, 1999: 64).

## Tinea manuum

Tinea manuum (*Figure 17.5*) is a fungal infection caused by *Trichophyton rubrum* (du Vivier, 1993; Rook, 1979: 13.16). The patient may present with complaints of scaling or peeling of the palms, finger and/or dorsum of the hands. On examination the skin feels very dry. The flexural creases of the palm are accentuated and have a white, powdery filling. Tinea manuum usually affects one hand only, and fails to spread to the other hand. Fingernails may also be affected and it is often associated with similar infection in the feet or groin, i.e. tinea pedis or tinea cruris.

Skin scrapings, cleared in an aequeous solution of potassium hydroxide containing 40% dimethyl sulphoxide may be viewed under the microscope for diagnosis. The presence of fungal hypae confirms tinea manuum. In the laboratory, *T. rubrum* is cultured from skin scrapings (Hunter et al, 1995).

Treatment entails oral antifungal agents such as terbinafine 250 mg for 2–6 weeks; or longer if the nails are involved. Alternatively, topical Whitfield's ointment or imidazole cream, e.g. clotrimazole or econazole, may be applied twice a day for 2–3 weeks (Leppard and Ashton, 1999: 209–15).

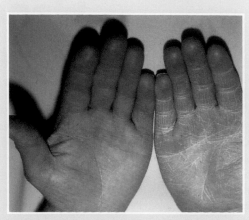

**Figure 17.5. Tinea manuum.**

## Table 17.1. Differential diagnosis

| Tinea manuum | Primary contact irritant dermatitis of the hand |
|---|---|
| Dry, scaling or peeling. Skin creases creases have white powdery filling | Ill-defined itchy, pink, rough, fissured patches. Sometimes blisters and weeping |
| Usually unilateral | Usually bilateral |
| Commonly palmar lesions | Backs of the hands more often affected than the palms. Often starts under a ring. |
| Often signs of tinea elsewhere, e.g. tinea pedis or tinea cruris | Often history of atopic eczema as a child or other eczematous tendencies. |
| Often fungal nails affected with dystrophic changes | Horizontal linear ridging of the nails if the posterior nail fold is involved. |
| No allergenic factors | Often allergenic factors that may feature at other sites too or be related to work |
| Treatment with antifungal agent, usually orally | Treatment with a topical corticosteroid and moisturizing ointments. Patch testing to isolate an allergen. Avoidance of the allergen or irritant |

## References

British Medical Association, Royal Pharmaceutical Society of Great Britain (2002) *British National Formulary 43*. March. BMA and RPSGB, London

du Vivier A (1993) *Atlas of Clinical Dermatology*. 2nd edn. Gower Medical Publishing, London

English J (2000) Contact dermatitis. *Medicine* 28(12): 62

Hunter J, Savin J, Dahl M (1995) *Clinical Dermatology*. 2nd edn. Blackwell Science, Oxford: 39

Leppard B, Ashton R (1999) *Treatment in Dermatology*. Radcliffe Medical Press, Oxford

Rook A, Wilkinson D, Ebling F (1979) *Textbook of Dermatology*. 3rd edn. Blackwell Scientific Publications, Oxford

## Test Your Knowledge

This 55-year-old man complained of an irritating, scaly rash on his hands. Although he had worked as a carpenter all his life he had never had any previous problems of this kind. It affected mainly the back of hands and his wrists. He had bought 1% hydrocortisone cream at the chemist but no improvement had been achieved after applying it for 1 week.

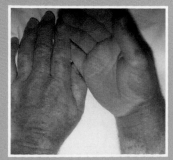

### Questions
1. What is the most likely diagnosis?
2. What investigations would you pursue?
3. What treatment would you recommend?

# Insect bites/ Bullous pemphigoid

Blisters occur in a number of different conditions. They may have genetic causes, such as epidermolysis bullosa, physical causes such as heat, irradiation or contact with irritant substances. Or they may be inflammatory infections such as bullous impetigo or herpes simplex, eczema or insect bites. Some are drug reactions or have immunological causes, e.g. pemphigoid, systemic lupus erythematosus or dermatitis herpetiformis (Collier and Wojnarowska, 2000).

This chapter discusses two specific problems that need to be differentiated: bullous insect bite reactions and bullous pemphigoid. Treatment of the latter is specific and quickly relieves the patient. Failure to recognize the problem will subject the patient to prolonged distressing symptoms and the risk of more serious complications.

## First diagnosis: Bullous pemphigoid

Bullous pemphigoid is an autoimmune disease that occurs in elderly people. It is rare before the age of 50 years but may, very occasionally, occur in childhood. It is more common in women and its incidence in the UK is 1.8 per 100 000 people. Two target antigens have been identified that can induce dermal-epidermal separation in normal human skin (Chan, 2002). It is thought that IgG immunoglobulins (anitbodies) and T lymphocyles attach components of the basement membrane (DermNetNZ2010a)

Bullous pemphigoid is reported to have been precipitated by ultra-violet irradiation, x-ray therapy and some drugs such as frusemide, non-steroidal antiinflammatory drugs, penicillamine and antibiotics (Chan, 2002).

Du Vivier (1993) explains that crops of large, tense, fluid-filled blisters develop on normal or reddened skin. They start as small vesicles that coalesce as they rapidly enlarge to form bullae. *(Figure 18.1)*. These blisters are firm and tend not to rupture easily. The condition is extremely itchy. The rash usually starts on the limbs, often the inner thighs, spreading down the legs and often affecting the arms and trunk. Bullae are the most common type of presentation but sometimes an itchy, urticarial rash may precede their development *(Figure 18.2)*.

The blisters become haemorrhagic and leave denuded, eroded skin and scabs when they break *(Figure 18.3)*. Healing occurs without scarring when treatment is quickly instituted. In a few patients blistering and ulceration may develop in the mucous membranes of the mouth.This may lead to problems of dysphagia and difficulties in taking food and fluids.

If untreated, the condition may persist for many months or years with spontaneous remissions and exacerbations. It may finally settle after 2–5 years.

It is always important to make a positive confirmation of pemphigoid because treatment, once started, may have to continue for months or years (du Vivier, 1993). Biopsy of a fresh lesion will show a split at the level of the basement

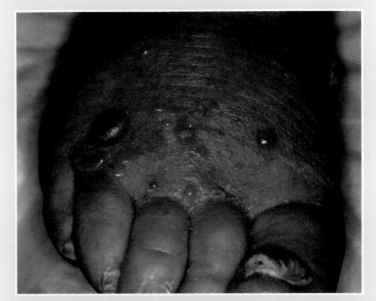
*Figure 18.1. Bullae and vesicles of bullous pemphigoid.*

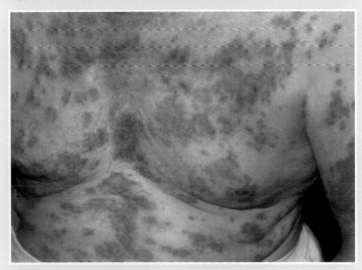
*Figure 18.2. Urticarial rash.*

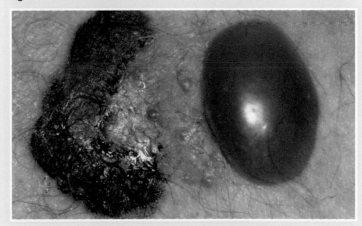
*Figure 18.3. Eroded skin, haemorrhagic effects and blistering.*

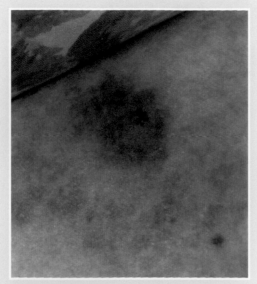

*Figure 18.4. Insect bites: Urticarial weal with central papule.*

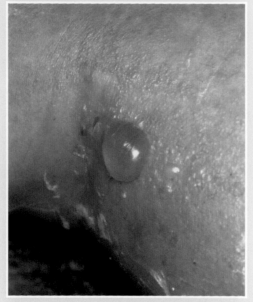

*Figure 18.5. Blisters after insect bite.*

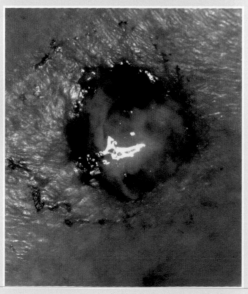

*Figure 18.6. Secondary infection of an insect bite.*

membrane, often with a mixed inflammatory infiltrate at the base that is rich in eosinophils. It is best to avoid biopsy of lesions of the lower leg because false negative results are more likely to occur at this site.

Direct immunofluorescence of the perilesional skin shows a linear band of immunofluorescence at the basement membrane zone. Blister fluid may also be sent for immunofluorescence.

Serology demonstrates Immunoglobulin G (IgG) or C3 antibody to the basement membrane in 75% of patients.

## Complications

Secondary infection, in which the clear blister fluid becomes purulent and yellow crusts form, often occurs (Chan, 2002; du Vivier, 1993). Death may follow in debilitated patients.

Elderly and debilitated patients may also develop urinary or pulmonary infections from secondary septicaemia. Immobile or bed ridden patients are at risk of deep vein thrombosis or pulmonary embolus.

Bullous pemphigoid has occasionally been found to be associated with a malignancy and this is thought to be more likely in cases with oral lesions.

Corticosteroid-induced osteoporosis is a concern for pemphigoid patients if they are treated with an oral corticosteroid dose of 7.5 mg a day for more than 3 months or if they have sustained a low trauma fracture at some time (British Medical Association and Royal Pharmaceutical Society of Great Britain, 2002: 373).

## Treatment

Severe cases may require hospitalization for initiation of corticosteroid treatment (du Vivier, 1993). Oral corticosteroids are usually required in doses of 30–60 mg of prednisolone. Once the condition is under control (usually after about 10 days), the dosage may be gradually reduced (e.g. 5 mg every 5th day), to the lowest dose that will prevent exacerbations. This maintenance dose may need to be continued for months or years before spontaneous remission is finally achieved. Occasionally, in mild cases, a potent topical corticosteroid may be sufficient to control the condition.

Azathioprine is sometimes also prescribed because it is thought to have a steroidsparing effect.

Antibiotics may be required in those cases with secondary infection of the lesions. For localized infection, topical antibiotics such as fusidic acid may suffice but, for more widespread problems, oral or intravenous antibiotics may be required.

Patients with the disease and on oral corticosteroids and especially those at risk of developing osteoporosis, require additional protection with a bisphosphonate such as alendronate, etidronate or risedronate (British Medical Association and Royal Pharmaceutical Society of Great Britain 2002: 374).

## Second diagnosis: Insect bites

Insect bites can be acquired from a variety of different sources. Dogs, cats, hedgehogs and birds frequently carry fleas that may attack humans and cause symptoms. Fleas, as well as bed bugs, breed in cracks, floorboards, soft furnishings and fitted carpets and may survive for months

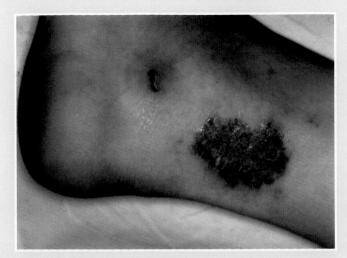

Figure 18.7. Eczema 9 months after insect bite.

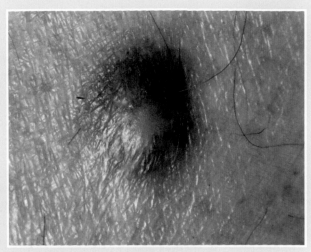

Figure 18.8. Dermatofibroma.

before attacking an unsuspecting human, especially in centrally heated premises. Many other insects and 'midges' may cause minor lesions and irritations, while wasps and bees may produce severe reactions in a few sensitive people. Ticks in the UK may carry Lyme disease. Travellers abroad are vulnerable to mosquitos bites that may transmit malaria, or ticks that cause Rocky mountain fever and sandflies with leishmaniasis (du Vivier, 1993: 14.8)

The main symptom of an an 'insect bite' is itching at the site. Urticarial weals may occur and these often have a central papule *(Figure 18.4)*, vesicle or blister *(Figure 18.5)*. Sometimes blisters may be quite large. These bullous lesions are particularly common on the legs of children. The lesions tend to be asymmetrical and are most common on the lower legs and ankles. Mites or fleas that colonize domestic animals tend to cause papular or urticarial lesions in areas that correspond to the way the animal is held in contact, e.g. on the abdomen, lower chest, thighs and forearms. Reaction to the bite is usually rapid or felt the next day.

It is not usually difficult in to diagnose an insect bite. The patient may give a history of contact with pets or of walking in the woods or playing in the fields or garden in the previous 48 hours. Bites may affect any age group, but, in an older person with bullous lesions, confusion could arise with bullous pemphigoid, which may be excluded by skin biopsy, direct immunofluorescence and/or serology. Should a biopsy be indicated, histology would confirm a diffuse infiltrate of lymphocytes, plasma cells and eosinophils that is consistent with a an insect bite.

## Complications

Secondary infection of bites with purulent discharge *(Figure 18.6)* is not uncommon, and a spreading surrounding cellulitis must be distinguished from a simple urticarial reaction. Eczema may develop at the site of the bite and persist for many months afterwards unless it is treated *(Figure 18.7)*.

Dermatofibroma *(Figure 18.8)* presents as a raised, firm papule with a smooth surface. It is often a deeply pigmented red-brown or brown. It may be confused with

a malignant melanoma. Dermatofibroma may be a single or multiple and it occurs most commonly on the lower limbs. It is thought to represent a reaction to a past insect bite (du Vivier, 1993: 8.2).

Angioneurotic oedema *(Figure 18.9)* or anaphylaxis (duVivier, 1993: 16.9–16.10) is a severe reaction that may occur after some bites such as wasp or bee stings. Severe urticarial rashes, oedematous areas or life threatening laryngeal oedema develops rapidly.

## Treatment

Topical hydrocortisone cream applied to the bite area has a soothing effect and eases the irritation and discomfort.

Some practitioners recommend a topical antihistamine or a local anaesthetic cream or spray, but these are best avoided because they may lead to sensitivity reactions in a few people (British Medical Association and Royal Pharmaceutical Society of Great Britain, 2002: 13.3). In cases of troublesome inflammation and itching a course of oral antihistamine such as fexofenadine or chlorpheniramine may be helpful (British Medical Association and Royal Pharmaceutical Society of Great Britain, 2002: 29)

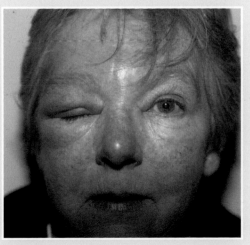

Figure 18.9. Angioneurotic oedema.

Topical antibiotics such as fusidic acid may be applied to a localized infection. An oral antibiotic such as amoxycillin may be used for more florid or widespread infections.

In severe anaphylactic reactions intramuscular adrenaline (epinephrine) is required. Patients who know they are prone to problems of DermatologyClinic this kind may carry a preassembled syringe (e.g. EpiPen) which they can quickly administer themselves. (British Medical Association and Royal Pharmaceutical Society of Great Britain, 2002: 159–60).

Blisters may have a variety of diagnoses, including insect bites and bullous pemphigoid. Effective treatment requires careful and accurate differential diagnosis (*Table 18.1*).

## References

British Medical Association, Royal Pharmaceutical Society of Great britain (2002) *British National Formulary* 44. September. BMA and RSPGB, London

Chan L (2002) Bullous pemphigoid. http://emedicine.com/derm/topic64. htm (accessed 10 November 2002)

Collier P, Wojnarowska F (2000) Blistering diseases. *Medicine* **28**

DermNetNZ2010a Bullouspemphigoid_2010 www.dermnetnz.org/immune/pemphigol.html (accessed 30.07.2010)

DermNetNZ2010b (12): 68–72. The Medicine Publishing Co Ltd

du Vivier A (1993) Blistering disorders of the skin. In: *Atlas of Clinical Dermatology*. Gower Medical Publishing, London: 17.2–17.4

## Table 18.1. Differential diagnosis

| | Bullous pemphigoid | Insect bites |
|---|---|---|
| **Age** | Occurs in the elderly, rare under 50 years | May occur at any age |
| **Symptoms** | Troublesome skin irritation | Irritation at the site of the bite or bites |
| **History** | May be preceded by urticarial rash Crops of large, tense blisters | History of contact with animals or recent exposure in country or garden |
| **Site** | Most commonly starts on the inner thigh before spreading to other parts contact with pets | Commonly on the lower legs or at sites of contact with pets |
| **Diagnosis** | Requires histological confirmation of the diagnosis | Biopsy is rarely required |
| **Treatment** | Oral corticosteroids are usually required | Symptomatic treatment with a mild topical corticosteroid |
| **Complications** | Complications related to secondary infection may be serious | Complication of secondary infection Anaphylaxis rare Eczeme Dermatofibroma |
| **Cause** | Autoimmune disease | Insect bites and stings |

## Test Your Knowledge

This 79-year-old man gave a history to intense generalized itching of the skin of the trunk and limbs in the previous 3 weeks. In the last week he had noticed a red rash on his thighs and lower abdomen. He felt generally unwell and was extremely worried. He sought help when he suddenly developed a mass of haemorrhagic blisters affecting mainly his left thigh. His general health was fair for his age but he had been on treatment for hypertension for several years.

### Questions
1. What is the likely diagnosis?
2. How would you make the diagnosis?
3. What treatment and advice would you give?

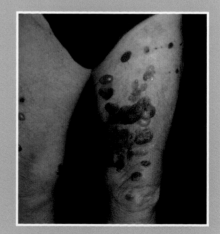

# Urticaria

Itching is a common symptom of urticaria and angioedema. This group of problems may be associated with a number of different factors, some of which may be allergy. Occasionally, the allergic and physical urticarias may lead to more serious problems of anaphylaxis and a potential threat to life.

## Aetiology of urticaria

Urticaria is common both in children and adults and is more common in people who are atopic, who may also have such problems as eczema, asthma and/or hay fever. Urticaria is the result of the release of histamine and other substances following degranulation of mast cells in the skin in response to certain stimuli. The result is vasodilatation and increased vascular permeability (DermNet NZ, 2009h).

### Autoimmune ordinary urticaria

In about a third of cases there is evidence of histamine-releasing antibodies, which cause degranulation of the mast cells and basophils by activating immunoglobulin E (IgE). This is associated with autoimmune problems, contact urticaria, anaphylaxis, urticarial vasculitis or C1 esterase inhibitor deficiency (Grattan and Humphreys, 2007).

### Non-immunological urticaria

Non-immunological urticaria describes those cases in which degranulation of mast cells and basophils occurs independently of IgE receptor activation. Some drugs such as codeine, salicylates or the non-steroidal anti-inflammatory drugs (NSAIDs) may provoke this type of urticaria (Grattan and Humphreys, 2007).

### Idiopathic chronic ordinary urticaria

Idiopathic chronic ordinary urticaria refers to a form of urticaria for which a specific cause cannot be found, in spite of thorough investigation.

### Angioedema

As with urticaria, angioedema may occur as an acute allergic response, within 1–2 hours of exposure to an allergen. It may also occur as a non- allergic reaction to a drug such as an angiotensin-converting enzyme (ACE) inhibitor. Often no precipitating factor is found (idiopathic) or it may follow trauma, exercise, emotional stress or alcohol. Some patients have a rare hereditary form of angioedema, which may not present until the teenage years.

## Presentation

The clinical features and different types of urticaria presented may indicate an underlying cause and suggest to the health professional the best approach to management of the case and, if necessary, investigation. The following are a number of the different types of urticaria that may be seen in the surgery.

### Ordinary acute urticaria

In ordinary acute urticaria there is the rapid onset of itchy blotches, blisters or weals (*Figure 19.1*), which vary in size and shape. On examination the weals are smooth and raised and may appear red around the edges, with central pallor (*Figure 19.2*). The lesions may last for anything from a few minutes to a few hours before fading completely.

Such a presentation may cause problems for the health professional who may see no evidence of the problem by the time the patient reaches the surgery. It is then necessary then to rely on the history.

Urticaria and angioedema may be seen as isolated symptoms or they may both occur at the same time.

### Angioedema

Episodes of angioedema present with the rapid development of oedema in the subcutaneous tissues which usually subsides within 24 hours. This may occur

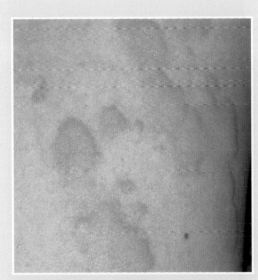

*Figure 19.1. Urticarial rash.*

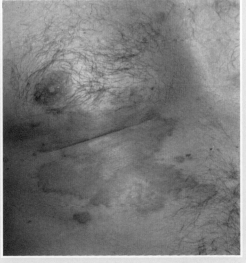

*Figure 19.2. Urticarial rash, red at the edges.*

at any site with swelling, such as in this patient with angioedema of the eyelid and tissues around the eye (*Figure 19.3*). Sometimes it may involve the mucous membranes, causing the sudden swelling of the lips (*Figure 19.4*), tongue, throat or genitals. Serious problems may ensue if the airway is compromised (DermNet NZ, 2009a).

### Physical urticaria

Urticaria may also be triggered by certain physical stimuli, as opposed to those that occur unexpectedly or as an allergic response.

### Pressure urticaria

In pressure urticaria, weals are rapidly induced by pressure on the skin. This may result from the pressure of tight clothes, standing or walking, scratching or drawing the blunt end of a pencil across the skin (dermographism)

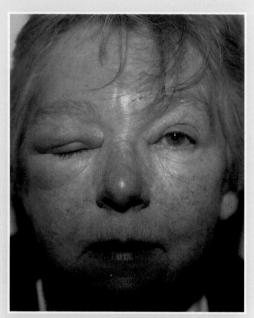

*Figure 19.3. Angioedema of the eye.*

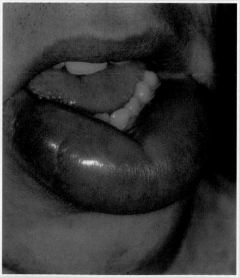

*Figure 19.4. Angioedema of the lip following a wasp sting*

(*Figure 19.5*). The weals so produced may last for a few hours or up to 3 days.

Pressure urticaria tends to particularly affect patients aged between 20–40 years, and many will also have problems of chronic urticaria or angioedema. Occasionally life will be so badly affected that a patient may not be able to continue work in a manual capacity if this involves pressure on the skin.

The cause of pressure urticaria is unknown. However, it is thought to be an autoimmune disease in which mast cells play an important part (Kirby et al, 2009).

### Thermal urticaria

Thermal urticaria may be induced by contact with cold things such as ice cubes or exposure to cold winds. It is uncommon and may be a hereditary problem, idiopathic or related to a blood problem such as leukaemia or an infection, e.g. from a virus.

Thermal urticaria may cause serious problems if bathing in cold water when hypotension, faint or anaphylaxis may result from rapid transudation of fluid into the skin. Symptoms may be delayed in hereditary cases for up to 9–48 hours and symptoms may continue for 24–48 hours.

Acquired problems rapidly show symptoms within a few minutes, and the urticaria settles after 1–2 hours (DermNet NZ, 2009c).

### Aquagenic urticaria

Aquagenic urticaria is a very rare form of urticaria in which water, of any temperature, may also produce weals within about 15 minutes of taking a bath or shower. The rash settles after about 2 hours. Unlike other forms of urticaria, it is thought to be the result of a hypersensitivity to the ions in the water rather than a histamine-releasing allergic reaction (Parker et al, 1992).

### Solar urticaria

Ultraviolet light from the sun or sun beds may cause urticaria to develop within a few minutes. It may quickly settle or sometimes last several hours. It may occur at any age, is thought to be an allergic reaction, but is not common. Areas used to exposure are less likely to react in this way (DermNet NZ, 2009g).

### Cholinergic urticaria

Cholinergic urticaria may follow exposure to exercise or emotional stress that induces sweating. The urticarial reaction that follows within a few minutes comprises small itchy weals, surrounded by red flares, as in this boy who had cycled to the surgery on a hot day (*Figure 19.6*). The rash may occur anywhere on the body but tends to be greatest on the trunk and arms. These patients often also have problems of pressure urticaria (DermNet NZ, 2009b).

### Papular urticaria

Papular urticaria is a common condition which is thought to be a reaction to insect bites. The patient may be unaware of the initial bite but develops crops of itchy red spots that may develop into blisters. The legs are most commonly affected as in this patient who had been out for a country walk a few days before (*Figure 19.7*). Fleas, which often infest family pets, are frequently to blame, but any insect bite may cause this problem in some patients, while others, even in the same family, may appear to be unaffected.

The lesions may take some days or longer to clear but scars often remain if the lesions have been scratched (DermNet NZ, 2009e).

## Contact urticaria

Contact urticaria should be suspected if there is an immediate reaction to contact with an offending substance. It differs from allergic contact urticaria in which the reaction may be delayed for a few hours or days. Patients complain of itching, tingling, burning and weals, which usually resolve in 24 hours.

Two types of contact urticaria occur (DermNet NZ, 2009d), namely:

- *Non-immunological contact urticaria*, in which there is a rapid but short-lasting reaction to things such as stinging nettles, cosmetics or vegetables; it may occur at the first contact with the substance
- *Immunological contact urticaria*, which usually occurs in atopic patients who are prone to allergies and will have had previous exposure to the allergen such as latex rubber gloves (*Figure 19.8*), antibiotics, or metals such as nickel or parabens. Apart from localized reactions, severe cases may have other generalized symptoms such as wheezing, nausea, vomiting, hoarse throat or anaphylaxis, which may be life-threatening.

## Urticarial vasculitis

The patient with urticarial vasculitis develops red patches or weals, resembling urticaria, which may be painful, burn or itch. The lesions may have a white centre and petechiae. When examined microscopically, this presentation is found to be a form of vasculitis. The rash persists for more than 24 hours before resolving spontaneously, but leaves post-inflammatory hyper-pigmentation. Patients may also suffer systemic symptoms of angioedema, abdominal pain, joint pain and/or fever.

The cause of urticarial vasculitis is unknown but has been linked to systemic lupus erythematosus, leukaemia, some malignancies, viral conditions such as hepatitis or drugs such as ACE inhibitors, penicillin, sulphonamides or the thiazide diuretics (DermNet NZ, 2009i).

## Chronic urticaria

Chronic urticaria presents in the same way as acute urticaria, with rash and sometimes other systemic symptoms, but the patient continues to have further bouts of the eruption for more than 6 weeks, sometimes years. It is often difficult to track down an actual cause for the urticaria, but a long list of possible suspects has been mooted. These include drugs, food or food additives, substances in contact with the skin, infections such as hepatitis B or herpes simplex, autoimmune problems or genetic factors as in hereditary angioedema (Hogan, 2009).

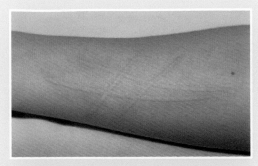

*Figure 19.5. Dermographism.*

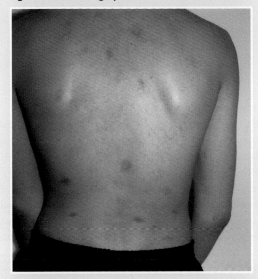

*Figure 19.6. Cholinergic urticaria.*

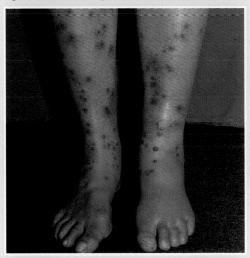

*Figure 19.7. Papular urticaria.*

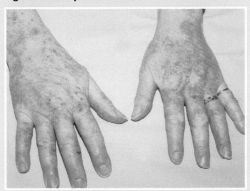

*Figure 19.8. Latex allergy.*

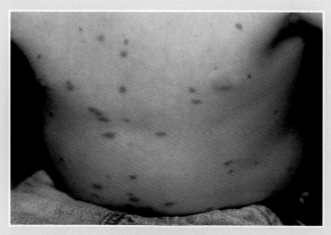

Figure 19.9. Urticaria pigmentosa in a child.

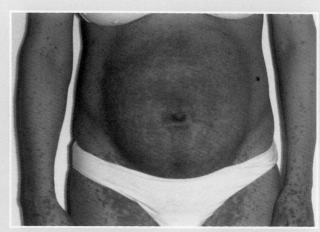

Figure 19.10. Pregnancy urticaria.

### Urticaria pigmentosa

Urticaria pigmentosa occurs in patients in whom there is an excessive accumulation of mast cells in the skin. These release histamine when rubbed or scratched causing urticarial weals (Darier's sign). Symptoms may be aggravated by aspirin, codeine, alcohol and anticholinergics. It may occur in children, often starting in the first few months of life. The lesions may gradually increase in number and are often mistaken for insect bites. As in this child the multiple 'spots' have a brownish colour (*Figure 19.9*).

In children the condition gradually lessens and has usually cleared by the teens. Some may not develop the condition until adult life. It may then persist for years with troublesome 'itch' and unsightly appearance.

There may also be the problem for adults of systemic mastocytosis affecting other organs in the body. If it is suspected, tests of liver function and urinary histamine levels and X-rays of the skull and long bones can be done to confirm it.

### Pregnancy urticaria

Pruritic urticarial papules and plaques of pregnancy (PUPPP) usually develops in the third trimester of pregnancy and is thought to be a reaction to stretch marks. Very itchy, small pink papules appear that coalesce, forming urticarial-type plaques. They start around the umbilicus and spread to the thighs, buttocks arms and legs (*Figure 19.10*). Spontaneous resolution usually follows within a few weeks of delivery. The rash poses no problem to the fetus. Emollients may help symptoms, together with antihistamines and topical steroids if necessary (DermNet NZ, 2009f).

## Investigations

The actual diagnosis of urticaria is usually a clinical one based on the history and/or findings on examining the patient. Where there is doubt about the cause or symptoms are persistent, a number of investigations are available (*Table 20.1*). Complicated problems may require advice from a dermatologist.

## Management

General advice should be given regarding minimizing or avoiding any recognized causes of the urticaria. Medical red alert tags should be recommended for those who may have a life-threatening reaction, e.g. severe reactions to wasp stings.

### Antihistamines

Antihistamines are helpful in most types of urticaria, although they seem to have little effect in pressure urticaria. They may be used to treat an episode or be used prophylactically to prevent another attack. Currently licenced for use in the UK are the non-sedating anitihistamines: cetirizine, desloratadine, fexofenadine, levocetirizine, loratadine and mizolastine, although cetirizine may induce drowsiness in higher doses and mizolastine should be avoided in cardiac patients (Joint Formulary Committee, 2009: 3.4.1). Some of these drugs can be obtained over the counter.

| Table 19.1. Tests that may help diagnose or confirm a diagnosis of forms of urticaria | |
| --- | --- |
| **Test** | **Use** |
| Full blood count Erythrocyte sedimentation rate | Vasculitic urticaria Severe or persistent chronic urticaria |
| Thyroid function test Thyroid antibiodies | Urticarial vasculitis Severe or more persistent chronic urticaria |
| IgE-specific (RAST) Skin prick tests | Acute episodic urticaria Contact urticaria |
| Serum C4 | Hereditary and acquired C1 esterase inhibitor deficiency Angioedema without weals Urticarial vasculitis |
| Skin biopsy | Urticarial vasculitis Urticaria pigmentosa |
| Physical challenge (exposing the individual to the suspected cause, e.g. ice) | Contact urticaria |

IgE = immunoglobulin E; RAST = Radioallergosorbent test
From: Grattan and Humphreys, 2007.

## Table 19.2. Differential diagnosis of types of urticaria

| Type of urticaria | Presentation | Duration of symptoms | Investigations if necessary (history often suggests cause) |
|---|---|---|---|
| Acute ordinary urticaria | Itchy, blotchy, smooth, raised weals or blisters Central pallor, red round edges | Few minutes to few hours | IgE Skin prick test |
| Angioedema | Oedema in subcutaneous tissues | Rapid onset. Usually settles within 24 hours | IgE Skin prick test |
| Pressure urticaria | Weals follow pressure on skin | Few hours to 3 days | Scratch test |
| Thermal urticaria | Urticarial response to cold | Acquired: onset 2–5 minutes, lasts 1–2 hours Hereditary: onset 9–48 hours, lasts 24–48 hours | Application of ice cube to skin for 1–5 minutes FBC, check for underlying problem |
| Aquagenic urticaria | Urticarial rash after contact with water, e.g. bath or shower | Onset within 15 minutes and continues for up to 2 hours | |
| Solar urticaria | Urticarial rash after exposure to UV light | Onset within few minutes of exposure. May quickly subside but can persist for some hours | Phototesting |
| Cholinergic urticaria | Urticarial rash related to sweating: small itchy, burning weals with red flare around | Onset within few minutes and may last just over an hour | |
| Papular urticaria | Itchy red spots and blisters, in reaction to insect bites | May last up to a few weeks. Leave scars if scratched | |
| Contact urticaria | Non-immunological: may occur at first contact. Immunological: follows previous exposure to allergen Generalized problems and anaphylaxis a risk | Rapid onset within 1 hour, quickly settles | IgE, specific IgE or skin prick tests |
| Urticarial vasculitis | Painful, burning urticarial rash in fixed area. Red patches with white centre and petechiae Post-inflammatory hyperpigmentation | Usually lasts more than 24 hours | FBC, ESR, TFT and skin biopsy |
| Chronic urticaria | Typical urticarial rash | Repeated episodes continue for over 6 weeks | FBC, ESR, TFT |
| Urticaria pigmentosa | Multiple, brownish spots which urticate when rubbed Adults: may have systemic mastocytosis | Children: gradually improves and usually better in teens Adults: may continue for years | Usually clinical diagnosis/ Darier's sign Skin biopsy LFT, urinary histamin levels, X-ray of skull and long bones if systemic features |
| Pregnancy urticaria | Occurs in third trimester of pregnancy. Small pink papules coalesce to form urticarial plaques. Start at umbilicus and spread | Resolves spontaneously within few weeks of delivery | |

ESR = erythrocyte sedimentation rate; FBC = full blood count; IgE = Immunoglobulin E; LFT = liver function test; TFT = thyroid function test; UV = ultraviolet

Antihistamines are best avoided in pregnancy, if possible, but none have yet been shown to be teratogenic in humans (Grattan and Humphreys, 2007).

### Corticosteroids

Corticosteroids may be given orally as a short course, e.g. prednisolone 50 mg daily for 3 days to adults, if it is felt necessary to shorten an episode of urticaria (Grattan and Humphreys, 2007). Topical steroids may also ease symptoms.

### Adrenaline

In cases of anaphylaxis or severe laryngeal oedema, first-line management is as follows:

- Secure the airway
- Lay the patient flat with the legs raised or in the recovery position, if unconscious
- Give adrenaline 1 in 1000 intramuscularly, with an initial dose of 0.5 ml
- Depending on the response, repeat this dose at 5-minute intervals for adults.

Intramuscular or slow intravenous chlorphenamine 10 mg is a useful addition after giving the adrenaline. Parenteral corticosteroids are used in cases of severe laryngeal oedema or anaphylaxis, although their effect is not immediate. Further treatment with bronchodilators may be necessary depending on the patient's condition (Joint Formulary Committee, 2009: 3.4.3).

For patients' use in an emergency, fixed-dose epinephrine (adrenaline) auto-injectors (EpiPen) can be carried by patients or their parents if it is felt that they might be faced with an emergency situation. They deliver an adrenaline dose of 300 µg for adults and 150 µg for children weighing 15–30 kg (Grattan and Humphreys, 2007).

## Further help

It is important to assess a patient's symptoms with a careful history and examination in order to make the correct diagnosis and offer appropriate treatment (*Table 19.2*). Alternative treatments to those discussed above and more specialist advice may be necessary in patients where the diagnosis is in doubt; where further tests are required to determine an allergic cause; where antihistamines are not giving sufficient relief; where there are abnormal markers for C1 esterase inhibitor deficiency; in suspected vasculitic urticaria; underlying disease; pregnancy; or if symptoms are affecting a child's school attendance.

## References

DermNet NZ (2009a) Angioedema. www.dermnetnz.org/reactions/angioedema.html (accessed 10 December 2009)

DermNet NZ (2009b) Cholinergic urticaria. http://dermnetnz.org/reactions/cholinergic-urticaria.html (accessed 10 December 2009)

DermNet NZ (2009c) Cold urticaria. http://dermnetnz.org/reactions/cold-urticaria.html (accessed 10 December 2009)

DermNet NZ (2009d) Contact urticaria. http://dermnetnz.org/reactions/contact-urticaria.html (accessed 10 December 2009

DermNet NZ (2009e) Papular urticaria. http://dermnetnz.org/arthropods/papular-urticaria.html (accessed 10 December 2009)

DermNet NZ (2009f) PUPPP. http://dermnetnz.org/reactions/puppp.html (accessed 10 December 2009)

DermNet NZ (2009g) Solar urticaria. http://dermnetnz.org/reactions/solar-urticaria.html (accessed 10 December 2009)

DermNet NZ (2009h) Urticaria. http://dermnetnz.org/reactions/urticaria.html (accessed 10 December 2009)

DermNet NZ (2009i) Urticarial vasculitis. http://dermnetnz.org/vascular/urticarial-vasculitis.html (accessed 10 December 2009)

Grattan C, Humphreys F (2007) Guidelines for the evaluation and management of urticaria in adults and children. *Br J Dermatol* **157**: 1116–23

Hogan DJ (2009) Urticaria, chronic. http://emedicine.medscape.com/article/1050052-overview (accessed 10 December 2009)

Joint Formulary Committee (2009) *British National Formulary* 58. September. BMJ Group and RPS Publishing, London

Kirby JS, Kim EJ, Levin RM, Heymann WR (2009) Urticaria, pressure. eMedicine. http://emedicine.medscape.com/article/1050387-overview (accessed 10 December 2009)

Parker RK, Crowe MJ, Guin JD (1992) Aquagenic urticaria. *Cutis* **50**(4): 283–4

## Test Your Knowledge

This 60 year old woman came to the surgery concerned about the very itchy rash that had appeared overnight—as she said 'It seems to come and go in different places'. On examination smooth, raised pink weals of varying sizes and shapes could be seen. She maintained that she had never had such a problem before but that she had been prescribed trimethoprim two days before for a urinary infection, but, she added 'I have had the drug before but it has never caused me any problem.'

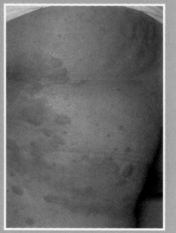

### Questions

**1.** What is the likely diagnosis?

**2.** How would you treat the current xacerbation and what would you prescribe?

**3.** What advice would you give her for the future?

# Erythema multiforme

Both urticaria (hives) and erythema multiforme are conditions that frequently present in the surgery. The patient complains of sudden onset of a rash. The sometimes florid and bizarre rash of erythema multiforme can be confused with that of urticaria. If care is taken in the history taking and examination it should be possible to make the right diagnosis and advise the patient about immediate management and ways in which he/she might be able to avoid a recurrence.

## Erythema multiforme

### Aetiology

Erythema multiforme is a hypersensitivity reaction that affects the skin and sometimes the mucous membranes. The reaction may be triggered by many factors including many bacterial and viral infections or chemical agents. Sulphonamides, antibiotics or non-steroidal anti-inflammatory drugs (NSAIDs) are often implicated but one of the most common antecedents is herpes simplex. Eythema multiforme is more common in men. It may affect people of any age but is unusual under 3 years or over 50 years of age (Foster, 2001).

The minor form of erythema multiforme mainly affects the skin only, while the major form (Stevens-Johnson syndrome) is more severe, and involves at least two mucous membranes and often internal organs also.

## Presentation

A patient with erythema multiforme minor complains of a rapidly spreading rash of macules and papules (*Figure 20.1*) that may burn but tend not to itch. The lesions may coalesce and sometimes blister. A particular feature in those cases related to herpes simplex are annular red or purple lesions that have a slightly raised centre and are thus known as target lesions. (*Figure 20.2*). The rash is symmetrically distributed and often occurs on the forearms, lower legs, backs of the hands, palms and soles of the feet. Sometimes there may be mild ulceration in the mouth. The patient is not 'ill' and the condition usually resolves in 3 weeks. A few patients may suffer recurrent attacks of erythema multiforme (du Vivier, 2002).

Erythema multiforme major (Stevens Johnson syndrome) is a much more serious condition. The patient is usually febrile with more severe changes in the skin and rash blisters. These blisters rupture, often with haemorrhage and necrosis (*Figure 20.3*). Any mucous membranes may be affected and the lips may be oedematous, bleeding and crusted (*Figure 20.4*). Other organs such as the lungs, gastrointestinal or genitourinary tract may also be involved and it is common for a purulent conjunctivitis to occur (Foster, 2001).

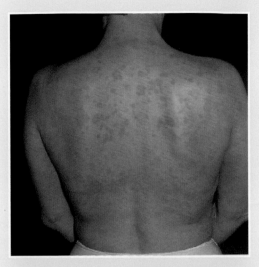

*Figure 20.1. Erythema multiforme rash on the back.*

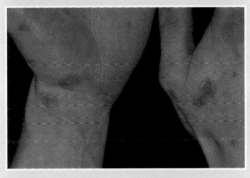

*Figure 20.2. Target lesions on the wrists.*

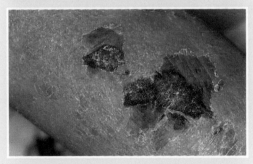

*Figure 20.3. Erythema multiforme major (Stevens Johnson Syndrome): necrotic erosion on the arm after rupture of blisters.*

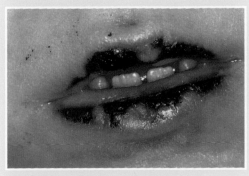

*Figure 20.4. Erythema multiforme major: oedematous, bleeding crusted lips.*

## Table 20.1. Differential diagnosis of urticaria and erythema multiforme

| | Urticaria | Erythema multiforme (EM) |
|---|---|---|
| Cause | Hypersensitivity reaction to foods, drugs, pollens, insect stings or latex | Hypersensitivity reaction to drugs and bacterial and viral infections |
| Age | Any age | Rare under 3 years or over 50 years |
| Symptoms | Rapid onset. Crops of itchy, blotchy rash, raised pink or white weals. Irregular margin. Quickly disappears without trace | Rapid onset. Non-itchy macules, papules that become confluent. Target lesions. Clears spontaneously within 3 weeks |
| Complication | Angioedema Anaphylaxis | EM major (Stevens Johnson syndrome): blisters, mucous membrane and other organ involvement |
| Treatment | Antihistamines—oral or by injection Corticosteroids—very occasionally | EM minor: symptomatic only EM major: hospital admission |

### Diagnosis

The diagnosis of erythema multiforme should be considered in any 'well' patient presenting with a bizarre rash. Erythema multiforme means a 'red rash of many shapes'. The classic appearance of target lesions usually leaves little doubt about the diagnosis. However, the blistering type of erythema multiforme may be confused with bullous pemphigoid, in which case skin biopsy and immunofluorescence, if positive, should confirm pemphigoid and exclude erythema multiforme (du Vivier, 2002).

### Management

Erythema multiforme minor is a self-limiting condition that requires usually symptomatic treatment only. The patient can be reassured that it is not catching and should resolve in 3 weeks. Mouth ulcers usually quickly settle without specific treatment. The patient should be advised not to take any drug that might have caused the problem. A few patients have recurrent episodes of erythema multiforme. If the history suggests that herpes simplex precedes the episodes a 5-day course of aciclovir (acyclovir) for recurrences of herpes simplex may abort an attack or repeated attacks may be reduced if long-term aciclovir (400 mg twice daily for 6 months) is given.

In cases of erythema multiforme major, the patient is usually ill and will require hospitalization for intravenous fluids and management of the extensive blistering and raw, painful erosions (du Vivier, 2002).

### Conclusion

The rash of erythema multiforme, which is sometimes florid and bizarre, may be confused with that of urticaria (*Table 20.1*). Therefore a careful history and examination is required to ensure the right diagnosis is made and enable useful advice to be given to the patient about management and ways to avoid a recurrence.

### References

du Vivier A (2002) Urticaria and angiooedema. *Atlas of Clinical Dermatology*. 3rd edn: 374–8

Foster J (2001) Erythema multiforme. April. www.emedicine.com/ EMERG/topic173.htm (accessed 28 November 2003)

## Test Your Knowledge

This 8-year-old child presented with a widespread pink, blotchy, non-itchy rash on the face, trunk and limbs. Examination showed numerous macules of varying size and shape. She was normally well but had had a urinary tract infection 2 weeks earlier that had required treatment with trimethoprim. She had never had any problems like this before.

### Questions

1. What is the likely diagnosis?
2. What particular features of the rash and history of the problem would make you reach this conclusion?
3. How would you advise the patient and her mother?

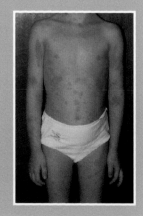

# Atopic eczema

Atopic eczema is an intensely itchy, inflammatory disease of the skin, also known as dermatitis. It is associated with eczematous lesions, dry skin and lichenification (thickening of the epidermis, with exaggeration of the normal creases) (Edelstein and Sinert, 2009). In many cases the diagnosis will be obvious but sometimes it may be necessary to investigate the possibility of either an underlying or an alternative diagnosis. The possibility that eczema is caused by contact with a substance that the person is allergic to, or results from contact with irritant substances, must also be considered.

The effects of atopic eczema can be great for both the patient and their family. In addition to the discomfort of the disease, the patient may suffer sleep loss, embarrassment, poor work or school attendance, and difficulties in obtaining or maintaining employment. The patients' families must watch their suffering and, particularly with children, be closely involved in the management of the condition and the correct application of treatments. Every patient's condition must therefore be assessed not only on the severity of the disease but also on the impact it has on their lives and those around them (National Collaborating Centre for Women's and Children's Health (NCC-WCH), 2007).

## Atopic eczema

The definitive causes of atopic eczema are uncertain, however, it is frequently seen in other members of the same family, which suggests a genetic component. Research has suggested that it is inherited by a maternal gene located on chromosome 11 (Ruiz et al, 1992). Environmental factors, such as dust mite, pollution and early exposure to infections, may also be causative (Bath-Hexall and Williams, 2006). In addition, atopic eczema is one of a triad of atopic problems with asthma and allergic rhinitis.

Some facial features may be noted in children with allergic and/or eczematous tendencies. These features— or atopic facies—include dark circles under the eyes (known as allergic shiners) and an extra fold under the lower eyelids (known as Denni-Morgan lines) (Carlson and Hering, 1981; Dr Paul, 2009) (*Figure 21.1*).

Atopic eczema is extremely common, affecting between 15–20% of school children and 2–10% of adults in the UK (Bath-Hexall and Williams, 2006). It most commonly starts in infancy and in 75% of cases will have manifested by the age of 5 years. In the majority of cases (60–70%), remission will occur by the age of 15 years (Edelstein and Sinert, 2009).

Although eczema can first appear in adult life, development at this stage is more likely to be related to another cause (Edelstein and Sinert, 2009). In the natural course of the disease, relapses and remissions are common and may occur frequently. Although infection, allergens, soap powders and stress may be blamed, these flares can often occur for no obvious reason (Bath-Hexall and Williams, 2006).

## Presentation

The symptoms, distribution and signs of atopic eczema vary with age. In the acute phase, the itchy rash may be inflamed and weeping, and blisters may occur. In the sub-acute phase, the itchy skin may sting or burn and appear scaly and

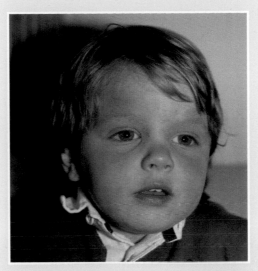

*Figure 21.1. Atopic facies.*

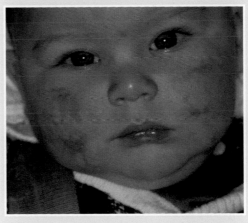

*Figure 21.2. Eczematous rash on the cheeks of 6-month old child.*

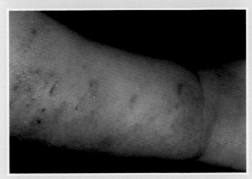

*Figure 21.3. Eczematous rash on the arm of a toddler.*

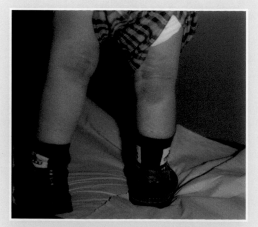

*Figure 21.4. Flexural eczema on a 2-year old.*

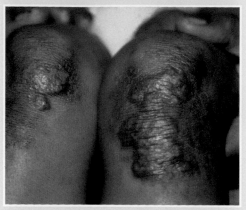

*Figure 21.5. Eczematous change and hyper-pigmentation on the extensor surface of the knees.*

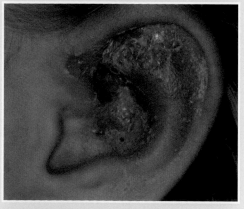

*Figure 21.6. Eczema of the ear lobe in a 4-year old.*

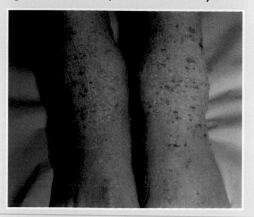

*Figure 21.7. Thickening dryness, scaling and lichenification in an adult.*

fissured. In the chronic phase the skin may be thickened, fissured and excoriated.

### Infants

Atopic eczema does not usually develop before the age of around 4 months. The first signs of the condition are often seen on the face, with a dry, scaly rash on the cheeks (*Figure 21.2*). A similar, more generalized rash may also appear, often excoriated from scratching.

### Toddlers and pre-school children

The rash and itching may be even more troublesome at the toddler and preschool stage. Extensor surfaces of the joints, such as knees, elbows and wrists (*Figure 21.3*) are likely to be involved. With increasing age, the flexural creases are more likely to develop eczematous change and the skin becomes lichenified as a result of constant scratching and rubbing (*Figure 21.4*).

### School-aged children

The extensor pattern of eczema distribution may continue into school age. When the condition subsides the child may be left with unsightly post-inflammatory hyperpigmentation that can take a long time to fade (*Figure 21.5*).

The involvement of the flexural creases of the knees and elbows tends to continue, and other areas such as the scalp, neck and ear lobes (*Figure 21.6*) may be affected. Pompholyx eczema—characterized by an itchy vesicular or blistery rash on the hands/or feet—may also occur. The majority of cases will have cleared on reaching the teenage years, however, some people will experience further eczematous problems in adult life (Edelstein and Sinert, 2009).

### Adults

Atopic eczema in adulthood may follow the same pattern as in childhood but is more likely to affect localized areas and show thickening, dryness, scaling and lichenification of the skin from repeated scratching and rubbing (*Figure 21.7*).

### Diagnosis

When presented with a patient complaining of itchy skin and an eczematous type of rash, the possibility that it has been triggered by some underlying cause, which requires further investigation or different treatment, must be considered. The diagnosis of atopic eczema can usually be made if a good history is taken. Specific factors that may indicate an atopic eczema diagnosis are listed in *Table 21.1*.

There are a number of potential causes of atopic eczema, including (NHS Institute for Innovation and Improvement, 2008):

* Infection
* Seasonal temperature changes
* Allergens in the atmosphere, such as house dust, mite or pet dander
* Stress
* Contact with allergens or irritant substances.

A good history will normally suggest a cause, so it is usually unnecessary to conduct laboratory tests to confirm the diagnosis. However, patch testing may sometimes be

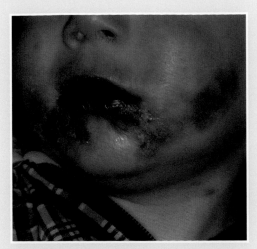

*Figure 21.8. Streptococcal-infected eczema.*

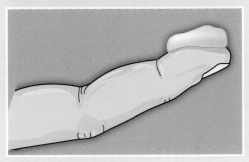

*Figure 21.9. The fingertip unit.*

| Table 21.1. Diagnostic factors for atopic eczema |
| --- |
| Onset of symptoms before age of 2 years |
| Personal and/or family history of eczema |
| Asthma or hay fever |
| Atopic facies |
| Dry and itchy skin |
| Aggravation by wearing wool |
| Dermographism (exaggerated skin response to scratching) |
| Obvious signs of eczematous skin change |
| Dry, cracked lips |
| History of exacerbations and relapses |
| Involvement of the face and extensor surfaces in young children |
| Flexural eczema - sometimes with lichenification |

helpful in confirming an allergic cause. If further investigation is required, a specialist should be involved.

## Complications

Exacerbations of atopic eczema are common and should be dealt with as detailed below. Secondary bacterial infection is always a risk and is often an underlying reason for relapses. *Staphylococcus aureus* or *Streptococcus* are the most common bacteria involved. It is important that patients and their carers know how to recognize symptoms when they occur; namely rapid worsening of the eczema that is not responding to the basic approaches and the presence of weeping areas, pustules, crusting and/or fever (*Figure 21.8*). A viral infection such as herpes simplex (eczema herpeticum) may cause widespread problems, with grouped vesicles or 'punched-out' lesions developing in the rash (NHS Institute for Innovation and Improvement, 2007).

## Management

When suggesting a programme of treatment, it is helpful to give the patient a written plan to follow. Such a plan will vary depending on the severity of the eczema. Patients and parents —particularly of young children — need careful instruction, and often require actual demonstration of how and when to apply medications. Readily available access to a professional, if the condition is not responding to treatment, is also required.

## Trigger factors

Management of the condition must consider potential trigger factors—such as soaps, detergents, infection, contact allergens or foods—which may be causing exacerbations of the disease. Recommendations of what to avoid can then be made. General advice to avoid potential trigger factors includes (Krafchik, 2008):

- Wearing cotton clothing
- Avoiding wearing wool next to the skin
- Washing clothes in a mild detergent without softeners or bleach
- Reminding the family that central heating dries the atmosphere, and of the benefits of humidifiers in reducing skin drying.

If the cause of the trigger or allergy is obvious, no further investigations will be necessary. However, if there is doubt, referral to a dermatologist to arrange patch testing for contact allergies may be advisable.

## Emollients

Daily and plentiful application of an unperfumed emollient to keep the skin well moisturized is a key aspect of management (Joint Formulary Committee, 2009). Emollients include aequeous cream, emulsifying ointment, liquid or white soft paraffin oilatum, and emollients with added antimicrobials such as benzalkonium or chlorhexidine.

## Oral antihistamines

Oral antihistamines may be helpful in relieving itching, particularly sedating antihistamines such as chlorphenamine or promethazine which are taken at night. Non-sedating antihistamines such as fexofenadine (for use in those over 6 years of age) or loratadine (for use in thos over 2 years of age) may be suitable in the daytime (Joint Formulary Committee, 2009).

## Topical steroids

Topical steroids are an important part of the treatment of eczema that is not controlled by emollients. They are used for their anti-inflammatory properties (NCC-WCH, 2007). The potency of the preparation required depends on the severity of the eczema; more potent ointments may be necessary to get the condition under control but should not

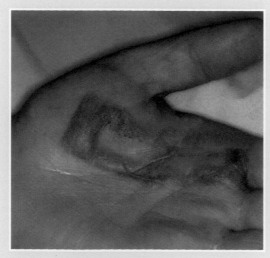

**Figure 21.10. Elastoplast allergy.**

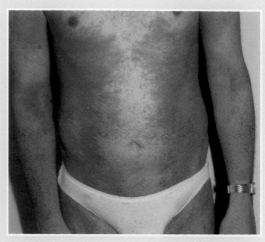

**Figure 21.11. Generalized eczema following use of shaving cream containing lanolin.**

be used for more than 7–14 days. Once the condition is improved, weaker preparations may be sufficient, however, preparations of more than 1% hydrocortisone should not be used on the face. Steroids are available as ointment or cream preparations, but ointments, being greasy, help more than the creams in keeping the skin well moisturized.

Topical steroids should be thinly applied twice a day; one fingertip unit should be sufficient to cover an area twice the size of the palm of an adult hand (*Figure 21. 9*). The Joint Formulary Committee (2009) recommends quantities for application on the various regions of the adult body (*Table 21.2*). Once the exacerbation has settled and the patient is weaned on steroids of decreasing potency, the emollient programme should be continued (Krafchik, 2008)

### Tar-based treatments

Tar-based treatments have been used over the years for their antimicrobial and antipruritic effects, and their ability to reduce scaling. They are a cheap option, however, some of their side effects have led to a preference for use of alternative applications. Their disadvantages include an unpleasant smell, stinging and skin irritation, light sensitivity, and staining of skin, clothes and/or the bath. Tar is often mixed with other ingredients—such as salicylic acid, sulphur or steroids—to produce shampoos, lotions, bath oils, creams and ointments. It is sometimes recommended that bandages are used to cover the area and

prevent staining. Tar-based treatments are best applied at night and left on for at least 2 hours. They should not be used on raw or blistered skin (DermNet NZ, 2009b; Joint Formulary Committee, 2009)

### Immunomodulatory drugs

Immunomodulatory drugs are available for use in cases that fail to respond to full treatment with topical steroids or where steroids' side effects, such as skin atrophy, are problematic. Topical pimecrolimus or tacrolimus address allergy and inflammation, and may be used over the age of 2 years, but their use should be initiated by a dermatologist (Novak et al, 2005).

### Other treatments

Other possible treatments include phototherapy, ciclosporin, azathioprine and oral corticosteroids. These may be recommended by a specialist in dermatology.

### Treatment of infections

When infection occurs, a swab should be taken and sent to the laboratory for culture and sensitivities. Localized areas may respond to a topical antibiotic such as fusidic acid. Oral flucloxacillin is the preferred antibiotic for more severe or generalized infection. Erythromycin may be used if the patient is allergic to penicillin. For herpes infection, a systemic antiviral such as aciclovir is necessary.

## Differential diagnosis

There are a number of conditions that may present with eczematous change, but for which there is another underlying cause that must be treated if the condition is to resolve. These include:

- Contact eczema
- Lichen simplex
- Discoid eczema
- Plaque psoriasis
- Scabies
- Seborrhoeic dermatitis
- Tinea corporis.

| Table 21.2. Recommended doses of topical steroid in eczema* | |
| --- | --- |
| Face and neck | 15–30 g |
| Both hands | 15–30 g |
| Scalp | 15–30 g |
| Both arms | 30–60 g |
| Both legs | 100 g |
| Trunk | 100 g |
| Groin and genitalia | 15–30 g |

*For 2-week period. From: Joint Formulary Committee, 2009

The common problems of contact and irritant dermatitis are considered below, and *Table 21.3* summarizes the differences between these forms and atopic eczema.

### Contact eczema

#### Allergic contact eczema

An eczematous reaction can occur after direct contact with a substance to which the patient is allergic, such as nickel in jewellery or rosin in an elastoplast dressing (*Figure 21.10*). The reaction may occur a few hours after contact but may take several days to subside. Occasionally in severe cases, the reaction may extend beyond the point of contact or be more generalized. For example, the man in *Figure 21.11* reacted to a lanolin-containing shaving cream on his face but developed a widespread rash.

When uncertainty exists about the cause, patch testing for allergies should elucidate the problem. Latex allergy produces an urticarial reaction rather than an eczematous one within minutes of contact and fades relatively quickly (DermNet NZ, 2009d). Once the aggravating factor is removed the reaction will settle, but may be helped by the use of emollients, topical steroids and oral antihistamine if itching is a problem. Severe reactions may require oral corticosteroids (Watkins, 2006; DermNet NZ, 2009a). Once developed, any of these allergies are usually lifelong and the allergens should be avoided in future.

#### Irritant contact dermatitis

Eczematous reactions may result from overuse of irritant substances, such as detergents or soaps (*Figure 21.12*).

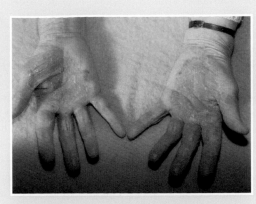

*Figure 21.12. Irritant contact dermatitis.*

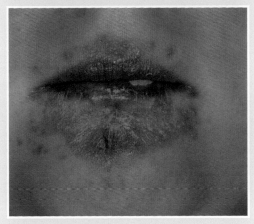

*Figure 21.13. Lip licking dermatitis.*

## Table 21.3. Differential diagnosis of eczema

| | Atopic eczema | Irritant contact eczema | Allergic contact eczema |
|---|---|---|---|
| **Cause** | Uncertain<br>Maternal genetic link<br>Atopy<br>Environmental trigger factors | Overuse of irritant substances on skin | Contact with allergens such as nickel or rosin |
| **Presentation** | Dry and/or itchy skin<br>Personal and/or family history of eczema, asthma or hay fever<br>Aggravated by wool<br>Dermographism<br>Onset of symptoms before 2 years<br>Atopic facies<br>Eczematous rash<br>Dry, cracked lips<br>Affecting face and extensor surfaces in young children<br>Flexural eczema, sometimes with lichenification<br>Exacerbations and relapses | Dry, itchy, scaly skin in area of contact with irritant substance | Eczematous rash<br>Possible presence of blisters<br>Development in minutes, hours or days after contact |
| **Complications** | Infections—bacterial or viral<br>Eczema herpeticum | Secondary infection | Secondary infection |
| **Management** | General advice and information on eczema and use of treatments<br>Support for families<br>Emollients<br>Topical steroids<br>Occasional systemic steroids<br>Tar-based treatments<br>Antihistamines<br>Specialist advice<br>Immunomodulatory agents<br>Phototherapy, ciclosporin, azathioprine<br>Antibiotics when infection occurs | Flushing with water for chemical burns<br>Emollients<br>Topical steroids<br>Antibiotics when infection occurs<br>Protect from further contact with the offending substance | Patch testing as required to confirm allergy<br>Emollients<br>Topical steroids<br>Oral steroids in severe cases<br>Antibiotics when infection occurs |

Other substances such as bleaches, acids or alkalis may also cause problems. For example, saliva is alkaline and contributes to the development of 'lip licking dermatitis' (*Figure 21.13*).

Patch testing in these types of problem do not assist diagnosis, although it is possible for contact and irritant eczema to coexist. The patient must be advised to avoid further contact with these substances and to protect the area if possible. The plentiful use of emollients will help to moisturize the area and topical steroid ointments will ease symptoms. If secondary infection occurs, antibiotics may be necessary (Watkins, 2006). In cases of actual chemical burn, the area should the flushed with water and, if available, specific antidote should be used (DermNet NZ, 2009c).

## Conclusions

Atopic eczema is a common problem for which patients commonly seek advice from professionals. Health professionals advice and support is crucial if patients are to learn how to practise the basic moisturizing of the skin with emollients, and know when added corticosteroids preparations are required to keep the condition under control. Also crucial is the need to recognize complications so that earlier intervention may avoid more serious results or the need for hospitalization.

## References

Bath-Hextall F, Williams H (2006) Eczema (atopic). BMJ Clinical Evidence [online], 1 July. BMJ Publishing Group Limited

Carlson RE, Hering PJ (1981) Allergic shiners. *JAMA* **246**(8): 835

DermNet NZ (2009a) Allergic contact dermatitis. http://dermnetnz. org/dermatitis/contact-allergy.html (accessed 25 October 2009)

DermNet NZ (2009b) Coal tar. http://dermnetnz.org/treatments/ coaltar.html (accessed 25 October 2009)

DermNet NZ (2009c) Irritant contact dermatitis. http://dermnetnz. org/dermatitis/contact-irritant.html (accessed 25 October 2009)

DermNet NZ (2009d) Urticaria. http://dermnetnz.org/reactions/ urticaria.html (accessed 27 October 2009)

Dr Paul (2009) Allergy signs in children. www.drpaul.com/library/ ALLERGYSIGNS.html (accessed 25 October 2009)

Edelstein J, Sinert R (2009) Dermatitis, atopic. http://emedicine. medscape.com/article/762045-overview (accessed 25 October 2009)

Krafchik B (2008) Atopic dermatitis. http://emedicine.medscape. com/article/1049085-overview (accessed 25 October 2009)

Joint Formulary Committee (2009) *British National Formulary* 58. September. BMA and RPS Publishing, London

National Collaborating Centre for Women's and Children's Health (2007) Atopic eczema in children: Management of Atopic Eczema in Children from Birth up to the Age of 12 Years. Clinical guideline 57. August. National Institute for Health and Clinical Excellence, London

NHS Institute for Innovation and Improvement (2007) Treatment of Infected Eczema. www.cks.nhs.uk/eczema_atopic/management/ detailed_answers/management_of_infected_eczema/treatment_ of_infected_eczema (accessed 25 October 2009)

NHS Institute for Innovation and Improvement (2008) Clinical knowledge summaries: Eczema—atopic—identifying trigger factors. http://tinyurl.com/yhvkctm (accessed 26 October 2009)

Novak N, Kwiek B, Bieber T (2005) The mode of topical immunomodulators in the immunological network of atopic dermatitis. *Clin Exp Dermatol* **30**(2): 160–4

Ruiz R, Kennedy D, Price J (1992) Higher risk of infantile atopic dermatitis from maternal atopy than from paternal atopy. *Clin Exp Allergy* **22**(8): 762–6

Watkins J (2006) Irritant v contact dermatitis. *Practice Nursing* **17**(1): 28–31

## Further information

**British Association of Dermatologists**
www.bad.org.uk
4 Fitzroy Square, London W1T 5HQ
Has patient advice leaflets on atopic eczema

**National Eczema Society**
www.eczema.org
Hill House, Highgate Hill, London N19 5NA

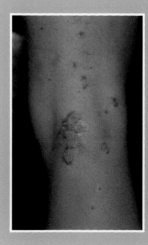

# Test Your Knowledge

This 16-year old boy had suffered with atopic eczema since infancy. Over the years the condition had been kept under relatively good control, owing to the dedicated support of his family. This support involved ensuring that he persisted with repeated emollients to moisturize the skin, and the addition of steroid creams to the treatment regime when the condition became more troublesome. More recently, as he is now considered to be 'grown up', he has been left to deal with his eczema management independently. Unfortunately, as he was about to take his GCSE exams, his eczema deteriorated and was rapidly spread over his body.

### Questions
1. What is the likely cause of this exacerbation?
2. How would you treat the current exacerbation?
3. What advice would you give him for the future?

# Compulsive itch

It may all start with something as simple as an insect bite or sting. The patient naturally responds to the intense irritation that may follow by scratching, which in turn may lead to skin damage and secondary infection, or at times be followed by an eczematous reaction that may in itself be itchy. More scratching will follow and the so called 'itch-scratch-itch' cycle may follow, leading to further skin damage, excoriations and lichenification (Oakley, 2009).

Other causes of itching are numerous and include dry skin, eczema, urticaria, specific skin conditions such as lichen planus or pemphigoid, reactions to certain medications, generalized conditions such as jaundice, diabetes or uraemia, or psychological disturbances. (NHS Choices, 2009). When faced with an itchy, scratching patient it will be important to fully assess the patient and recognize any underlying cause that may need to be dealt with. This will require a full history and examination, and possibly certain investigations, in order to narrow down the various possibilities and at the same time decide on the most appropriate treatment.

In this chapter a few conditions will be considered in which health professionals encounter a constantly scratching patient where an underlying cause may not be obvious.

## Lichen simplex
### Presentation
Lichen simplex is a relatively common problem that develops as the result of repeated rubbing or scratching of an area, in response to an itch or out of habit. It occurs most commonly in people between 30–50 years and is more common in women and those with atopic tendencies (Hogan et al, 2009a). It affects only those areas that are accessible to the patient, thus common sites are the scalp or nape of the neck (*Figure 22.1*), the extensor surfaces of the forearms or wrists, inner thighs, knees or lower legs (*Figure 22.2*), vulva, scrotum or buttocks (*Figure 22.3*).

The patient may present with one or more well demarcated, scaly, erythematous plaques. Often signs of scratching and excoriations may be obvious (*Figure 22.4*) and after time, lichenification and hyperkeratosis may develop, together with changes in pigmentation, especially hyperpigmentation (*Figure 22.5*). The trauma to the area always carries the risk of secondary infection cellulitis and pus.

## Nodular prurigo
### Presentation
The actual cause of nodular prurigo is still unknown but 80% of patients have a personal or family history of atopic problems. It may also be associated with renal or liver dysfunction, HIV, trauma or skin infection or in patients with anxiety or psychiatric problems. It usually is seen in women after middle age and may distress the patient to the extent that life is dominated by the itch and normal living and work interfered with (Hogan et al, 2009b).

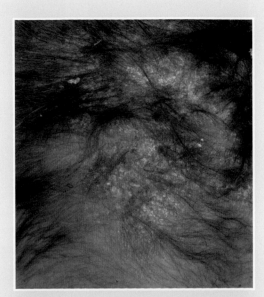
*Figure 22.1. Lichen simplex at the back of the neck.*

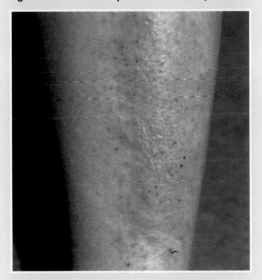
*Figure 22.2. Lichen simplex on the shin.*

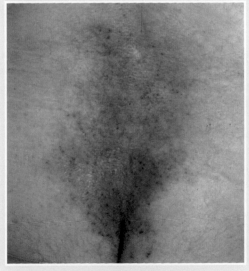
*Figure 22.3. Lichen simplex on the back.*

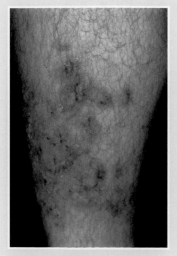

Figure 22.4. Lichen simplex with scratch marks and excoriations.

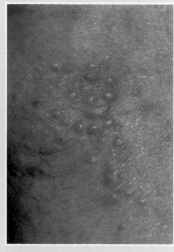

Figure 22.6. Nodular prurigo:multiple small nodules.

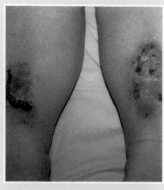

Figure 22.8. Neurotic excoriations with angulated lesions.

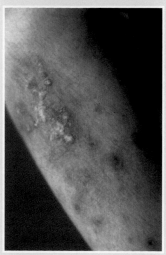

Figure 22.5. Lichen simplex with hyperpigmentation that could be mistaken for lichen planus.

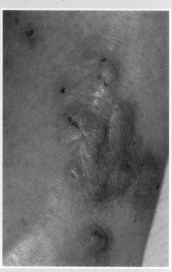

Figure 22.7. Nodular prurigo with excoriations and crusting.

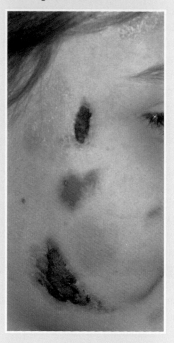

Figure 22.9. Bizarre lesions of dermatitis artefacta.

The patient complains of persistent, unrelieved itching in specific areas. On examination anything from a few to hundreds of discrete nodules or papules may be seen (*Figure 22.6*). These may vary in size from 3–20 mm and occur most commonly on the extensor surfaces of the limbs or trunk. Sometimes there may be obvious signs of excoriation (*Figure 22.7*) and crusting of the lesions. Often the patient seems to be obsessed by the itching and constantly scratches when explaining the problem.

## Self trauma
### Neurotic excoriations
Neurotic excoriations are said to be caused by repeated, conscious scratching and picking. The awareness of what he/she is doing differentiates from a patient with dermatitis artefacta, in which similar damage may occur but the patient appears to completely ignorant of the fact that he/she is causing the problem.

Sometimes there may have been some initial problem to stimulate the patient's behaviour. Lesions develop, particularly on the extensor surfaces of the limbs, the face and upper back which are, of course, within reach of the patient. Usually the lesions are symmetrically distributed erosions and/or ulcers with angulated borders (*Figure 22.8*). The patient will be left with unsightly scars, especially if he/she receives inadequate treatment.

Neurotic excoriations are more common in women and often starts in the teenage years, or in young adults with personality disorders, or social or emotional stresses to which the patient is reluctant to admit (Scheinfeld, 2010).

### Dermatitis artefacta
As in the patient in *Figure 22.9*, dermatitis artefacta presents with bizarre-looking lesions that look like no other dermatological problem. Odd geometrically-shaped lesions are seen in a patient who is apparently completely unaware, or at least denies, that he/she is causing the problem. It occurs most frequently in the teenage years and in young adults and most commonly there is some underlying problem in the patient's life. As with other itchy conditions in which the skin is traumatized, secondary infection of the lesions is always a threat.

## Parasitophobia

A patient may repeatedly present with complaints of itching and sensations of something crawling under or biting the skin. The patient is convinced that his/her body has been invaded by parasites or some insect that is leading to these symptoms. In an effort to solve the problems the patient may have taken extreme measures, sought a number of second opinions, hygienists or exterminators with visits requested for the pest controller to 'decontaminate' the house.

In the surgery, the patient will demonstrate the 'bites', excoriated lesions and residual scars (*Figure 22.10*), which the patient claims are the result of infestation, but in fact, are just the result of repeated scratching. To prove his/her point, the patient often brings the 'proof'—the substance produced when scratching—in a matchbox (*Figure 22.11*). Microscopically these are found to be merely fragments of skin, hair or dried blood.

In psychological terms, the cause of these delusions of parasitosis is classified as a monosymptomatic hypochondriacal psychosis (Ngan, 2009).

## Investigations

When presented with an itchy patient, depending on the symptoms and signs, it may be possible to make certain assumptions about the cause of the problem or even, in some cases, make a positive diagnosis. However, there will be times when specific tests will be required to confirm suspicions or to help the health professional come to the right conclusion.

A good history of the condition is crucial, together with information about the patient's general state of health and knowledge of any medications that the patient may have been prescribed or bought over the counter. Also, particularly in a patient whose rash may be related to one of the problems discussed in this article, the health professional needs to explore the patient's situation both at work and at home, and decide whether stress or some underlying personality disorder should be considered.

Following this, there are a number of possible tests available that may throw light on the true diagnosis and the most appropriate test needs to be selected:

- Full blood count to exclude any haematological problems
- Serum electrolytes and urea to assess renal function
- Liver function tests
- Thyroid function
- Urine and fasting glucose to exclude diabetes mellitus
- Serum immunoglobulin E (IgE)—a raised level would suggest atopic tendencies that are commonly associated with lichen simplex or nodular prurigo
- HIV testing if this is felt to be appropriate
- Skin scrapings to exclude fungal infection that might cause or be associated with the rash. Scraping from a 'burrow' could demonstrate scabies to be the cause of the rash or to reassure a patient with parasitophobia that no 'mites' are found
- Skin biopsy for solitary lesions that could be malignant and to differentiate other problems that might present in a similar way to lichen simplex such as lichen planus, psoriasis or T-cell lymphoma (Hogan et al, 2009a)
- Patch testing if an allergy is suspected (Oakley, 2009).

## Management of Pruritus

Unsurprisingly, if a specific cause is found for the irritation, appropriate treatment should be offered. However, in managing the conditions discussed in this article, the following approaches can be used alongside liberal use of emollients for itchy, dry skin (*Table 22.1*).

Everything must be done to help the patient to understand that the problem develops or is aggravated by scratching and rubbing, which may also leave a legacy of scars. Help must then be given to find ways of counteracting the habit. Fingernails should be kept short and gloves worn at night when scratching may occur during sleep.

### Topical steroids

Topical steroids are the first-line treatment as they not only help to reduce the inflammation and itch, but also help to soften keratotic areas. Initially, potent steroids may be required to get the condition under control. However, the health professional needs to be aware of the skin-thinning effect of potent topical steroids and their use should be limited to thicker-skinned areas, with 3-week courses and never normally used on the face. (Joint Formulary Committee, 2009). Long-term use of a mild topical steroid may need to be continued.

### Oral antihistamines

Oral antihistamines, particularly sedating antihistamines such as diphenhydramine or hydroxyzine may be helpful in anxious patients, especially at night.

### Antidepressants

In some cases, antidepressants such as amitriptyline may help due also to its antihistamine effects; doxepin is recommended (Hogan et al, 2009a).

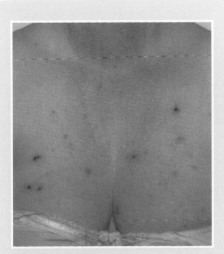

Figure 22.10. Presentation of parasitophobia —'bites', excoriations and scars.

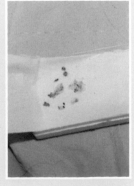

*Figure 22.11. Matchbox presentation of parasitophobia: microscopic skin particles and dried blood.*

## Topical antibiotic

Where lesions become infected a topical antibiotic such as fusidic acid or an oral antibiotic will be necessary (Hogan et al, 2009a).

In addition, some treatments may be appropriate to certain conditions.

## Lichen simplex

The potent effect of topical steroids can be increased if these are used under occlusion. Not only does it then act more effectively locally but the necessary dressing acts as a barrier to scratching. If response is inadequate, it is suggested that the immunomodulators tacrolimus or pimecrolimus may be beneficial (Kelekci et al, 2008) or, where all else fails, local botulinum toxin injections have been tried (Heckmann et al, 2002).

## Nodular prurigo

The outlook for cure of nodular prurigo is not particularly good and spontaneous remission is unusual. Somehow, the patient must learn to get out of the 'itch-scratch' cycle.

Topical, intralesional or occasionally oral corticosteroids do sometimes help to ease the itching but are not always beneficial. Other agents such as topical menthol, phenol or local anaesthetics such as lidocaine ointment may improve the itch as well as oral antihistamines. In severe cases, ultraviolet light treatment may help. Where all else fails topical immunomodulators such as tacrolimus and pimecrolimus have been used with some success.

## Self trauma

The outlook in cases of neurotic excoriations or dermatitis artefacta is poor, unless the patient is prepared to accept the need to deal with the underlying psychological illness. Involvement of a psychologist or psychotherapist can be helpful if the patient is willing to take this step. However, is usually necessary to gain a good rapport and the confidence of the patient before embarking on discussions and helping underlying problems.

Topical antibiotics such as fusidic acid, often combined with a topical steroid may help to treat or reduce secondary infection and irritation (Koo and Ting, 2009).

## Parasitophobia

The management of patients with this problem is extremely difficult and the outlook often poor, although occasionally a spontaneous 'cure' may occur. The aim is to involve psychiatric help but this requires the patient to accept that he/she has a psychiatric problem. It may take time to gain the patient's trust and to help him/her to understand that other help and advice is needed. Every step must be taken to exclude infestation or other problem, and this may need also a dermatological even an entomological opinion.

Failure to work in this way with the patient may lead him/her to seek advice elsewhere and be faced with repetition of all the previous tests, thus delaying positive treatment. With specialist supervision antipsychotic drugs may be beneficial, and if the patient is seen to be depressive, antidepressant drugs may be useful.

## Table 22.1. Causes, presentation and management of compulsive itching

| | Cause | Presentation | Management |
|---|---|---|---|
| **Lichen simplex** | More common in women, 30-50 years Repeated rubbing and scratching in response to initial insult, insect bite or habit Often associated atopic tendencies | Well-demarcated scaly Scratch marks in areas accessible to patient Later lichenification, hyperkeratosis and hyperpigmentation | General approach plus: Topical steroids under occlusion Topical immunomodulators Botulinum toxin |
| **Nodular prurigo** | Cause unknown. Often atopic personal or family history Associated with some generalized problems such as liver, renal, thyroid, HIV or anxiety | Most common in middle-aged women Persistent itching. Discrete nodules from few to hundreds. Usually on extensor surfaces: limbs or trunk | General approach plus: Intralesional steroids Topical menthol, phenol or local anaesthetics Ultraviolet light Topical immunomodulators |
| **Self trauma: Neurotic excoriations** | More common in teenage or young women with personality disorders or stress | Constant scratching and picking, patient aware he/she is causing the problem Symmetrically distributed erosions or ulcers in areas within reach. Angulated borders, scars. | General approach plus: Aim to deal with psychological problems but must first gain the confidence of the patient Topical or oral antibiotics if secondary infection |
| **Dermatitis artefacta** | Usually teenagers or young adults Underlying emotional or psychological problems | Bizarre lesions, erosions with geometric shapes Patient unaware that they are damaging themselves | Bizarre lesions, erosions with geometric shapes Patient unaware that they are damaging themselves |
| **Parasitophobia** | Delusional problem of infestation by parasites | Itching, sensations of 'things' crawling under the skin and scratch marks | General approach plus: Encourage psychological help and antipsychotic/ antidepressant drugs. |

*Acknowledgments: The author has received written permission to publish the slides contained here*

## References

Heckmann M, Heyer G, Brunner B, Plewig G (2002) Botulinum toxin type A injection in the treatment of lichen simplex: an open study. *J Am Acad Dermatol* **46**(4): 617–9

Hogan J, Mason S, Bower SM (2009a) Lichen simplex chronicus. http://emedicine.medscape.com/article/1123423-print (accessed 19 February 2010)

Hogan D, Blower S, Mason SM, Mason SH (2009b) Prurigo nodularis. http://emedicine.medscape.com/article/1088032-print (accessed 19 February 2010)

Joint Formulary Committee (2009) *British National Formulary* 58. September. BMA and RPS Publishing, London

Kelekci HK, Uncu HG, Yilmaz B et al (2008) Pimecrolimus 1% cream for pruritus in postmenopausal diabetic women with vulvar lichen simplex chronicus: a prospective non-controlled case series. *J Dermatolog Treat* **19**(5): 274–8

Koo J, Ting P (2009) Dermatitis artefacta: Differential diagnoses and workup. http://emedicine.medscape.com/article/1121933-diagnosis (accessed 19 February 2010)

Ngan V (2009) Delusions of parasitosis. http://dermnetnz.org/arthropods/parasitophobia.html (accessed 19 February 2010)

NHS Choices (2009) Causes of itching. www.nhs.uk/Conditions/Itching/Pages/Causes.aspx (accessed 19 February 2010)

Oakley A (2009) Symptoms of skin disease. www.dermnetnz.org/doctors/principles/symptoms.html (accessed 19 February 2010)

Scheinfeld NS (2010) Neurotic excoriations. http://emedicine.medscape.com/article/1122042-print (accessed 19 February 2010)

# Test Your Knowledge

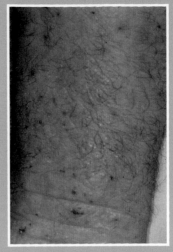

This 69-year-old man had appeared in the surgery on and off over the previous 11 years. What at first appeared to be a mild patch of eczema on his wrist had never settled. Apart from slightly dry skin he had no other dermatological problems. The stresses of his life in the catering trade had gone since his retirement a couple of years before. He had hoped that his changed lifestyle might have eased the problem, but now he sat there, almost in tears, continually scratching away at his right wrist, desperate that 'something must be done'.

He said that nothing he had tried before, such as emollients or topical 1% hycrocortisone cream, had improved the situation.

## Questions

1. What is the likely diagnosis?
2. Would you recommend any investigations?
3. What treatment would you suggest?

# Scabies

Patients often come to the surgery complaining of itching. In many cases there will be an obvious cause. For example, patients with eczema, lichen planus, urticaria or some other disease will usually have something to show for it. The rash may be distinctive or easily described, even if, as in urticaria, it may have gone by the time they attend.

Many other patients who complain of itch may have very little to see when examined. Often the only evidence is scratch marks, a few traumatized spots or a relatively insignificant non-descript rash. The distress is made clear. Often patients will say, 'It is driving me mad.' Sometimes the difficulty is being caused or self-perpetuated by scratching.

Clinicians must do their best to relieve the symptoms of itch and decide whether there is an underlying medical problem or cause that can be treated. Scabies is an example of an extremely itchy skin condition with few specific physical signs, but an acurate diagnosis and treatment is important.

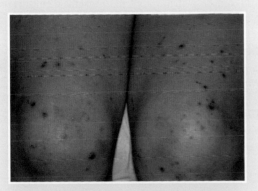

*Figure 23.1. Scabies: excoriated, papular rash.*

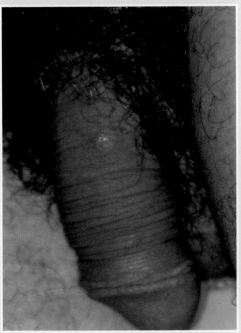

*Figure 23.2. Scabies: itchy nodule on the penis.*

## Scabies
### Aetiology

Scabies is caused by a small mite (*Sarcoptes scabei*) that burrows under the skin (DermNet NZ, 2005). It is transmitted from person to person by prolonged skin contact. Sometimes it is sexually transmitted. It may survive away from its host for a few days and is occasionally passed on in contaminated bedding or clothing.

The male mite dies after mating and the fertilized female burrows into the epidermis and lays her eggs. They hatch a few days later. She dies about a month later.

The affected individual does not react immediately to the mites but develops a sensitivity to them and their faeces. After about 4–6 weeks the patient responds with intense irritation (Binder and Sciammarella, 2005).

### Presenting symptoms

The predominant symptom of scabies is itching. The intensity of the itch gradually increases over a few weeks. The trunk and limbs are usually affected but the face and scalp are rarely involved. The itch tends to be worse at night time. Often there may be other members of the same family or a friend who is similarly affected. This will give a helpful clue to the diagnosis.

### Examination

On examination a generalized rash of papules may be found that are often excoriated by scratching (*Figure 23.1*). In certain areas, such as the axillae, between the fingers, groins or the shaft of the penis, itchy nodules may be seen that are, in an itching patient, very suggestive of scabies (*Figure 23.2*).

In infants, blisters on the sides of the feet, palms and soles are characteristic of scabies (*Figure 23.3*). In some cases the patient has an inflammatory, allergic response to the mite (*Figure 23.4*). Others may have problems of an eczematous reaction and/or secondary infection of the lesions (du Vivier, 2002a).

This child (*Figure 23.5*) had had problems of itching for several years. He had seen the doctor on several occasions and a diagnosis of eczema was made. Finally it was realized that the underlying problem was scabies. Once accurately diagnosed, his symptoms cleared in response to the correct treatment.

Some patients with lowered immunity, mental retardation or sensory loss may present with more severe symptoms of thick, keratotic scaly lesions on the hands and feet. This may be followed by a generalized scaly rash that is often misdiagnosed as eczema but may be Norwegian (or crusted) scabies (so called because it was first described in Norway).

Norwegian scabies may cause particular problems in places such as nursing or rest homes because, as the scales are shed, the mites can easily spread to other residents.

### Diagnosis

The diagnosis depends on the finding of one or more burrows, which take the form of an 'S'-shaped papule about 3–5 mm in length (*Figure 23.6*).

The burrows are best looked for along the sides of the fingers or feet, nipples, buttocks or genitalia. If the roof of the burrow is scraped off, mixed with potassium hydroxide and looked at under the microscope, the scabies mite and/or eggs should be visible, confirming the diagnosis.

### Management

It is extremely important that the treatment of scabies includes the treatment of any other close contacts or contacts with overt symptoms. In closed communities this may cause great problems, because contacts include not only all the inmates but also staff, visitors and their families. All the contacts must be treated at the same time. Failure to be thorough will ensure that the problem recurs.

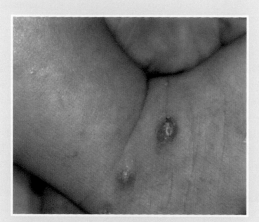

**Figure 23.3. Blisters on the foot of a 3-month-old baby.**

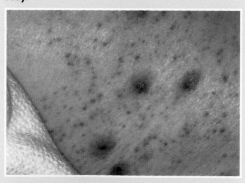

**Figure 23.4. Allergic response to the scabies mite.**

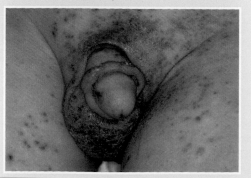

**Figure 23.5. Eczematous response in a child with scabies.**

The treatment choices for scabies are:

* 5% permethrin cream
* Malathion lotion.

The cream or lotion should be applied to the whole body, being careful to include the skin between the fingers and toes. The face and the scalp need not be treated. The treatment should be applied at night and left on for 24 hours before washing or bathing. Bed linen and clothes should also be washed and ironed. It is recommended that this treatment should be repeated a week later (Joint Formulary Committee, 2005: section 13.10.4).

Topical antibiotics, such as fusidic acid cream may be required for problems of localized secondary infection of the lesions. A systemic antibiotic such as flucloxacillin would be necessary for more widespread infection.

The itching eczematous reaction may not settle immediately. Topical calamine lotion, hydrocortisone cream, crotamiton and/or a sedating antihistamine such as promethazine or alimemazine may help to ease the discomfort while awaiting resolution.

If the treatment fails, it may be assumed either that the treatment has not been properly applied, that there are still contacts with the problem, or that the wrong diagnosis has been made.

## Nodular prurigo

*See Chapter 22 on Compulsive itch for information on Nodules prurigo.*

## Delusional parasitophobia

*See Chapter 22 on Compulsive itch for information on Delusional parasitphobia.*

## Other causes of generalized Pruritus

There are a number of other medical conditions that may be associated with generalized Pruritus associated with no obvious reason (*Table 23.1*).

An examination may reveal scratch marks and excoriations but no specific underlying rash. Depending on the findings of the general examination, a number of investigations may be necessary. These may include:

* Full blood count
* Electrolytes and urea

| Table 23.1. Possible causes of generalized Pruritus |
| --- |
| Iron deficiency anaemia |
| Uraemia |
| Obstructive jaundice |
| Hypo- or hyperthyroidism |
| Lymphoma |
| Carcinoma |
| HIV |
| Dry skin |
| Lice |
| Psychological |

## Table 23.2. Differential diagnosis of scabies

| | Scabies | Nodular prurigo | Delusional parasitophobia |
|---|---|---|---|
| Cause | • *Sarcoptes scabei* (mite) | • Unknown | • Delusional state |
| Presentation | • Generalized itching<br>• Burrows<br>• Rash of papules and nodules<br>• Excoriation<br>• Itching partner or friend | • Itching<br>• Thickened skin, nodules<br>• Post-inflammatory hypo- or hyper pigmentation | • Anxious patient<br>• Obsessed by the itch<br>• Brings 'evidence' to the surgery that have negative findings |
| Site | • Trunk, limbs, axillae, genital areas (nodules<br>• Infants: soles, palms, sides of feet | • Localized or generalized within reach of patient's hands | • Generalized |
| Complications | • Secondary infection<br>• Eczema<br>• Norwegian scabies | • Secondary infection | • Secondary infection |
| Investigations | • Skin scraping from burrow roof to make scabies mite and eggs visible | • Exclude scabies<br>• Exclude other causes of Pruritus | • Exclude scabies<br>• Exclude other causes of Pruritus<br>• Histology of patient's 'evidence' |
| Management | • Permethrin 5% cream<br>• Malathion lotion<br>• Treat patient twice, 2 weeks apart<br>• Treat all contacts<br>• Hospital admission for severe cases | • Topical steroid<br>• Steroid containing tape<br>• Sedative antihistamine at night<br>• Occlusive bandages | • Gain trust<br>• Psychotrophic drug |

- Liver function tests
- Autoimmune profile
- Chest X-ray, including a check for lymphadenopathy
- HIV ELISA test.

### Management

Abnormal findings from the investigation should suggest how the condition should be managed. In cases of dry skin the patient should be advised about the application of plenty of emollients or crotamiton 10%. In other cases, symptomatic treatment of Pruritus is the same as in scabies, i.e. topical steroid cream or ointment, and a sedative antihistamine at night, if necessary.

### References

Binder WD, Sciammarella J (2005) Scabies. *eMedicine* 14 November. www.emedicine.com/EMERG/topic517.htm (accessed 20 February 2006)

DermNet NZ (2005a) Scabies. 14 August. www.dermnetnz.org/arthropods/scabies.html (accessed 20 February 2006)

DermNetNZ (2005b) Delusions of parasitosis. 17 December. www.dermnet.org.nz/arthropods/parasitophobia.html (accessed 20 February 2006)

du Vivier A (2002a) Infestations of the skin. In: *Atlas of Clinical Dermatology*. 3rd edn. Churchill Livingstone, London: 331–4

du Vivier A (2002b) Psychological disorders of the skin. In: *Atlas of Clinical Dermatology*. 3rd edn. Churchill Livingstone, London: 668

Mason S, Hogan D (2003) Prurigo nodularis. *eMedicine* 29 October. www.emedicine.com/DERM/topic350.htm (accessed 20 Feb)

### Conclusions

Scabies is an extremely itchy and irritating skin condition that can be treated but it has few physical signs. An acurate diagnosis is important to distinguish it from other itchy presentations (*Table 23.2*) so that it can be treated effectively.

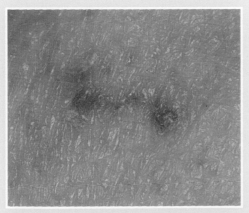

*Figure 23.6. Burrow of the scabies mite, Sarcoptes scabei*

# Test Your Knowledge

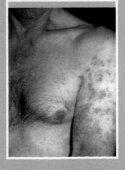

This man had been itching for months. He tried soothing his itch with calamine lotion and later moved on to some betamethasone cream that his wife had used when she had eczema, but nothing seemed to help. When his granddaughter started to itch she went to the GP who diagnosed scabies. He had visited her a few weeks before he started to itch. She had responded well to her treatment. He therefore sought help and was prescribed permethrin which he applied to the itchy areas on one occasion. However, the condition got worse and on a second visit the GP decided that the problem must be one of eczema and treated him accordingly. However, there was still no improvement and the patient was back to see his doctor yet again.

### Questions

1. What is the likely diagnosis?
2. How would you confirm the diagnosis?
3. What treatment would you advise and why do you think that the patient had not responded to the previous advice?

# Infestations

Skin irritation is a common complaint in those afflicted by a variety of skin infestations and insect bites. Contact with fleas, bed bugs, lice, ticks (which can transmit Lyme disease), flies, wasps or bees is an everyday occurrence. Close contacts of people who have scabies may find that the mite has been transmitted to them when some weeks later they are troubled by an itchy rash.

Travel abroad may expose people to a variety of other parasites. For example, the beautiful sandy beaches of the Caribbean, and Central and South America are home to the hookworm larva and the troublesome larva migrans (Watkins, 2008).

In this chapter some of the other common infestations in the UK will be discussed.

## Fleas

There are a number of different species of flea (*Siphonaptera*). The adult lives by feeding from the blood of its host, whether it be animal or human. The most common variety in the UK is *Ctenocephalides* (cat and dog fleas) and *Pulex irritans* (human flea) (Buxton, 1947).

### Life cycle

The life cycle of the flea is about 3–4 weeks depending on the temperature and availability of food. The adult flea feeds on the blood of its host by piercing the flesh and sucking the blood. The female lays eggs in areas that are frequented by the host such as bedding, carpets or chairs. About 2 weeks later, the eggs hatch into small, worm-like larvae (*Figure 24.1*), which feed on organic matter in their surrounds. They pupate in the form of a cocoon from which the adult flea hatches. The adult then has the ability to leap considerable distances in its search for a host (Bohart Museum of Entomology, 2005).

### Presentation of bites

The patient develops clusters of irritating, inflammatory papules (*Figure 24.2*), which may become infected if the patient cannot resist the urge to scratch (*Figure 24.3*). Examination reveals a dark red spot with reddened surround. These often occur in the skin folds of the waist or the flexures, such as the axillae or behind the knees. Some patients will develop an urticarial allergic reaction to the bites (*Figure 24.4*).

One variety of flea, xenopsylla, that is carried by rats, may transmit the plague while other species transmit typhus, although in the UK such transmission has not occurred for many years (Bohart Museum of Entomology, 2005).

### Management

Patients should be advised to avoid scratching the bites and use an antiseptic soap or cream to discourage secondary infection. Topical hydrocortisone cream 1% or calamine lotion should ease the itch. Secondary infection may require the use of an antibiotic.

Other treatment is aimed at killing the adult fleas and destruction, as far as possible, of the eggs, larvae and pupae

that will live in the home in bedding, for example. Carpets must be vacuumed and the hoover bag thrown away, having first sprayed the whole house and all soft furnishings with an insecticide. The environment should be sprayed with an insect growth regulator such as pyriproxyfen or methoprene to kill the eggs and pupae that are resistant to insecticides. Any animals or birds should first be moved out as these substances are toxic to them. Old contaminated chairs are best discarded (Lydon Veterinary Centre, 2009). A pet should also be treated for tapeworm as this may have been transmitted to them via the fleas.

### Adulticides

Veterinary advice will be helpful in the use of adulticides. The insecticide, which quickly kills fleas, can be put on the neck and will then spread over the rest of the animal. This will need to be repeated on a monthly basis. Alternatively, there is an oral preparation for animals, nitenpyram, which will quickly kill adult fleas (Dobson et al, 2000).

Insect growth regulators such as nitenpyram are effective in preventing the eggs of fleas from hatching, thus reducing the need to repeatedly 'spring clean' the house. It can be fed to pets monthly. The flea ingests the substance as it feeds

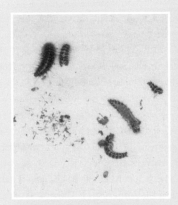

**Figure 24.1. Flea larvae found in the carpet of a patient with flea bites.**

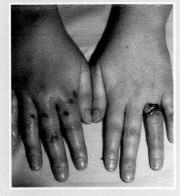

**Figure 24.3. Infected flea bites on the hands.**

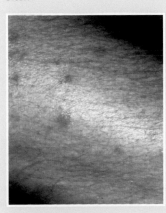

**Figure 24.2. Flea bites: inflammatory papules.**

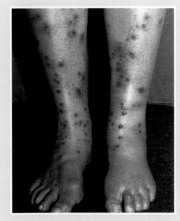

**Figure 24.4. Papular urticarial reaction to insect bites.**

## Table 24.1. Differentiating fleas and bed bugs

|  | Fleas | Bed bugs |
|---|---|---|
| Life cycle | Eggs hatch in 2 weeks<br>Larval 'worms'<br>Pupa<br>Adult<br>Life span up to 18 months (without food, few days only) | Eggs hatch in 10–20 days<br>Young adults moult 5 times to reach maturity<br>Life span >1 year |
| Host | Animal and human<br>Feed on blood of host | Human<br>Feed on blood of host |
| Appearance | Flattened wingless insects<br>Jump considerable distances | Small rust-coloured insects, flattened oval body<br>Reduced wings, 6–9.5 mm in size |
| Symptoms | Itching, inflammatory papules<br>Urticarial reactions | Bites appear as firm, white swellings |
| Complications | Secondary infection<br>Transmission of tapeworm | None |
| Management | *Bites:* Antiseptic soap, hydrocortisone 1% cream or calamine lotion<br>Antibiotics if infection<br>Vacuum carpets, launder bedding, furnishings<br>*Insects:* Insecticidal spray, adulticides to kill fleas<br>Insect growth regulators to stop eggs hatching | Insecticidal sprays<br>Thorough cleaning of home, bedding and clothing<br>Pest control help |

from its host and the nitenpyram prevents the eggs from hatching (Dobson et al, 2000).

If further advice is required or the fleas remain a persistent problem, direction to the local centre of the UK Pest Control Directory can be obtained on the internet (www.pestcontrol-uk.org).

## Bed bugs

Bed bugs (family *Cimicidae*) occur throughout the world. Their life is spent in dark places such as cracks, crevices and settees, near possible hosts. Their choice of residence is often in the vicinity of beds or chairs, leaving them only to feed at night on the blood of a human or animal host.

### Life cycle

Bed bugs are small, flattened, oval, rust-coloured insects with reduced wings, usually 6–9.5 mm in size (Brooks, 2006). The female, once mature, lays as many as two or three eggs a day. These hatch about 10–20 days later as small replicas of the adult (*Table 24.1*). They must undergo five moults, each after a further feed, to mature.

### Presentation of bites

The appearance of a bed bug bite differs from that of the flea in that it leaves a firm, white swelling. Fortunately, it does not transmit other disease.

Sometimes evidence of bed bugs' presence may be found in the blood spots left on sheets or, in cases of heavy infestation, an almond-like smell in the room.

### Management

Advice from the pest control unit may help in the choice of a pest control company to treat the home with an insecticidal spray. Cleanliness is important if bed bugs are to be avoided. Therefore carpets and soft furnishings should be vacuumed, all bed linen and clothing laundered, and cupboards, drawers and beds washed thoroughly in hot water.

The occupants, both human and animal, should be moved out for some hours until the job is done and surfaces are dry. An insecticidal spray may be sufficient to deal with any newly-hatched youngsters (Oldham Metropolitan Borough, 2008).

## Lice

Lice (family *Phthiraptera*) are small insects without wings that feed on human blood and attack humans only. Different species of lice affect different areas of the body:

- *Pediculus humanus capitis*, the head louse
- *Pediculus humanus humanus*, the body louse
- *Phthirus punis*, the pubic louse.

Transmission is by close contact with people affected by the infestation.

### Life cycle

Lice require a daily feed to survive and lay their eggs. Head lice hatch in 7–10 days, body lice in 5–7 days and pubic lice in 13–17 days. The hatched nymphs are the same as 'miniature adults' but must moult three times before reaching maturity, a process that may take up to 3 weeks. Life will then continue for a further month, during which time numerous eggs are laid (New York City Department of Health and Mental Hygiene, 2010).

### Presentation of infestation
#### Head lice

Patients complain of an itchy scalp. The diagnosis is confirmed by the discovery of small (2–3 mm) insects on the scalp (*Figure 24.5*), frequently behind the ears and nape of the neck.

Fleas will also be suspected if whitish eggs (nits) are seen clinging to the hairs. These may resemble dandruff, but cannot be flicked off.

Once the nymph has hatched, the empty shells may remain attached to the hairs for a long time (*Figure 24.6*). Repeated scratching may lead to sore areas on the scalp. Head lice cling on to fine hair only and therefore do not

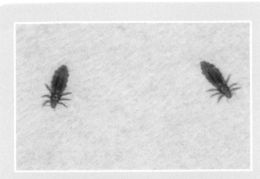

*Figure 24.5. Head lice.*

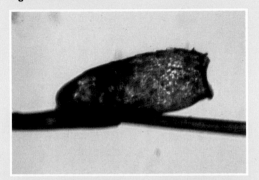

*Figure 24.6. Empty egg shell case of head lice.*

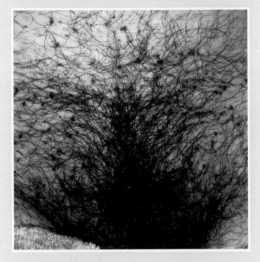

*Figure 24.7. Pubic lice.*

affect coarser hair elsewhere on the body. They are spread by close contact or the sharing of combs, brushes or hats.

## Body lice

The body louse is most at home in the seams and folds of unwashed dirty clothing. Fortunately they are uncommon in the UK and developed countries. The areas most commonly affected by the body louse are those areas covered by clothing.

Itching is not a particular feature in the early stages. Later, more severe itching may occur, resulting in visible marks from scratching, eczematous change, discolouration of the skin and allergic reactions in the form of urticaria (*Table 24.2*).

Although body lice may be just a nuisance in causing itching, they do occasionally carry other diseases, such as typhus, trench fever or epidemic relapsing fever, which can be transmitted to their host (Raoult and Roux, 1999).

## Pubic lice

Pubic lice (crabs) usually frequent the pubic or perianal areas of the body, but may also sometimes be found on facial hair such as moustaches or eyebrows. Adult lice are up to 2 mm in length but broader across, having a crab-like appearance. They may infect both humans and dogs.

The main symptoms are itching and small red spots that follow the bites. Once settled, the lice remain fairly static causing the hair to matt as faeces accumulate (*Figure 24.7*).

Public lice are not responsible for the transmission of any other disease but the close sexual contact that facilitates transmission means that there may be a risk of other sexually transmitted infections (STIs) in sexual partners.

## Management of head lice
### Wet combing

Wet combing of the hair involves thoroughly combing the wet hair and whole scalp with a fine-toothed plastic comb to remove the lice. This should take at least 30 minutes and should be repeated again every 4 days for at least 4 weeks. This method is time consuming and not always effective.

### Parasiticidal preparations

Parasiticidal preparations of malathion or pyrethroid may be effective if applied to the hair and scalp for at least 12 hours before washing off. This should be repeated again after 7 days. Problems have arisen because of the development of resistance of the lice to the treatment. If one preparation fails to work, a different one should be tried.

### Dimethicone

Dimethicone is a silicone oil, which is rubbed into the hair and scalp and left on for 8 hours. It coats the lice, thus suffocating and killing them. It has no effect on the nits so the treatment must be repeated after 7–10 days to catch them when they have hatched (Burgess et al, 2005).

## Management of body lice

All close members of the family and sexual partners should be treated. Sexual contacts should also be checked for other STIs.

Washing clothes in hot water and tumble drying or dry cleaning kill lice and eggs effectively. Lice require regular feeding, so that if clothing is not worn for some days, the lice will die.

The whole body should be treated with parasiticidal preparations such as malathion, phenothrin or permethrin. Treatment should be repeated after 7 days. If the response is poor, a different insecticide should be tried. Parasiticidals should not be used near the eyes.

An effort should be made to remove body lice from the hair. Forceps are useful for this. Coating the area with Vaseline or dimethicone can also be useful, particularly for the eyebrows, where parasiticidal preparations may cause problems if they get into the eyes.

Oral antihistamines may be prescribed to ease the itching, and to help prevent secondary damage to the skin from scratching.

## Table 24.2. Dermatolgy diffenretal diagnosis

| | Head lice | Body lice | Pubic lice |
|---|---|---|---|
| **Life cycle** | Eggs hatch in 5–7 days<br>Nymphs - 3 moults<br>Adult life span 30 days | Eggs hatch in 5–7 days<br>Nymphs: 16–18 days<br>(3 moults)<br>Adult life span 40 days | Eggs hatch in 7–8 days<br>Nymphs moult over<br>13–17 days<br>Adult life span 1 month |
| **Host** | Human only<br>Feed on blood of host | Human<br>Prefer dirty clothing in contact with the body<br>Feed on blood of host | Human, occasionally dogs<br>Feed on blood of host |
| **Appearance** | Small wingless insects 2–3 mm | Larger than head lice, longer body and antennae | Crab-like up to 2 mm long and wide |
| **Symptoms** | Itching scalp, sores<br>May find live lice and yellow/white eggs (nits) stuck to hairs | Itching, scratch marks, eczema, discoloured skin, urticarial rash in covered areas | Itchy, small red spots in pubic area or coarse-haired areas<br>In time, hair matts |
| **Complications** | Secondary infection | Secondary infection<br>Typhus, trench fever, epidemic relapsing fever | Secondary infection<br>Often sexual transmission to partner |
| **Management** | Wet combing<br>Parasiticides<br>Dimethicone | Treat all family and sexual contacts if affected<br>Oral antihistamines<br>Launder clothes in hot water<br>Destroy clothing and bedding if possible<br>Parasiticidal preparations<br>Dimethicone or Vaseline<br>Remove lice with forceps<br>Check patient and sexual contacts for STIs | Shave hair<br>Treat sexual partner(s)<br>Pediculicide and repeat after 7 days<br>Dimethicone or Vaseline<br>Launder clothing and bedding<br>Check patient and sexual contacts for STIs |

## Management of pubic lice

Once the diagnosis has been confirmed by the finding of a nymph or adult and/or the eggs stuck to the hair, all the hair from the affected region should be shaved.

A pediculicide such as permethrin, pyrethrin or malathion is used to kill the lice with close adherence to the instructions on the packet. The application should be washed off after 12 hours and the treatment repeated 7 days later when more eggs may have hatched (Joint Formulary Committee, 2010: 13.10.4).

## Conclusions

It is not uncommon for most of these infestations to be seen in general practice. Patients will request help and advice about how to handle the problem both for themselves and their families. There are times when a pest control advice service may need, but often, with guidance, patients can deal with an infestation themselves with preparations that are available over the counter. It is important for the practice nurse to be able to confirm a diagnosis and offer the necessary guidance.

## References

Brooks SE (2006) Bed bug. http://entnemdept.ifas.ufl.edu/creatures/urban/bed_bug.htm (accessed 28 April 2010)

Bohart Museum of Entomology (2005) Human skin parasites and delusional parasitosis. http://delusion.ucdavis.edu/delusional.html (accessed 25 April 2010)

Burgess IF, Brown CM, Lee PN (2005) Treatment of head louse infestation with 4% dimeticone lotion: randomised controlled equivalence trial. *BMJ* **330**(7505): 1423

Buxton PA (1947) *The Louse: An Account of the Lice which Infest Man, their Medical Importance and Control.* 2nd edn. Edward-Arnold, London

Dobson P, Tinembart O, Fisch R, Junquera P (2000) Efficacy of nitenpyram as a systemic flea adulticide in dogs and cats. *Vet Rec* **147**(25): 709–13

Joint Formulary Committee (2010) *British National Formulary* 59. March. BMJ Group and RPS Publishing, London

Lydon Veterinary Centre (2009) Which flea treatment? www.lydonveterinarycentre.co.uk/pet-care-flea-treatment.php (accessed 25 April 2010)

New York City Department of Health and Mental Hygiene (2010) Lice (pediculosis). www.nyc.gov/html/doh/html/cd/cdped.shtml (accessed 25 April 2010)

Oldham Metropolitan Borough (2008) Bed bugs: Facts online. August. www.oldham.gov.uk/ocfs-env-epeh47s.pdf (accessed 25 April 2010)

Raoult D, Roux V (1999) The body louse as a vector of reemerging human diseases. *Clin Infect Dis* **29**(4): 888–911

Watkins J (2008) Larva migrans. *Practice Nursing* **19**(8): 394

## Test Your Knowledge

This 30-year-old woman had been away for the weekend to Brighton with her husband. They had stayed in bed and breakfast accomodation where an added pleasure had been to make friends with the owner's three dogs. However, within a few hours of their return they had both noticed a problem of clusters of itchy red spots appearing on the face, neck and limbs. The problem had continued and some of the spots were papular and urticated in nature.

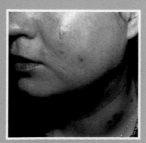

### Questions
1. What is the likely diagnosis?
2. How would you treat the patient?
3. Is there any further action you feel you should take?

# Genital

There are a number of skin conditions that may cause itching in the genital area. Among these are psoriasis, lichen planus, lichen sclerosis et atrophicus, eczema, dermatitis and scabies. Often, but not always, there will be other signs of the skin condition elsewhere on the patient's body which will give a clue to the cause of itching in the genital area.

As in all cases, a full history—not only of the initial complaint, but also of any other skin conditions or allergies from which the patient or his/her family has suffered, as well as a full examination—are crucial to reaching the correct diagnosis. In this chapter some of these problems will be discussed and their recognition and management examined.

## Folliculitis

Folliculitis in the pubic region commonly follows trauma, such as may occur if the area is shaved or scratched. Scratching may be due to some underlying problem. This trauma may damage the hair follicles and leave them liable to infection. This patient (*Figure 25.1*) had been scratching for some weeks and developed a troublesome folliculitis, with small inflamed spots around the hair follicles.

### Management

She was prescribed a course of flucloxacilln and advised to use a povidone-iodine antiseptic solution when bathing, together with mupirocin nasal ointment twice daily in case of nasal carriage of *Staphylococcus aureus*. In fact, she was living in a house with a number of cats affected by fleas. As it was suspected that the initial cause of the itch was flea bites, it was recommended that she contact her vet to ask advice about insecticidal sprays or powders to treat the animals, and also the home. She was reminded that the whole house would need to be treated including soft furnishings, carpets and gaps between floorboards, having thoroughly vacuumed the place first.

Where shaving causes the problem, and the patient intends to continue with this practice, she should be advised how to minimise the risk of problems in the future, by first clipping the hair with sharp scissors, then to always use a new safety razor, female shaving cream and shave in the direction of hair growth.

## Scabies

*See Chapter 23 for information on Scabies.*

## Psoriasis

Psoriasis is a common condition that may affect any part of the body and is sometimes itchy. Certain factors increase the chances of developing psoriasis, namely genetic, trauma, smoking, alcohol, stress and it may be induced by certain drugs (Lui and Mamelak, 2009). When it occurs in the genital area and other flexural areas, it takes on a different appearance, (National Psoriasis Foundation, 2010) The lesions tend to be smooth, red and dry and lacking the silvery scale seen on the body. (*Figure 25.2*). This picture demonstrates the rash normally seen in this area, and in this case, there are silvery plaques extending on to the buttocks. Similar plaques on the elbows and knees, if present, and/or nail changes such as pitting, onycholysis and/or salmon patch (*Figure 25.3*), a personal and/or family history of psoriasis can help confirm the likelihood of the problem. Secondary infection with *Candida* in the perineum is common (Watkins, 2010a).

### Management

Treatment in the genital region must be moderated, owing to sensitivity of the skin in this area. A weak topical steroid will usually help to control symptoms but a more potent preparation may be required, if the response is not satisfactory, but for a few days only. As the skin is this area is 'thin', stronger preparations should be used with care and steroid creams discontinued, once the psoriasis has cleared.

Alternative treatments include calcipotriol or the topical calcineurin inhibitors that do not thin the skin. Should candida have compounded the problem, it must be treated with an anti-fungal agent, such as clotrimazole.cream (Dermnet NZ, 2010).

## Genital lichen sclerosis et atrophicus

Lichen sclerosis et atrophicus is a chronic inflammatory dermatosis that may affect not only the genital area but also other areas of the body. The cause is unknown but it is frequently associated with autoimmune disorders, particularly thyroid disease. (Dalziel and Shaw, 2010). It may present at any age and is not uncommon in children. It may be symptomless but often causes problems with severe vulval itching and soreness. Excoriations are

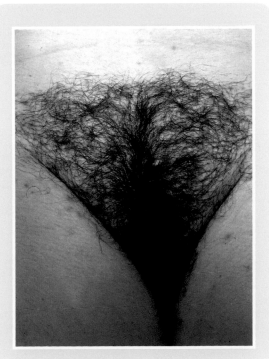

***Figure 25.1. Folliculitis in a patient with fleas.***

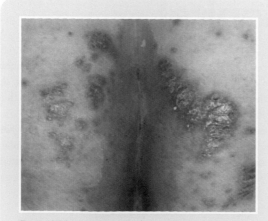

**Figure 25.2. Psoriasis in the natal cleft.**

common. When occurring in the genital area in women, it usually affects the vulva and in time may lead to obliteration of the labia minora and stenosis of the introitus (*Figure 25.4*) thus causing serious problems in passing urine and dyspareunia. On examination, the skin is smooth with white plaques and at times blisters, which may be haemorrhagic (*Figure 25.5*). This could lead to suspicion

of sexual abuse, particularly if this is seen in a child. Secondary infection of the lesions is always a possibility and also, there is said to be a 5% lifetime risk of patients with lichen sclerosis et atrophicus developing a vulval squamous cell carcinoma. On the whole, the prognosis is good in children, in whom lichen sclerosis et atrophicus may resolve spontaneously, but for some adults, it may continue as a chronic problem. (Meffert, 2009).

### Management

If necessary a punch biopsy of the skin lesion will confirm the diagnosis, and careful watch should be kept for any lesion causing concern of malignancy. Any persistent or suspicious ulcer or lump should be biopsied to exclude this problem. Also, because of the frequency of thyroid disease in patients with lichen sclerosis et atrophicus, thyroid function should be checked, The first approach to the treatment of lichen sclerosis et atrophicus is topical steroids which should ease symptoms and sometimes help it to resolve. Initially a more potent steroid such as clobetasol propionate is recommended. Once things are under control, a weaker topical steroid or emollient should be used. If there is concern about continued use of a potent topical steroid, a topical calcineurin inhibitor could be substituted, although there are still questions about

## Table 25.1. Differential diagnosis

| | Cause | Presentation | Management |
|---|---|---|---|
| **Folliculitis** | Infection of hair follicles<br>May follow scratching of shaving | Small, inflamed spots around hair follicles | Povidone-iodine antiseptic solution in bath<br>Antibiotic such as flucloxacillin<br>Advice about underlying cause<br>Intranasal mupirocin if concern about nasal carriage of infection |
| **Scabies** | *Sarcoptes scabei* (mite)<br>Skin-to-skin contact or from infected bedding or clothing | Itching<br>Burrows<br>Erythematous papules and vesicles<br>Microscopy scraping from burrow | Treat patient and all contacts<br>Keep away from school until first treatment completed<br>Wash bedding and clothes at 50°C (minimum)<br>Apply permethrin to whole body and wash after 8–10 hours<br>Malathion if cannot tolerate permethrin<br>Ivermectrin on named-patient basis only |
| **Psoriasis** | Genetic links and environmental factors<br>Inflammatory skin condition with hyperproliferation of cells in the epidermis | Smooth, red, dry rash in perineal area, may itch<br>Plaques elsewhere on the body or nail changes help to suggest the diagnosis | Topical steroids: a more potent steroid may be required for a few days but return to weak preparation as soon as possible<br>Emollients<br>Calcipotriol<br>Topical calcineurin inhibitors<br>If added *Candida*: antifungal cream |
| **Lichen sclerosis et atrophicus** | Cause unknown but often associated with autoimmune disease | May be symptomless<br>Vulval itching, excoriations, obliteration of labia minora, stenosis introitus, dyspareunia, dysuria<br>Smooth white plaques or blisters, may be haemorrhagic<br>Risk of secondary infection and malignant change | Skin biopsy if diagnosis in doubt or concern about malignancy<br>Topical steroids: initially potent, then weak<br>Sedating antihistamine at night<br>Intralesional steroids, ultraviolet light<br>Antidepressants or sedatives |
| **Dermatitis** | Irritant or allergic reaction | Inflamed, itchy rash<br>Blisters or scaling | Avoid cause<br>Emollients<br>Topical steroids<br>Topical calcineurin inhibitor<br>Patch testing for allergies |
| **Lichen simplex** | Repeated scratching | Itching<br>Thickened skin or excoriations | Skin biopsy if diagnosis in doubt<br>Emollients<br>Topical steroids: initially potent, then weak<br>Sedating antihistamine at night<br>Intralesional steroids, ultraviolet light<br>Antidepressants or sedatives |

the safety of them for long term use or in young children. Occasionally, in difficult cases, isotretinoin or acitretin have been tried and reported to be beneficial (Meffert, 2009). There may be times when the health professional feels that referral to a specialist in vulval problems should be made either for confirmation of the diagnosis or advice regarding treatment. While awaiting the appointment, emollients and mild topical steroid may help in the meantime.

## Dermatitis

The patient presents with a well demarcated, inflamed itchy rash in which there may be blisters and/or scaling.

Irritant dermatitis is caused by contact with irritants substances such as detergents, water, urine, faeces or friction. A common manifestation of this is nappy rash in babies (*Figure 25.6*).

Allergic dermatitis is due to contact with a substance to which the patient may be allergic such as perfumes, soaps, washing powders or detergents or rubber latex that may be in condoms or rubber gloves. This may be by direct contact or it could be transferred by the fingers, if the patient has been handling something to which she is allergic. The rash is similar to that caused by an irritant substance. Initially it is limited to the area of contact, but in severe cases, may extend to other areas.

### Management

As the rash is similar in both irritant and allergic dermatitis, it may be difficult to advise unless allergy testing is performed. However, although this may provide some indication, irritant dermatitis may coexist with an allergy. In either case, the patient must be advised to avoid any possible causative factors. A good history and careful observation should help indicate the most helpful advice. For example, a young baby lying constantly in a wet, dirty nappy would obviously require more frequent changing and as much time as possible without a nappy on, if the condition is going to clear.

As regards actual care, emollient creams and topical steroids are the mainstay of treatment. Antibiotics such as flucloxacillin or erythromycin may be required, if secondary infection occurs or an antifungal agent such as clotrimazole, if the common problem of *Candida* is involved (DermNet NZ, 2010).

## Lichen simplex

The problem of lichen simplex was addressed by Watkins (2010a). The itch-scratch cycle in which the patient repeatedly scratches and area of skin, leads to gradual thickening of the skin which is often excoriated, in the same way as this may occur at other sites of the body.

### Management

The obvious advice to a patient with that problem is to stop scratching Unfortunately this advice is not as easy to follow as it sounds. It may be helpful to apply plenty of emollients. Topical steroids do ease the itching. Initially, potent preparations may be necessary, in order to get the itch under control. A sedating antihistamine may be helpful to reduce the risk of a patient scratching at night. Skin biopsy may be helpful if there is any doubt about the diagnosis.

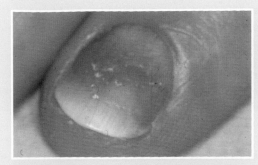

*Figure 25.3. Psoriatic nail: pitting, salmon patch and onycholysis.*

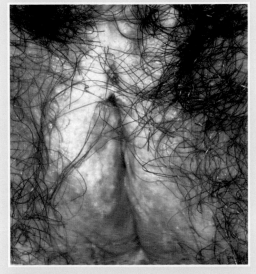

*Figure 25.4. Lichen sclerosus et atrophicus with problems of the stenosis of the introitus.*

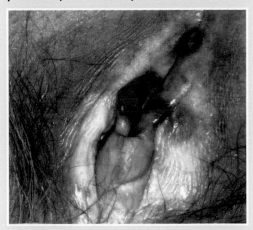

*Figure 25.5. Lichen sclerosus et atrophicus vulva.*

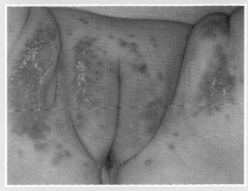

*Figure 25.6. Irritant nappy rash.*

Occasionally, in persistent cases, intra-lesional steroids or ultraviolet light may be effective, and for those with depression or problems of stress, a sedative, anti-depressant and/or counselling may be beneficial (Skinsight, 2006).

## Conclusions

There are a number of different skin conditions that may cause the patient to complain of itching in the genital region. A correct diagnosis is necessary in order to be able to give the patient the appropriate treatment and advice. This diagnosis will not be reached unless a good history is taken and thorough examination made. Only then can the patient hope to be able to gain relief from this distressing and embarrassing problem.

## Test Your Knowledge

This 66 year old woman had been aware if itching around the anus for some time. Eventually she had managed to take a look at the area and she was worried because she noticed that the skin there was white. Her general health was good and she had never previously suffered with any skin problems. On examination the peri-anal whiteness was clear but there were also some skin changes and excoriations affecting the vulva.

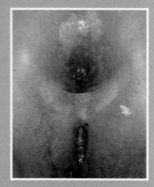

### Questions

1. What is the likely diagnosis?
2. How could you confirm the diagnosis and what problems could be associated with the condition, now or in the future?
3. How would you advise this patient?

## References

Dermnet NZ (2009) Flexural Psoriasis http://dermnetnz.org/scaly/flexural-psoriasis.html (accessed 1 June 2010)

DermNet NZ (2010) Allergic contact dermatitis http://dermnetnz.org/dermatitis/contact-allergy.html (accessed 1 June 2010)

DermNet NZ (2010) Irritant contact dermatitis. http://dermnetnz.org/dermatitis/contact-irritant.html (accessed 1 June 2010)

Dermnet NZ (2010) Scabies http://dermnet.org.nz/arthropods/scabies.html (accessed 1 June 2010)

Feline Advisiory Bureau (2008) Tackling fleas on cats. www.fabcats.org/owners/fleas/info.html (accessed 1 June 2010)

Joint Formulary Committee (2010) *British National Formulary* 59. March. BMJ Group and RPS Publishing, London

Lui H, Mamelak AJ (2009) Plaque psoriasis. http://emedicine.medscape.com/article/1108072-overview (accessed 18 June 2010)

Meffert J (2009) Lichen sclerosis et atrophicus. http://emedicine.medscape.com/article/1123316-overview (accessed 18 June 2010)

National Psoriasis Foundation (2010) Specific locations: genitals www.psoriasis.org/netcommunity/sublearn03_loc_genitals (accessed 1 June 2010)

Palo Alto Medical Foundation (2009) Pubic hair removal. www.pamf.org/teen/health/skin/pubichairremoval.html (accessed 1 June 2010)

Patient UK (2007) Scabies. http://www.patient.co.uk/health/Scabies.htm (accessed 1 June 2010)

Skinsight (2006) Lichen simplex chronicus. www.skinsight.com/adult/lichenSimplexChronicus.htm (accessed 1 June 2010)

Watkins J (2010a) Pruritus, part 3: Compulsive itch. *Practice Nursing* **21**(3): 132–38

Watkins J (2010b) Pruritus, part 4: Infestations. *Practice Nursing* **21**(5): 247–52

# Tinea corporis

Tinea corporis may present frequently in the surgery. While it may seem easy to diagnose, other conditions such as granuloma annulare, the herald spot in pityriasis rosea, and discoid eczema may easily be confused with it. It is important to make a correct diagnosis because management of these conditions is different *(Table 26.1)*. Failure to recognize and treat tinea corporis not only allows the condition to spread, but also increases the risk that the patient will pass it on to others (Wandsworth, 2002).

## Tinea corporis

### Aetiology

Tinea corporis is a superficial dermatophyte infection of the skin. The species of fungus most commonly associated with this infection are *Trichophyton rubrum*, *T.mentagrophytes*, *Microsporum canis* and *Epidermophyton floccosum*. The infection may be acquired from other infected humans, farm animals, household pets or the fomites with which they have been in contact (Lesher and Zember, 2004).

Close skin contact with lesions can spread infection, but the fungus can also survive on furniture and clothes and be acquired from these or from contaminated clippers, brushes and combs (Wandsworth, 2002). Tinea corporis occurs at any age but is more common in children.

### Presentation

The patient presents with an itchy, annular rash with a well defined margin. The lesion may be inflamed and raised. It grows rapidly, developing scales, crusts and papules *(Figures 26.1–26.2)*. As it grows in size there is resolution at the centre *(Figure 26.3)*. The lesions may be single or multiple and affect any part of the body *(Figure 26.4)*. In

## Table 26.1. Differential diagnosis

| | Tinea corporis | Granuloma annulare | Pityriasis rosea herald spot | Discoid eczema |
|---|---|---|---|---|
| **Cause** | Fungal infection:<br>• Trichophyton rubrum<br>• T. mentagrophytes,<br>• Microsporum canis | • Unknown<br><br>• Sometime associated with diabetes mellitus | Unknown | Unknown |
| **Age** | More common in children | More common in females children and young adults | Children and young adults | • Men aged 50–70 years<br><br>• Young atopics |
| **Presentation** | Annular rash, well defined margin, itchy, increases in size with central resolution | • Localized: well defined, annular red plaque. Border of flat topped papules<br><br>• Perforating: papules with central umbilication<br><br>• Generalized: multiple annular pink/brown or skin-coloured macules and papules | Single oval or round patch 1–2 cm diameter.<br>Salmon coloured, central wrinkling with darker edge and collarette of scale | • Single or multiple, itchy papules/vesicles leading to crusting<br><br>• Becomes dry and scale<br><br>• Secondary infection is common |
| **Site** | Any part of the body | • Localized: backs of hands, feet, ankles and limbs<br><br>• Perforating: hands and fingers<br><br>• Generalized: trunk and limbs | • Usually on the trunk<br><br>• Occasionally neck or extremities | • Most common on lower limbs and dorsum of hands<br><br>• Arms and trunk less often |
| **Investigations** | Skin scrapings for micoscopy/culture | • Skin scrapings – negative<br><br>• Biopsy if necessary<br><br>• Check urine/blood for glucose | • Skin scrapings negative<br><br>• Very occasionally biopsy<br><br>• Diagnosis clear when further rash develops | • Skin scrapings – negative<br><br>• Swab to check for secondary infection |
| **Management** | • Topical antifungals: imidazole, terbinafine cream, benzoic acid ointment<br><br>• Oral terbinafine<br><br>• Isolate until treatment working | Usually spontaneous resolution<br><br>If treatment necessary:<br>• Localized: intralesional steroids. Potent topical steroids<br><br>• Generalized: systemic steroids methotrexate, isotretinoin, PUVA | • No treatment normally required<br><br>• Topical calamine lotion<br><br>• Occasionally topical or oral steroids | • Topical emollients<br><br>• Oral antihistamines<br><br>• Potent topical steroids with antibiotic<br><br>• Occasioanally systemic steroids and/or antibiotic |

Key: PUVA = psoralen plus ultraviolet light therapy

some patients the rash may simulate an allergic reaction, e.g. to a watch strap, or an inflamed lesion may be confused with impetigo or herpes simplex.

The source of the fungal infection may stem from other tinea-infected areas, such as the clefts between the toes (Athlete's foot) *(Figure 26.5)* or the groin (tinea cruris *(Figure 26.6)*. Changes in these areas help confirm suspicions about the diagnosis and indicate a need for treatment.

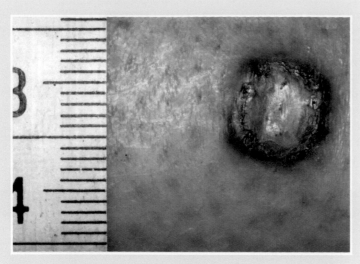

**Figure 26.1. Tinea corporis: raised, inflamed border with papules and crusting.**

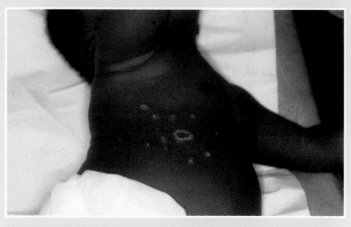

**Figure 26.2. Spreading tinea coporis in a baby: dry, scaly border.**

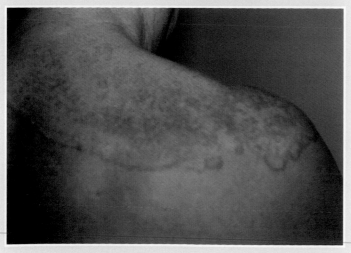

**Figure 26.3. Tinea corporis of the shoulder showing central clearing.**

In cases of ***tinea incognito*** the appearance of the rash is different: the margin of the lesion is less obvious, and the lesion more extensive, less scaly, and more pustular and itchy *(Figure 26.7)*.

Tinea incognito is usually the result of inappropriate treatment. It is not uncommon for a fungal rash to be incorrectly treated with a topical steroid cream. This may occur because either the patient has tried this approach before seeing a health professional, or a health professional has misdiagnosed the problem and issued the wrong prescription. Investigation and treatment of tinea incognito is the same as for tinea corporis (DermNet NZ, 2004b).

### Infectivity

The incubation period for tinea is 10–14 days. Close skin contact with another person could spread the disease. It is therefore recommended that the patient is isolated until treatment has begun and is seen to be working. There is no need to isolate contacts unless they are showing signs of the disease (Stockport Health Authority, 1999).

### Investigations

To investigate the lesion, skin scrapings should be taken from the active border of the lesion. To confirm a diagnosis of tinea the skin scrapings should be mixed with potassium hydroxide. When looked at under the microscope the scrapings should demonstrate branching hyphae if tinea is present (Lesher and Zember, 2004). Skin scrapings can also be sent to the laboratory for culture, which again should confirm the diagnosis. However, the result may take some time to come through.

### Management

The cure rate for tinea is 70–100% with topical or systemic treatment, but reinfection is always possible if a reservoir such as a nail infection or tinea pedis or cruris remain (Lesher and Zember, 2004). In cases of tinea incognito, any topical steroid should be discontinued.

### Topical treatment

Effective topical treatment for localized lesions includes imidazole creams, e.g. econazole, ketoconazole, clotrimazole or miconozole, applied twice daily for at least 2 weeks. Terbinafine cream is also effective if applied once or twice a day for up to 2 weeks, but it is more expensive. Compound benzoic acid ointment (Whitfield's ointment) has also been used as a topical treatment for many years. Although it is cheap, it is less cosmetically acceptable to patients (Joint Formulary Committee, 2004: 585).

### Systemic treatment

Terbinafine 250 mg daily for 4 weeks is the drug of choice for tinea corporis if systemic treatment is required. Systemic treatment is usually indicated for widespread infection, the immunocompromised or those that have not responded to topical treatment. However, it should be discontinued if there are any signs of liver toxicity. Imidazole antifungals, e.g. fluconazole or itraconazole, may also be used but these have been associated with liver damage and should not be used in any patient with a history of liver disease.

Griseofulvin 0.5–1 g daily for 4–6 weeks can be prescribed but is contraindicated in severe liver disease and pregnancy. Men should not father children within 6 months of using this treatment and it should be avoided in pregnancy and while breast feeding (Joint Formulary Committee, 2004: 307).

## Granuloma annulare

### Aetiology

The cause of granuloma annulare is unknown. It can occur at any age but is most common in females, children and young adults. It may be associated with diabetes mellitus, particularly in the generalized form of the condition (Lichenstein, 2005).

### Presentation

Different forms of granuloma annulare may be seen. They are usually symptomless but may be tender when knocked.

*Localized granuloma annulare* may develop anywhere on the body but the most common sites for lesions are the backs of the hands, feet, ankles and limbs. Patients present with a well-defined red plaque that is annular, with a border of flat-topped papules (*Figure 26.8*), which often mimic the rash of tinea.

*Perforating granuloma annulare* presents typically on the hands and fingers. Small, superficial papules develop with central umbilication *(Figure 26.9)*.

*Generalized granuloma annulare* presents with multiple lesions that may appear over the trunk and limbs. The annular shape of the lesions may be somewhat distorted. The lesions may also be skin coloured, pink or brown macules and papules *(Figure 26.10)* (Du Vivier, 2002). This form of granuloma annulare may sometimes be associated with diabetes mellitus (DermNet NZ, 2004a).

### Investigations

The diagnosis of granuloma annulare can normally be made from the history and clinical examination. Skin scraping for fungal elements and culture will be negative, thereby distinguishing the condition from tinea corporis.

If necessary, a skin biopsy will confirm the diagnosis (Lichenstein, 2005). If there is a possibility of associated

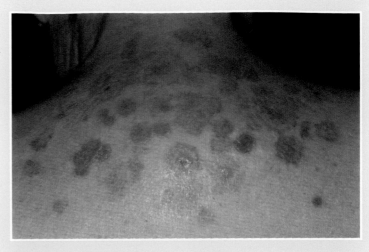

*Figure 26.4. Multiple lesions in tinea corporis.*

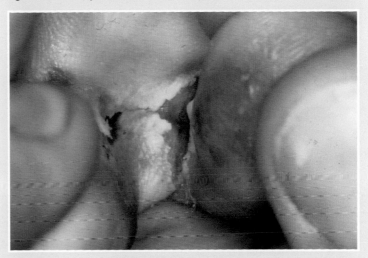

*Figure 26.5. Interdigital tinea pedis, often associated with tinea corporis.*

diabetes mellitus, a urine and/or blood test should be taken to check for glucose (Lichenstein, 2005).

## Management

Treatment is not usually necessary because spontaneous resolution can usually be expected within a few months or sometimes years. If necessary, the localized form may

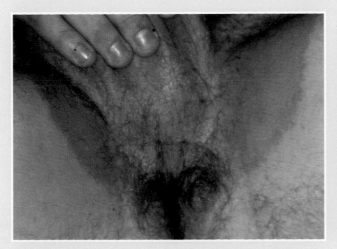

*Figure 26.6. Tinea cruris, often associated with tinea corporis.*

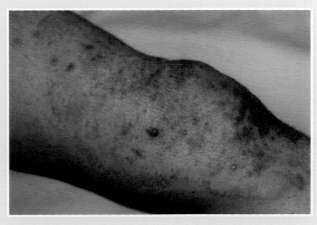

*Figure 26.7. Tinea incognito with a less obvious margin and pustules.*

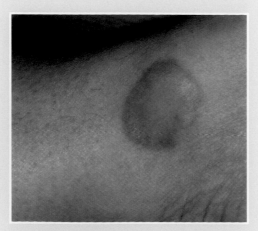

*Figure 26.8. Localized granuloma annulare.*

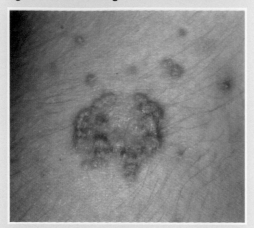

*Figure 26.9. Perforating granuloma annulare.*

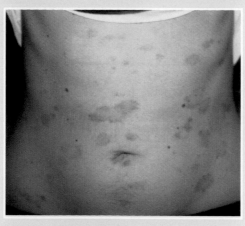

*Figure 26.10. Generalized granuloma annulare.*

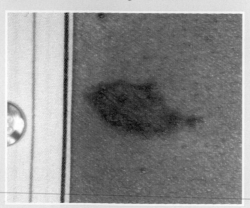

*Figure 26.11. Herald patch of pityriasis rosea.*

respond well to intralesional steroids. In the generalized forms, potent topical steroids may be helpful. Topical imiquimod and topical calcineurin inhibitos have occassionally been found to help. Other preparations that have been tried are systemic steroids, methotrexate, dapsone, isotretinoin or psoralen plus ultraviolet light (PUVA) photochemotherapy. However, the possible side effects of these treatments must be weighed against the need to treat something that is essentially harmless (DermNet NZ, 2004a).

## Herald patch of pityriasis rosea
### Aetiology
No specific cause has been found for pityriasis rosea but it has been suggested that the rash is a reactive response to a viral infection (DermNet NZ 2010). A few drugs such as penicillamine and isotretinoin have been thought possibly to be implicated and it is more common in patients with stopy, seborrhoeic dermatitis and acne vulgaris. It occurs most commonly in children and young adults (Lichenstein, 2004).

### Presentation
It is the initial 1–2 cm diameter 'herald patch' that may be confused with tinea corporis. A single oval or round patch presents, usually on the trunk but occasionally on the neck or limbs. The lesion has a central, wrinkled area that is salmon coloured, with a darker outside edge and intervening 'collarette of scale' *(Figure 26.11)*. The diagnosis becomes clear within the next 10 days, when more generalized but smaller patches appear over the chest and abdomen *(Figure 26.12)*. Atypical pityriasis rosea occurs in about 20% of cases where the herald patch may not occur. In addition, the rash may be distributed peripherally and be severe with urticaria, vesicular, pustular or purpuric lesions (Lichenstein, 2004).

### Investigations
A skin scraping for fungal elements will prove negative if pityriasis rosea is present, ruling out the possibility of tinea corporis (Lichenstein, 2004). Occasionally, a skin biopsy may be necessary to confirm the diagnosis (Lichenstein, 2004).

### Infectivity
Infectivity does not appear to be a problem, and children and adults can usually continue with their normal work and school lives (Lichenstein, 2004).

### Management
Pityriasis rosea is a harmless, self-limiting condition that normally requires no treatment (Lichenstein, 2004). Topical or calamine lotion may soothe if there is any associated irritation of the skin. In more severe cases, topical or oral steroids can be used.

## Discoid eczema
### Aetiology
The cause of discoid eczema (nummular dermatitis) is still unknown. It may sometimes be triggered by local trauma, venous stasis and/or dry skin. It is more common in men aged 50–70 years. It may also occur in teenagers and young adults who also suffer with atopic eczema (Sams, 2004).

## Presentation

The patient presents with a history of papules or vesicles that become crusted, weeping, single or multiple plaques with an erythematous base. Between the lesions the skin is normal (*Figure 26.13*). Secondary infection with staphylococci often occurs and, in time, the lesions become dry and scaly. Because they are itchy, excoriation results if the patient scratches. The areas most commonly affected are the backs of the hands but often the limbs and trunk are involved (Sams, 2004).

## Investigation

A skin scraping should be taken to exclude the possibility of tinea corporis. A swab should be taken from the area to check for culture, sensitivities and the possibility of secondary infection (Sams, 2004).

## Management

Topical emollients to help the dry skin and an antihistamine for the itch may be useful. A potent topical steroid may first be required to get the condition under control before moving down the scale of strengths. This may need to be combined with a topical antibiotic such as fusidic acid, because sepsis is so common. Severe cases may initially require systemic steroids and antibiotics (Du Vivier, 2002: 50). Discoid eczema may be difficult to treat and control. Severe and persistent problems may require specialist advice.

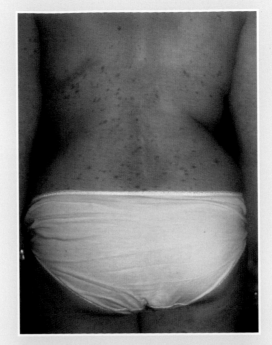

*Figure 26.12. Rash of pityriasis rosea.*

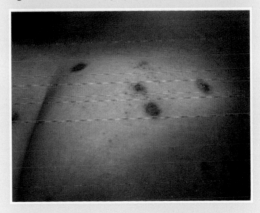

*Figure 26.13. Discoid eczema on the buttock.*

## References

Chuh A, Chan H, Zawar V (2004) Pityraiasis rosea—evidence for and against an infectious aetiology. Epidemiol Infect 132(3): 381–90

DermNet NZ (2010) Pityriasis Rosea. http://dermnetnz.org/viral/pityriasis-rosea.html (accessed 30 July 2010)

DermNet NZ (2004a) Granuloma annulare. http://dermnetnz.org/ dermal-infiltrative/granulomaannulare. html (accessed 29 March 2005)

DermNet NZ (2004b) Tinea incognito. http://dermnetnz. org/fungal/tinea-incognito.html (accessed 29 March 2005)

du Vivier (2002) The skin and systemic disease. Atlas of Clinical Dermatology. 3rd edn. Churchill Livingstone: 533–40

Joint Formulary Committee (2004) British National Formulary 48. September. British Medical Association and Royal Pharmaceutical Society of Great Britain, London

Lesher JL, Zember G (2004) Tinea corporis. eMedicine. www.emedicine.com/derm/topic421. htm (accessed 22 March 2005)

Lichenstein R (2004) Pityriasis rosea. eMedicine. www.emedicine.com/emerg/topic426.htm (accessed 29 March 2005)

Lichenstein R (2005) Granuloma, annulare and pyogenic. eMedicine. www.emedicine.com/emerg/topic 753.htm (accessed 29 March 2005)

Sams HH (2004) Nummular dermatitis. eMedicine. www. emedicine. com/derm/topic298. htm (accessed 29 March 2005)

Stockport Health Authority (1999) Infection Control and Cross Infection Guidelines for Nurseries. 3rd edn. Control of Infection Unit. www.infectioncontrol. org.uk/nsect1.html (accessed 29 March 2005)

Wandsworth Primary Care Trust (2002) Ringworm. South West London Health Protection Unit. www.wandsworth-pct.nhs.uk/ pdf/factsheets/Ringworm.pdf (accessed 29 March 2005

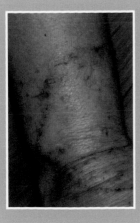

# Test Your Knowledge

This 60-year-old woman first had been to her doctor complaining of a rash on her neck. She was prescribed topical fusidic acid for what was thought to be a bacterial skin infection. When it did not improve and another area was developing on her foot, the doctor considered a diagnosis of eczema. She was then given a course of oral flucloxacillin and topical fusidic acid with hydrocortisone. Still there was no improvement and by the time she returned to the surgery, not only had this additional annular patch appeared on her wrist, but her grand-daughter, who had come to stay with her, was also showing signs of the same problem. She had a patch on one arm. The lesions were increasing in size and she was really concerned.

## Questions

1. What is the likely diagnosis?
2. What investigations would you do?
3. What advice would you give to the patient?

# Nails 1: A pointer to disease

In everyday life we meet, say hello, and shake hands without much thought to the state of the other person's hands. In the surgery, however, meeting provides an opportunity to assess the patient as he/she walks through the door. As we take the patient's hand, a look at the nails may reveal signs of an underlying problem or hidden disease.

The nails may help direct the clinician's attention to the possibility of a specific condition or help confirm a diagnosis that may be suggested by another rash, sign and/or symptom. Of course, not all changes in the nails may be obvious; toenails may also be affected.

## Anxiety

Nail biting (*Figure 27.1*) is particularly common in children and occurs in as many as 50% between the ages of 10–18 years (Sekula, 2000). Many of these will spontaneously cease the habit in adult life, although in some it may persist. It may be a bad habit that the patient finds difficult to change but sometimes it is associated with depression, anxiety and compulsive disorders for which the patient may require professional help (Gibson, 2006).

Nail biting in itself does not lead to any long-term problems (as long as it does not affect the cuticles) but it may encourage conditions such as paronychia or pariungual warts.

### Median nail dystrophy

Repeated scratching of the nail plate or picking at the cuticle may result in the development of a longitudinal depression along the nail (usually the thumbnail) with transverse ridging that is sometimes known as the 'Christmas tree effect'. The lunula becomes enlarged.

Median nail dystrophy may be the result of a conscious or unconscious action, but commonly patients with median nail dystrophy (or habit tic deformity) have an underlying psychological problem (*Figure 27.2*).

### Management

Discussion of these problems with the patient may help reveal difficulties that the patient may be glad to talk about. It offers a chance to decide, with the patient, what further help (if any) he/she would like in order to deal with the problem, whether in the form of antidepressant or anxiolytic medication, counselling or psychiatric help (Sekula, 2000).

## Psoriasis

Nail changes are common in psoriasis. They usually occur in association with skin involvement, but may occur isolation. It is most commonly associated with psoriatic arthritis and may be seen in over half of these cases (Ngan, 2006). There are three signs that might call attention to the condition. The first of these is pitting, where small pits may be seen, spread uniformly or randomly across the nail plate (*Figure 27.3*). The changes

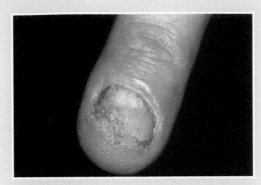

*Figure 27.1. Finger of a nail biter.*

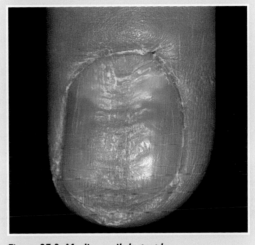

*Figure 27.2. Median nail dystrophy.*

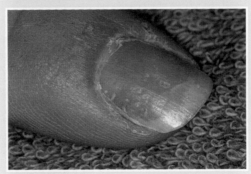

*Figure 27.3. Pitting in the nail of a patient with psoriasis.*

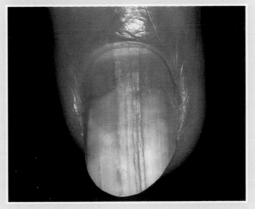

*Figure 27.4. Onycholysis in a patient with psoriasis.*

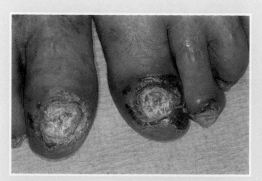

**Figure 27.5. Psoriasis: acrodermatitis continua of Hallopeau of the toes.**

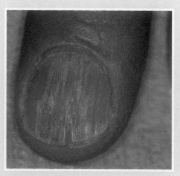

**Figure 27.6. Longitudinal ridging in a patient with lichen planus.**

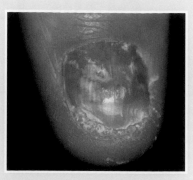

**Figure 27.7. Lichen planus: thickening and darkening of the nail.**

are often symmetrical and the lunula is often involved. Although pitting is most commonly seen in psoriasis it may occur in other conditions such as alopecia areata, eczema, Reiter's syndrome and pemphigus (Family Practice Notebook, 2000).

The second sign is onycholysis, frequently seen in psoriasis. It may suddenly appear with separation of the free edge of the nail plate from the underlying nail bed (*Figure 27.4*). The separated nail whitens. Although this is common in psoriasis, it may also be found in a number of other conditions such as eczema, lichen planus, periungual warts, fungal infections of the nail, iron deficiency anaemia, thyrotoxicosis and sarcoidosis.

Onycholysis may also develop after exposure to ultraviolet light in a patient on a photosensitizing drug such as tetracycline or psoralen with ultraviolet A (PUVA).

A late sign is psoriatic nail dystrophy. In severe cases the nail becomes thickened, opaque and discoloured. Unlike the changes in fungal infections, there are symmetrical changes, usually of all the nails. Sometimes it is associated with acrodermatitis continua of Hallopeau, in which sterile pustules occur around the nail (*Figure 27.5*).

### Management

Nail clippings should be taken to exclude the possibility of tinea, which would be treatable with an antifungal preparation such as terbinafine. This would need to be continued for up to 3 months or longer (Joint Formulary Committee, 2006: 5.2). Occasionally a nail biopsy may be necessary to confirm the diagnosis as similar changes may be found associated with other conditions.

The treatment of nail psoriasis is generally unsatisfactory and the use of any treatment must depend on the severity of the condition and the concern of the patient. There is no cure. Even if there is improvement either spontaneously or with medication, the condition may well relapse at a later date. Possible approaches are to apply calcipotriol twice daily to the nail folds. This may help but will need to be continued for a long time.

Other choices are topical potent corticosteroids, intralesional triamcinolone, topical fluorouracil cream to the matrix for 6 months, PUVA or systemic methotrexate, retinoids or ciclosporin. All have attendant risks. The severity of the problem must always be weighed against the possible side effects of any treatment (Ngan, 2006).

### Lichen planus

In 10% of cases of lichen planus, the nails may be affected. Usually there are other cutaneous or buccal signs of the condition. However, this may not always be the case. The nail plate is thinned and longitudinal lines or depressions are seen in the nail plate (*Figure 27.6*). Onycholysis may also occur and/or the nail may thicken or darken (*Figure 27.7*). In cases where there is severe damage, the nail becomes atrophic and in some cases adhesions may form between the skin and the dorsal nail

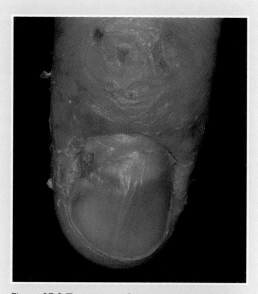

**Figure 27.8. Transverse ridging in a patient with eczema.**

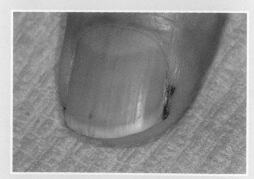

**Figure 27.9. Splinter haemorrhages in a patient with rheumatoid arthritis.**

fold, with partial destruction of the nail (pterygium formation). If the atrophic nail is shed there may be no regrowth. Two or three finger nails are likely to be affected but occasionally the toes are also involved. (DermNetNZ, 2006). Longitudinal ridging may also occur in other conditions such as alopecia areata, psoriasis and fungal infection of the nail.

### Management

If treated early in the disease, a course of systemic prednisolone for 3 weeks may prevent permanent scarring and nail loss. To establish the diagnosis early, a biopsy may be required.

## Eczema

Eczema is an extremely common condition. When it involves the posterior nail fold it may affect the growth of the nail. As a result the affected nail or nails may be pitted, with irregular tranverse ridging. As is shown in *Figure 27.8*, there is obvious eczematous change around the nail in some places. In others, there may be a past history of such changes. In severe cases there may be actual temporary shedding of the nail (du Vivier, 2002).

### Management

If the eczema is treated and cleared with emollients and topical steroids, the nail will return to normal as the changes 'grow out'. The rate of growth may be variable but is at the rate of about 3 mm a month. A fingernail may take up to 6 months to regrow but toenails will take longer (Nail Solutions, 2006).

## Splinter haemorrhages

Small splinter haemorrhages may sometimes be seen under the nail (*Figure 27.9*). These may occur in normal healthy people, perhaps as the result of trauma, psoriasis, rheumatoid arthritis or fungal nail infection, but they may also be seen in bacterial endocarditis. The condition is more likely to occur in those with a previous history of rheumatic fever where there is damage of the heart valves, in cases of congenital heart defects or after valve replacement. The patient is likely to be unwell with fever, shortness of breath, chest pain and/or palpitations (Fawcett et al, 2004).

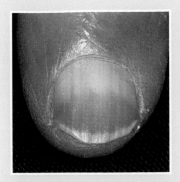

**Figure 27.10. Terry's half-and-half nails.**

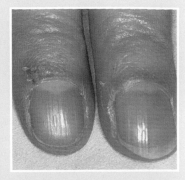

**Figure 27.11. Periungual erythema in a patient with dermatomyositis.**

### Management

Early diagnosis and treatment in hospital are crucial to the outcome in cases of bacterial endocarditis. Blood cultures, erythrocyte sedimentation rate (ESR), urine check, electrocardiogram (ECG), chest X-ray and echocardiogram may be necessary if infective endocarditis is suspected to confirm the problem.

## Terry's half-and-half nails

Terry's half-and-half nails present with changes that cause the proximal part of the nail to whiten. The lunula is obliterated (*Figure 27.10*). It is thought to be caused by 'a decrease in vascularity and increase in connective tissue in the nail bed' (Fawcett et al, 2004). All the fingers are usually affected. These changes are seen in about 10% of patients with renal failure and will revert to normal within 2–3 weeks of renal transplantation, but are not affected by dialysis (GP Notebook, 2003). Terry's nails may also be seen in cases of cirrhosis of the liver, chronic congestive heart failure and type 2 diabetes. Where the patient has not already been diagnosed, a full patient history and examination is required, as well as investigations of liver function, electrolytes and urea, and blood glucose. The appropriate specialist advice should be sought.

## Periungual erythema

Some patients suffering with connective tissue disorders may show signs of erythema around the nail fold at the

## Table 27.1. Medical conditions associated with nail changes

| Nail change | Associated medical conditions |
| --- | --- |
| Pitting | Eczema, psoriasis, alopecia areata |
| Transverse ridging | Eczema, psoriasis, paronychia |
| Longitudinal ridging | Lichen planus, psoriasis, habit tick deformity, alopecia, areata |
| Nail dystrophy | Psoriasis, fungal nail infection |
| Onycholysis | Psoriasis, trauma, lichen planus, eczema, periungual warts, fungal nail infection, iron deficiency anaemia, thyrotoxicosis, sarcoidosis, drug photosensitivity |
| Terry's half-and-half nails | Renal failure, cirrhosis of the liver, chronic congestive heart failure, type 2 diabetes |
| Splinter haemorrhages | Trauma, psoriasis, fungal nail infection, bacterial endocarditis |
| Periungual erythema | Lupus erythematosus, dermatomyositis, sarcoidosis, HIV |

base of the nail (*Figure 27.11*). This is caused by dilated blood vessels in this area. These changes may be seen in a number of different conditions including lupus erythematosus, dermatomyositis, sarcoidosis and HIV (Itin et al, 1998). Any patient with this sign should be referred to the doctor for full examination and investigation to ascertain any underlying associated condition.

## Conclusions

A number of conditions may be associated with changes in the nail (*Table 27.1*). Therefore it is important to consider the diagnosis carefully so that appropriate treatment can be given.

## References

DermNetNZ (2006) Lichen planus. www.dermnetnz.org/scaly/lichen-planus.html (accessed 5 December 2006)

du Vivier A (2002) Nail disorders: Eczema. *Atlas of Clinical Dermatology*. 3rd edn. Elsevier Science Ltd: 608

Family Practice Notebook. LLC (2000) Nail pitting. www.fpnotebook.com/DER159.htm (accessed 5 December 2006)

Fawcett R, Linford C, Stulberg D (2004) Nail abnormalities: Clues to systemic disease. *American Family Physician*. www.aafp.org/afp/20040315/1417.html (accessed 5 December 2006)

GP Notebook (2003) Terry's nails. www.gpnotebook.co.uk/cache/1832189976.htm (accessed 5 December 2006)

Gibson L (2006) Nail biting: Does it cause permanent damage? www.mayoclinic.com/health/nailbiting/AN01144 (accessed 5 December 2006)

Itin P, Courvouisier SM, Battegay M (1998) Erythema of the proximal nailfold in HIV-infected patients: frequency, relation to hepatitis C virus and HIV viral load. *Int Conf AIDS* 12: 574 http://gateway.nlm.nih.gov/MeetingAbstracts/102229783.html (accessed 5 December 2006)

Joint Formulary Committee (2006) *British National Formulary* 52. September. BMJ Publishing Group and Royal Pharmaceutical Society of Great Britain, London

Nail Solutions (2006) Nail anatomy and structure. www.nail-solutions.co.uk/Nail%20anatomy.htm (accessed 5 December 2006)

Ngan V (2006) Nail psoriasis. www.dermnetnz.org/scaly/nail-psoriasis.html (accessed 5 December 2006)

Sekula SA (2000) Self injury of the nails and hands. *Dermatology Online Journal* 6(1): http://dermatology.cdlib.org/DOJvol6num1/special/nail-injury/sekula.html (accessed 5 December 2006)

## Test Your Knowledge

This patient was worried about her nails. For some months she had noticed some changes and she was worried because her manager at work on the delicatessen counter at the supermarket was questioning whether she might have something 'catching'. She was otherwise well, but she had recently noticed some pain and stiffness in her fingers. There was no history of eczema, skin changes or alopecia.

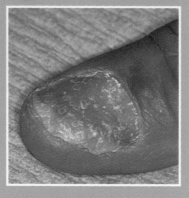

### Questions

1. What is the most likely diagnosis in this case?
2. What further examination or investigations might you pursue?
3. What treatment could you offer the patient to 'cure' her nails?

# Nails 2: The traumatized nail

In the previous chapter the way that a patient's nails can help clinicians indentify underlying problems in a patient's health was examined. This chapter follows a slightly different approach, looking at how trauma to the nails can create problems for the patient, and how the patient can learn to manage these problems or even prevent them from occuring.

## Leuconychia

A person suffering from leuconychia will see changes in the appearance of his/her nail. These changes are most commonly white spots, although streaks (*Figure 28.1*) or more extensive discolouration may appear, either spontaneously or following trauma to the nail matrix. One man had suffered torture 20 years earlier, but the changes had persisted (*Figure 28.2*). Similar total leuconychia may be observed in patients with renal failure, lymphoma or hypoalbuminaemia of chronic liver disease (when the nails affected are usually the thumb and index finger). Leuconychia may also be inherited through an autodominant gene (GP Notebook, 2003).

### Management

Simple leuconychia that may result from minor trauma is of no concern and should gradually grow out with the nail. Where an underlying medical condition is suspected, it should be followed up, investigated and managed appropriately.

## Onychogryphosis

Onychogryphosis (also known as Ram's horn or ostler's toe) is caused by hypertrophy of the nail. This, together with the fact that growth is slower on one side of the nail, leads to a gross, thickened and distorted nail deformity with darkening of the nail. The most common cause of this condition is trauma, either from a blow, stubbing the toe or the repeated banging of the nail against shoes. This frequently occurs in the elderly, especially if the nails are not trimmed regularly. Consequently, it is usually the big toenail that is affected. Often the nail lengthens so that it traumatizes the adjacent toes (*Figure 28.3*).

### Management

A chiropodist will usually be required to carefully cut and pare the affected nail, and footwear should be checked to ensure correct fitting. Occasionally, particularly in the young with only one affected toe, avulsion of the nail may achieve long-term relief (Neale and Adams, 1989).

## Ingrowing toenails

Ingrowing toenails (onychcryptosis) is a common problem that most commonly affects the big toe(s). It may be caused by ill-fitting shoes that compress the toes and cause the nail to curve into the skin. Other causes are cutting nails so that the edges penetrate the skin, or an association with fungal infections that may result in the thickening of the nail. Initially the end of the toe is slightly swollen and inflamed. These changes increase and the toe becomes painful. Pus may begin to form and drain. As the condition worsens, granulation forms in addition to the inflammation and pus (*Figure 28.4*). The lateral nail fold hypertrophies (*Figure 28.5*) and, if the infection is not controlled, it may lead to constitutional symptoms of fever.

### Management

Prevention of ingrowing toenails is better than cure. Patients should always be advised to cut nails straight across and not into the corners, to wear good fitting shoes, to observe good hygiene and to ensure that feet are kept clean and dry.

Treatment of ingrowing toenails depends on the severity of the problem. In the early stages, warm water soaks four times a day, good hygiene and the insertion of a cotton wick under the lateral groove at each soaking (raising the nail so that it no longer digs into the skin) may suffice.

As infection develops, topical treatments, e.g. fusidic acid, or oral antibiotics such as amoxycillin or flucloxacillin, may be required.

For more severe problems surgery is usually required, with lateral nail avulsion and matricectomy carried out under a ring block anaesthetic. Any pus should be drained, the nail cut straight across and electrocautery or phenol ablation used to destroy cells that might regrow any unwanted nail. An antibiotic ointment is applied and the

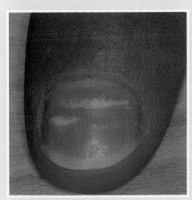

*Figure 28.1. Leuconychia.*

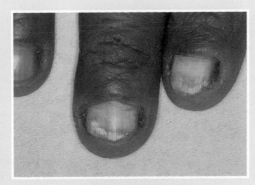

*Figure 28.2. Total leuconychia persisting 20 years after an episode of torture.*

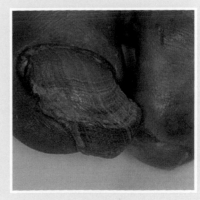

*Figure 28.3. Onychogryphosis.*

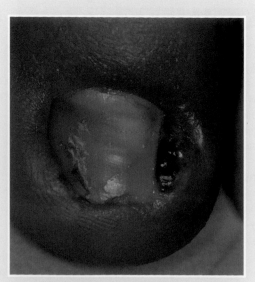

*Figure 28.4. Ingrowing toenail: inflammation and granulation at the nail fold.*

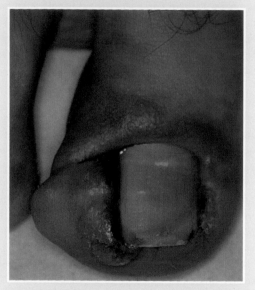

*Figure 28.5. Ingrowing toenail: gross hypertrophy of the nail fold.*

area should heal after a few weeks, during which time dressings and further application of the antibiotic ointment should be continued about twice a week (Ngan, 2006).

## Involution of the nail

In this condition there is a marked curving of the lateral, and/or medial edges of the nail, resulting in the nail bed becoming pinched between them (*Figure 28.6*). This may lead to inflammation or ulceration of the toe. It most commonly affects the big toe and may be the result of wearing tight-fitting shoes or a congenital problem that can sometimes affect other members of the family.

### Management

Mild cases may not require any specific treatment other than advice regarding footwear. The nail should be cut to meet with the shape and length of the toe. More severe cases may require the attention of a chiropodist, the use of a nail brace or partial nail avulsion (Neale and Adams, 1989: 132–3).

## Paronychia
### Acute bacterial paronychia

This superficial skin infection around the nails is usually associated with *Staphylococcus aureus*. Bacterial paronychia usually follows trauma, such as nail biting, stubbing the toes, over-enthusiastic pushing back of the cuticle or picking at a hangnail. The patient complains of the sudden onset of painful inflammation and swelling around the nail (*Figure 28.7*), with the development of a pus-filled blister that may later discharge. If the infection is under the nail, the nail may become distorted, loosened and detached (*Figure 28.8*). Normally only one nail is affected.

Severe cases run the risk of abscess formation, septicaemia or spreading of the infection to adjacent tendons and bones (Kantor, 2005).

### Chronic paronychia

Chronic paronychia is an infection of the nail fold by *Candida albicans* and sometimes by other microorganisms. It occurs most commonly in those who frequently immerse their hands in water and may sometimes be seen in diabetics, those with vaginal *Candida*, as a complication of eczema, or as a result of the repeated trauma of pushing back the cuticles. There is a gradual onset of swelling of the nail fold, which may be inflamed and tender and sometimes discharge small amounts of pus from under the cuticle. The nail plate becomes ridged and discoloured (*Figure 28.9*).

### Investigations

A swab taken from the proximal nail fold should confirm bacteria and/or *Candida* involvement on microscopy and culture. Nail clippings would be required to confirm a fungal infection if this is suspected.

### Management

Acute paronychia is extremely painful and the patient will require adequate analgesia such as paracetamol or ibuprofen to give relief. Hot water soaks (every 4 hours) will also help reduce the inflammation and pain, and promote the drainage of any pus. Oral antibiotics such as flucloxacillin may help abort progress if given before there has been pus formation. If pus is present and not draining, it can be released by incision through the nail fold or removal of part of the nail (Ellis et al, 1998).

With chronic paronychia, the patient should be advised to keep his/her hands dry and to wear cotton-lined rubber gloves for all wet work. A coating of flexible collodion to the nail fold may help act as a barrier to water and infection. Improvement may be achieved by the application of a topical antifungal lotion such as nystatin to the nail fold twice daily, or a course of an oral antifungal agent such as fluconazole may be tried. Progress is likely to be slow and recurrence of the problem is common (DermNetNZ, 2006).

## Subungual haematoma

Injury to the nailbed by a blow or crushing may result in a haemorrhage, with blood collecting under the nail. There will normally be a history of injury and it is easily recognized as a black, purple, red or brown area under the

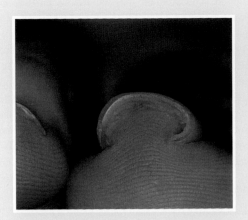

Figure 28.6. Involution of the nail.

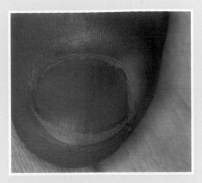

Figure 28.7. Acute bacterial paronychia with inflammation and early pus formation.

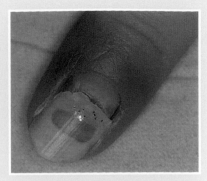

Figure 28.8. Paronychia: shedding nail 2 months after paronychia: new nail growth.

nail. In time the haematoma will move up the nail as it grows but the nail is usually lost after some weeks. However, it will regrow later (GP Notebook, 2003) (*Figure 28.10*).

In some cases the trauma may have been sufficiently severe to cause fracture of the underlying phalanx. Crush injuries are especially likely to be associated with a fracture of the terminal phalanx.

**Differential diagnosis**

There are times when there may be doubts about the diagnosis (*Table 28.1*). Many patients, in particular, the elderly, may have no recollection of any injury, but present with a problem of discolouration or a black streak under the nail (*Figure 28.11*). This should always raise suspicion of a malignant melanoma (Swetter, 2005). Other conditions

that may present with similar symptoms are a glomus tumour and Kaposi's sarcoma.

Subungual melanoma may present with diffuse discolouration or a longitudinal pigmented band within the nail plate. In melanoma, an additional concerning sign is spread of the pigment to the proximal or lateral nail folds (Hutchinson's sign). As the tumour thickens, the nail may become distorted and split. If there is any doubt about the diagnosis, a biopsy should be arranged urgently, as any delay will increase the risk of metastasis (du Vivier, 2002: 223–4).

**Management**

Treatment is not required if the patient is not in too much pain, and where the haematoma is enclosed with an intact nail and there is no laceration of the skin fold or nail

## Table 28.1. Differential diagnoses

| | Cause | Presentation | Management |
|---|---|---|---|
| Leuconychia | Spontaneous<br>Trauma<br>Chronic liver disease<br>Renal failure<br>Lymphoma<br>Genetic | White spots or streaks<br>Total leuconychia | No treatment required<br>Total leuconychia: investigate and manage underlying cause. |
| Onychogryphosis | Trauma | Thickening, darkening and distortion of the nail | Chiropodist<br>Avulsion of the nail if necessary |
| Ingrowing toenail | Ill-fitting footwear<br>Incorrect nail cutting | Swelling and inflammation of the toe<br>Granulation and pus formation<br>Lateral nail fold hypertrophy<br>Constitutional symptoms | Foot hygiene, sensible footwear<br>Warm water soaks<br>Antibiotics: topical or oral<br>Lateral nail avulsion under ring block anaesthesia |
| Involution of the nail | Tight shoes<br>Congenital | Marked incurving of nail edges<br>May cause inflammation and ulceration | Symptomless: no treatment<br>Problems: nail brace or partial nail avulsion |
| Bacterial paronychia | *Staphylococcus aureus*<br>Trauma<br>Nail biting | Sudden onset<br>Pain, inflammation and swelling of nail fold<br>Pus formation | Analgesics<br>Hot soaks<br>Incision of nail fold and drainage of pus |
| Chronic paronychia | *Candida albicans*<br>Wet hands | Gradual onset<br>Swelling and inflammation of nail fold<br>A little pus may be expressed | Keep dry<br>Flexible collodion over nail fold as barrier<br>Topical or oral antifungal agent |
| Subungual haematoma | Trauma | Discolouration under nail<br>Black, purple, red or brown | Mild: no treatment required<br>Check re-fracture<br>Under tension: trephine<br>Biopsy if possibility of malignant melanoma |

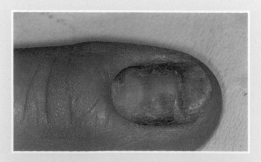

*Figure 28.9. Chronic paronychia.*

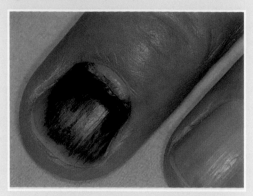

*Figure 28.10. Subungual haematoma.*

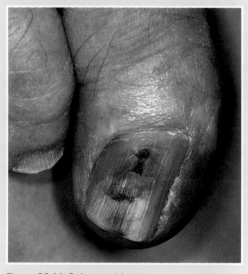

*Figure 28.11. Subungual haematoma: possible malignant melanoma.*

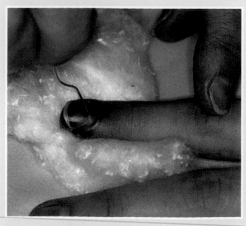

*Figure 28.12. Trephining a subungual haematoma with a heated paper clip.*

disruption. The problem may be left to resolve itself spontaneously and gradually 'grow out'. However, if the blood is under tension initially, it can be very painful.

This pressure can be released by trephining the nail with electrocautery or a red hot paper clip (*Figure 28.12*). A sharp instrument or pointed needle should be avoided because it may cause damage to the underlying soft tissue. Care should be taken where considering trephining if there is suspicion of an associated fracture, because this would convert a closed facture into an open one with all its attendant risks (Vaughn, 2006) .

## References

DermNet NZ (2006) Paronychia. www.dermnetnz.org/fungal/paronychia.html (accessed 7 December 2006)

du Vivier A (2002) Subungual melanoma. *Atlas of Clinical Dermatology.* 3rd edn. Elsevier Science Ltd: 223–4

Ellis H, Calne R, Watson C (1998) The nails. In: *General Surgery.* 9th edn. Blackwell Science: 39

GP Notebook (2003) Leukonychia. www.gpnotebook.co.uk/cache/-234487799.htm (accessed 7 December 2006)

GP Notebook (2003) Subungual haematoma. www.gpnotebook.co.uk/cache/1865744440.htm (accessed 7 December 2006)

Kantor J (2005) Paronychia. MedlinePlus Medical Encyclopedia. www.nlm.nih.gov/medlineplus/ency/article/001444.htm (accessed 7 December 2006)

Neale D, Adams I (1989) Common foot disorders. *Nail disorders.* 3rd edn. Churchill Livingstone: 131–2

Ngan V (2006) Ingrown toenails. www.dermnetnz.org/hair-nails-sweat/onychocryptosis.html (accessed 7 December 2006)

Swetter S (2005) Malignant melanoma. *eMedicine.* www.emedicine.com/derm/topic257.htm (accessed 7 December 2006)

Vaughn G (2006) Fingertip injuries. eMedicine. www.emedicine.com/EMERG/topic179.htm (accessed 7 December 2006)

Watkins J (2007) Nails part 1: A pointer to diagnosis. *Practice Nursing* **18**(1): 21–3

## Test Your Knowledge

This middle-aged woman was worried about her nail. For some months she had been aware of swelling, inflammation and tenderness around the posterior and lateral nail folds on one finger. Now the problem was starting up in another finger on that hand. At one edge there was occasional leakage of a small amount of pus

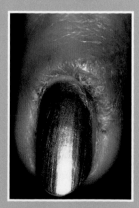

from time-to-time. She was a hairdresser and concerned that her boss at work had noticed that she had a problem and was afraid that some of her customers might be worried that she might have an infection that could be passed on to them.

### Questions

1. What is the likely diagnosis?
2. How could you confirm the diagnosis?
3. How would you manage the condition?

# Red faces

A variety of infectious diseases occur in childhood, such as measles, rubella and scarlet fever. Although children are the most often affected, non-immune adults are also at risk of these infections. Most remain common, but some, thanks to the advent of routine immunization, are rarely seen in the UK. However, unfounded fears about the measles, mumps and rubella (MMR) vaccination, have allowed immunity in the community to drop and some cases are beginning to occur.

Before the introduction of a single measles vaccine in 1968 (MMR was introduced in 1988), 545 050 cases of measles were notified in 1951 and 317 deaths occurred. This had dropped by the year 2000 to 2378 notified cases and only only death as a result of good uptake of the MMR vaccine.

Sadly, with the MMR scare and reduced uptake of the vaccine, a rise in the incidence of measles has occurred, with 3705 cases and one death in 2006 (Health Protection Agency (HPA), 2007a). It is therefore still important to be able to recognize and confirm the diagnosis of measles, as well as infectious diseases, when they present in the surgery.

This chapter concentrates on those infectious illnesses that may present with a facial rash, and discusses the additional signs, symptoms and investigations that may help reach the correct diagnosis.

## Measles

### Aetiology

Measles is a highly infectious condition caused by a paramyxovirus and spread by airborne droplets produced when coughing and sneezing. Lifelong immunity follows measles, but those who have not suffered the disease, or who have not been immunized, are at risk of getting the infection. A passive immunity is passed on to infants in the first few months of life only, if the mother has had the disease. The incubation period for measles is 9–18 days and exclusion from school should be observed for 5 days after the onset of the rash (HPA, 2007b). Measles is a notifiable disease.

### Clinical presentation

Prodromal symptoms usually begin 10–12 days after exposure. The patient becomes unwell, with fever, red eyes, cough and cold. Within a few days, bluish-white Koplik's spots can be seen on the mucous membranes in the mouth (*Figure 29.1*). This stage of the illness may last for as much as 10 days before the appearance of a non-itchy erythematous, maculopapular rash which begins behind the ears and the face (*Figure 29.2*) before spreading to the trunk and limbs. The child usually appears 'ill' with a high fever (*Figure 29.3*). The Koplik's spots disappear within a day or two of the rash developing. After about 3 or 4 days the rash fades but the cough may persist for up to 3 weeks (DermNet NZ, 2007b).

### Diagnosis

The history of the illness and the presence of Koplik's spots usually make the diagnosis obvious. However, measles is a notifiable disease and since it is now a rarity in the UK, laboratory confirmation is required for notification purposes. A salivary swab can be tested for measles-specific immunoglobulin M (IgM) or ribonucleic acid (RNA), within 6 weeks of the onset of the illness (Borton, 2007).

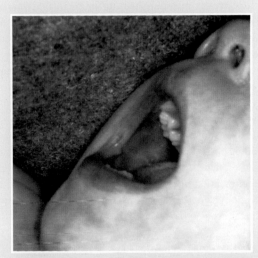

*Figure 29.1. Koplik's spots in the prodromal stage of measles.*

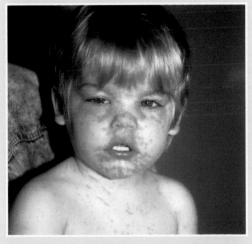

*Figure 29.2. Measles: Early rash on the face.*

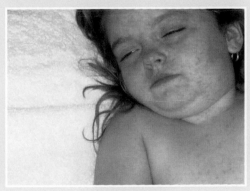

*Figure 29.3. 'Ill' child with measles.*

**Table 29.1. Incubation time and school exclusion recommendations**

| | Incubation time recommendation | School exclusion |
|---|---|---|
| Measles | 9–18 days | 5 days after onset of rash |
| Rubella | 15–20 days | 5 days after onset of rash |
| Scarlet fever | 1–4 days | 5 days after starting antibiotic |
| Fifth disease | 4–18 days | none |
| Roseola infantum | 10–15 days | none |

From: Health Protection Agency, 2007b

## Complications

Complications are common cases of measles, particularly in the weak, malnourished or immunocompromized. Diarrhoea may lead to dehydration, conjunctivitis and otitis media, with its risks of hearing loss. Chest infections are not uncommon and more serious problems of encephalitis and haemorrhagic measles occasionally occur.

## Investigations

All cases should have an salivary swab sample taken as soon as possible, and within 6 weeks of the onset of the disease, that should be sent to the Virus Reference Department at the Centre for Infections, even if the infection has been confirmed by the local laboratory (Health Profection Agency 2010)

## Management

Uncomplicated measles should be offered symptomatic treatment only, with fluids and paracetamol, but a watch should be kept for any possible complications that would require antibiotics or admission to hospital.

## German measles (rubella)
### Aetiology

Rubella is caused by an RNA virus of the togavirus family (Lombardo, 2007). Fortunately, it is rarely seen in the UK at present thanks to routine immunization. It is spread by droplet infection from an infected patient 1–3 days before the appearance of the rash and infectivity continues for a further 5 days after that (HPA, 2007b).

The incubation period for the disease is 15–20 days. Children with rubella should be excluded from school and other contact areas for 5 days. Rubella is a notifiable disease.

### Clinical presentation

Rubella is a mild illness, which may pass unnoticed in up to 50% of cases. If signs occur the patient may have a slight fever, sore throat and cold, but the individual does not usually appear to be badly ill. A pinky-red, maculo-papular rash begins on the face and then spreads to the neck (*Figure 29.4*), trunk and limbs and may last for about 5 days and, when marked, may resemble the rash of scarlet fever. One finding that would lead to suspected rubella are enlarged, tender occipital and posterior cervical glands (DermNet NZ, 2007b).

### Diagnosis

The usual approach to confirmation of rubella is by serology, in which the titre of serum rubella IgM is shown to rise from a lower level within 7–10 days of the onset of the illness and 14–21 days later (rubella diagnosis).

### Complications

In fit, healthy children and adults complications are rare but some patients, particularly adults, may complain of joint pains which will occasionally persist for months, or even years. The most serious problem is congenital rubella syndrome, which has a 50% chance of affecting a fetus if the mother develops rubella in the first trimester of pregnancy. It is hoped that most prospective mothers are immunized against rubella, but any

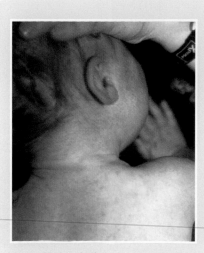

*Figure 29.4. Rubella.*

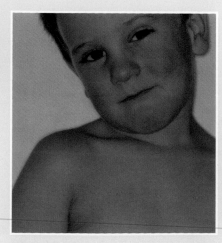

*Figure 29.5. Circumoral pallor in scarlet fever.*

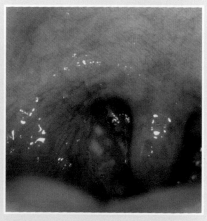

*Figure 29.6. Scarlet fever. Inflamed throat with tonsillar exudate.*

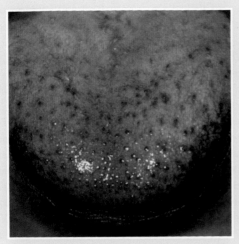

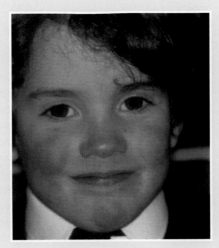

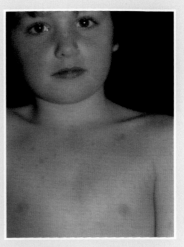

*Figure 29.7. White strawberry tongue in scarlet fever.*  *Figure 29.8. Red cheeks in Fifth disease.*  *Figure 29.9. Rash in Fifth disease.*

non-immunized mother in contact with a case or thought to develop the disease should be checked by serology and advised if shown to have had the disease. Problems that may arise in the child are:

- Low birth weight
- Microcephaly
- Deafness
- Seizures
- Mental retardation
- Cataracts
- Glaucoma
- Retinitis
- Heart defects
- Encephalitis
- Meningitis.

The risks and options of a termination should be discussed (Medline Plus, 2007).

**Management**

Symptomatic treatment is required for rubella, with fluids and paracetamol or ibuprofen if necessary.

## Scarlet fever

### Aetiology

Scarlet fever is the result of a bacterial infection with a group A β-haemolytic *Streptococcus*. The scarlet fever rash develops in those patients with the group A β-haemolytic *Streptococcus*, and who are sensitive to the toxin produced by it. Some may have a streptococcal infection but not develop a rash. The infection may be spread from an infected person by airborne droplets or by skin contamination from someone with a streptococcal skin infection, such as impetigo (DermNet NZ, 2007c). The incubation period for the condition is 1–4 days from contact with a case, and school exclusion is recommended for 5 days after commencing antibiotic

## Table 29.2. Diagnosis and management

|  | Measles | Rubella | Scarlet fever | Fifth disease | Roseola infantum |
|---|---|---|---|---|---|
| Cause | Paromyxovirus | RNA virus | Group A β-haemolytic Streptococcus | Parovirus B19 | HHV types 6 and 7 |
| Rash | Non-itchy, erythematous, maculopapular. Ears face, then trunk and limbs | Pinky red, maculopapular Face, neck then trunk and limbs | Erythematous Neck, trunk and limbs | Network pattern limbs and trunk | Pink papules. Maculopapular. Non-itchy |
| Diagnostic features | Prodromal symptoms. Cough. Koplik's spots | Occipital and posterior cervical glands | Sore throat Cervical glands Circumoral pallor Strawberry tongue Late peeling of the skin | Red hot cheeks Not 'ill' | Rash preceded by high fever 3–5 days Fever settles when rash appears |
| Diagnosis | Salivary swab | Serology | Throat swab ASOT | Clinical, serology if necessary | Clinical |
| Complications | Diarrhoea, dehydration Conjunctivitis Otitis media Encephalitis (rare) Heamorrhagic measles (rare) | Joint pains Congenital rubella syndrome | Rheumatic fever Otitis media Chest infection Nephritis Osteomyelitis Septicaemia | Rare Arthritis Aplastic crisis Intrauterine death Hydrops foetalis | Febrile convulsions Multisystem problems in immunocompromised |
| Management | Symptomatic Watch for complications | Symptomatic | Penicillin V or erythromycin for 10 days | Symptomatic | Symptomatic |

From: Health Protection Agency, 2007b

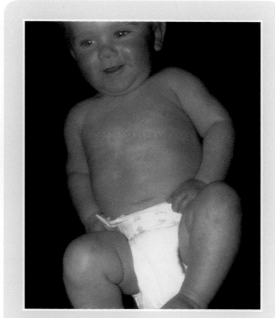

*Figure 29.10. Roseola infantum*

treatment (HPA, 2007b) (*Table 29.1*). Scarlet fever is a notifiable disease.

### Clinical presentation

Patients suddenly develop a fever, sore throat and enlarged cervical glands. The patient may feel unwell with headache, abdominal pain and vomiting In the next few days an erythematous rash appears, starting on the neck and below the ears, before spreading to the rest of the body. On the face the area around the mouth is pale (circumoral pallor) (*Figure 29.5*). The throat is inflamed and there may be exudate on the tonsils (*Figure 29.6*). The tongue is swollen, coated with prominent red papilla (white strawberry tongue) (*Figure 29.7*) The temperature gradually settles and after about 6 days, the rash fades and the skin peels (DermNetNZ, 2007c).

### Diagnosis

Diagnosis of scarlet fever can usually be made on the history and findings on examination. A throat swab sent for culture and sensitivities should confirm the presence of group A β-haemolytic *Streptococcus*. In the acute phase of the illness this is probably all that is necessary to confirm the diagnosis, but and antistreptolysin O test (ASOT) will demonstrate a recent group A streptococcal infection if a raise titre is found (*Table 29.2*).

### Complications

With treatment, complications are less likely to occur but untreated, the patient risks problems of rheumatic fever, otitis media, pneumonia, nephritis, osteomyelitis or septicaemia. Fatal results may ensue.

### Management

Treatment with penicillin V or if allergic to penicillin, erythromycin, for 10 days should clear the condition and reduce the risks of complications (Joint Formulary

Committee, 2007: Section 5.1). Otherwise symptomatic treatment with fluids, paracetamol and antihistamines or calamine lotion, if troubled by itchiness of the rash.

## Fifth disease
### Aetiology

Fifth disease, or erythema infectiosum, is a common infection that generally affects young children. It is caused by parovirus B19 and is spread by droplets from the respiratory tract. Outbreaks of the condition tend to occur in the late winter and early spring. The incubation period from the time of contact with the disease and its development is 4–18 days and school exclusion is not recommended because exclusion is ineffective, as transmission occurs before the patient is unwell (HPA, 2007b). Fifth disease is a mild condition with few complications, except occasionally in pregnancy. About 60% of adults are seropositive for parovirus B19 if tested. Many will be unaware of having had the disease (Zellmann, 2007).

### Clinical presentation

The main presenting symptom of Fifth's disease is hot red cheeks (*Figure 29.8*). Within a few days a network pattern of rash will develop on the limbs and then the trunk (*Figure 29.9*). The rash may persist intermittently for up to 6 weeks. The child usually remains well and apparently unaffected by the condition.

### Diagnosis

The diagnosis should be obvious from the history and signs found on examination. If necessary, as in the case of an exposed pregnant woman, a blood test can be done. If the result is seropositive for parovirus B19, it would suggest either present or past infection.

### Complications

Fifth disease rarely causes any problems. Occasionally adults might experience problems with arthritis and if the patient has a blood disorder, he/she might suffer an aplastic crisis. If it occurs in pregnancy, it does not seem to be associated with any congenital malformations, but intrauterine death or hydrops foetalis have occurred in the first half of pregnancy (DermNet NZ, 2007a).

### Management

Fifth disease is a mild condition that usually resolves spontaneously without treatment.

## Roseola infantum
### Aetiology

Roseola infantum is a common infection of childhood caused by human herpes virus (HHV) types 6 and 7. The infection is spread by droplets from the respiratory tract and affects young children between the ages of 6 months and 3 years of age. It rarely occurs in adults and it is thought that lifelong immunity results following infection. The incubation period from the time of contact with a sufferer is 10–15 days, but no quarantine period is recommended as the disease is not serious (HPA, 2007b).

## Clinical presentation

The child may initially present with sudden onset of a high fever, which persists for about 3–5 days with no other specific symptoms. As the fever subsides, the child will develop generalized pink papules or maculopapular non-itchy rash. It starts on the trunk, but may spread to face, neck and limbs (*Figure 29.10*) and fades over the following 2–3 days. Symptoms may be marked, as described, or minimal (DermNet NZ, 2006).

## Diagnosis

The diagnosis should be possible purely from the history and physical signs.

## Complications

Febrile convulsions may occur in the early stages of infection, when the child has a high temperature. However, almost without exception, the prognosis in roseola infantum is excellent, provided the child is immunocompetent. Immunocompromized children, however, may suffer rare multisystem complications involving the gastrointestinal system, central nervous system of the blood (White and Gorman, 2007).

## Management

Symptomatic treatment only is required for this condition with tepid sponging, paracetamol and plenty of fluids.

## References

Borton C (2007) Measles www.patient.co.uk/showdoc/40000391 (accessed 12 December 2007)

Centers for Disease Control and Prevention (2007) Rubella: Diagnosis. http://tinyurl.com/2tmzrb (accessed 12 December 2007)

DermNet NZ (2006) Roseola. http://dermnetnz.org/viral/roseola.html (accessed 12December 2007)

DermNet NZ (2007a) Fifth disease. http://dermnetnz.org/viral/fifth.html (accessed 12 December 2007)

DermNet NZ (2007h) Measles. http://dermnetnz.org/viral/morbilli.html (accessed 12December 2007)

DermNet NZ (2007c) Scarlet fever. http://dermnetnz.org/bacterial/scarlet-fever.html (accessed 12December 2007)

Health Protection Agency (2010) HPA Measles Guidelines http://hpa.org.au/topics/infectiousdiseasesAZ/measles (accessed 30 July 2010)

Health Protection Agency (2007a) Measles deaths—England and Wales, By Age Group, 1980–2006. http://tinyurl.com/3dlt47 (accessed 12 December 2007)

Health Protection Agency (2007b) Guidelines on the Management of Communicable diseases in Schools and Nurseries. http://tinyurl.com/2mem89 (accessed 12December 2007)

Joint Formulary Committee (2007) *British National Formulary* 54. September. BMJ Publishing Group Ltd and RPS Publishing, London

Lombardo C (2007) Rubella. *eMedicine*. www.emedicine.com/derm/topic380.htm (accessed 12December 2007)

Medline Plus (2007) Congenital Rubella. Medical Encyclopedia. http://tinyurl.com/2qnz53 (accessed 12 December 2007)

White S and Gorman C (2007) Roseola Infantum. *eMedicine*. www.emedicine.con/derm/topic378.htm (accessed 12December 2007)

Zellmann G (2007) Erythema Infectiosun (Fifth Disease). *eMedicine*. www.emedicine.com/derm/topic136.htm (accessed 12December 2007)

## Test Your Knowledge

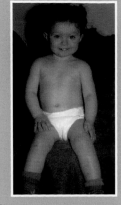

Jamie is 3 years old. His mother was concerned because she had noticed a slight maculopapular rash that morning. It had started on his face and was now spreading to the trunk and limbs. Jamie was only slightly 'off colour', with a low grade fever, but quite cheerful and happy in himself. His mother was particularly worried as she was 8 weeks pregnant and concerned that the problem might be contagious and affect the baby.

### Questions

1. What is the possible diagnosis?
2. What other signs would you look for to confirm it?
3. How would you discuss the problem with the mother and how could you help to confirm or refute her concerns?

# Red and spotty faces

Patients with blemishes on their faces tend to seek advice early. They are usually embarrassed by their problem and upset by the kindly (or otherwise) remarks of their friends and colleagues. Some of the symptoms that might bring patients to the surgery include spots, pustules or inflammation around the mouth or beard area. Alternatively, these symptoms are often noticed readily by the doctor or nurse when the patient presents.

Frequently the health professional will be able to offer a simple explanation, diagnosis and suggestions for treatment or management that may bring the condition

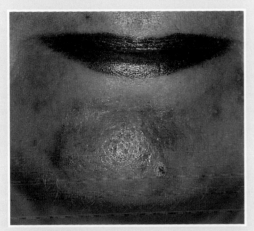

*Figure 30.1. Perioral dermatitis.*

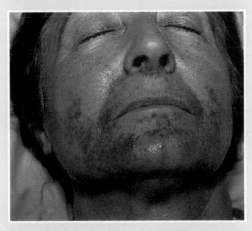

*Figure 30.2. Spreading perioral dermatitis in a woman who had tried to clear it with topical steroids.*

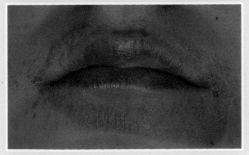

*Figure 30.3. Lip licking dermatitis in a child.*

under control. The following discussion will consider the management of perioral dermatitis, lip-licking dermatitis, sycosis barbae and seborrhoeic dermatitis (*Table 30.1*). Other conditions that may also include these symptoms are acne vulgaris and acne rosacea. These are not discussed here as they have been dealt with in Chapter 31.

## Perioral dermatitis
### Aetiology
Perioral dermatitis is a relatively common condition that occurs most commonly in women and only occasionally in men. The cause of the condition is unknown but it seems to be associated with poor hygiene and failure to adequately wash the face, regular use of face creams, e.g. moisturizers, or the use of make-up or sunscreens (DermNet NZ, 2004a). Another frequent association is the use of topical steroids to the area.

Patients who develop rashes may be prescribed corticosteroid creams or ointments or may decide for themselves that such a preparation is worth trying. They may find that the ointment works but that when they discontinue treatment the condition deteriorates. A return to the application may again control it but the patient may find that he/she requires an increasingly potent steroid to achieve a result, leading to an addictive cycle (Wells and Brodell, 1993).

### Presentation
The patient presents with groups of small, itchy or tender red spots around the mouth (*Figure 30.1*). Sometimes the rash may spread and become more extensive. The skin immediately around the lips is usually spared (*Figure 30.2*).

### Investigations
A diagnosis can normally be made from the appearance of the rash. If there is any suggestion of secondary infection, a swab should be taken from the area or a spot for culture in the laboratory.

### Management
Response to treatment is normally good, providing the patient cooperates with the advice given. The patient should be advised to discontinue the use of all face creams and topical steroids. It must be explained to the patient that the symptoms are likely to temporarily relapse when the steroids are stopped, but that the symptoms will never improve if the patient continues to use steroids (Sneddon, 1976).

Patients should wash the face only with plain water until the condition has cleared. The use of topical metronidazole or erythromycin may be helpful. For more severe or persistent cases, oral oxytetracycline, lymecycline, doxycycline, minocin or erythromycin may be prescribed for a period of 6–12 weeks (Kantor, 2004).

Even where treatment is effective, it is possible that the perioral dermatitis will recur. Recurrences should be addressed by repeating the treatment.

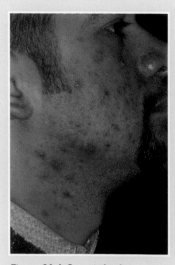
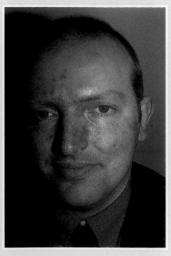

*Figure 30.4. Sycosis barbae.*     *Figure 30.5. Seborrhoeic dermatitis.*

## Lip licking dermatitis

### Aetiology

Lip licking dermatitis is sometimes observed in children who have a persistent habit of licking their lips. Often they suffer with an underlying atopic eczema and it may be regarded as a form of irritant contact dermatitis (Mortimer, 2004). It may also occur in adults, where it is more likely to be caused by an allergy related to the use of cosmetics such as lipstick or toothpaste (Lawrence and Cox, 2002).

### Presentation

The area around the mouth shows eczematous changes of scaling, fissuring and oozing (*Figure 30.3*).

### Investigations

Patch testing may be useful to isolate the offending substance if an allergy is suspected (Mortimer, 2004).

### Management

The patient should be discouraged from licking his/her lips, if possible, and he/she should avoid the use of any suspected allergen. Washing with a soap substitute, e.g. emulsifying ointment, as well as regular and frequent application of emollients or greasy ointments can help the condition.

If necessary, a mild topical steroid ointment may be applied, but preferably for a short time only. It is important to observe the recommendation that medium-strength and potent topical steroids should not be used on the face.

## Sycosis barbae

### Aetiology

Sycosis barbae (*Figure 30.4*) is a deep-seated staphylococcal folliculitis that occurs in the beard area and in men only. In some there may be an association with ingrowing hairs, particularly under the neck. This occurs more commonly in Afro-Caribbean men (du Vivier, 2002: 253–4), and may be aggravated by trauma from shaving (McMorran et al, 2003).

### Presentation

The patient presents with inflamed red and yellow spots and pustules in the beard area, with some inflammation of the surrounding skin. Close inspection may reveal a hair at the centre of each pustule. Sometimes there will be keloid formation as the lesions heal.

### Investigations

A swab for culture and sensitivities should be taken from the pustules and also from the nose, which may be acting as a carrier site (du Vivier, 2002: 644).

### Management

To manage the condition, good hygiene should be observed and the beard should be allowed to grow, especially in cases where there are ingrowing hairs. Oral antibiotics. e.g.

## Table 30.1. Diagnosis and management

| | Perioral dermatitis | Lip licking dermatitis | Sycosis barbae | Seborrhoeic dermatitis |
|---|---|---|---|---|
| **Age/sex** | Adults, usually women | Children Adults (contact dermatitis) | Adult men | After puberty, into old age |
| **Cause** | Topical steroids Poor hygiene Topical creams | Lip licking Contact dermatitis | Staphylococcal Folliculitis | Associated with *Pityrosporum ovale* Stress, illness and some drugs |
| **Presentation** | Small, itchy, tender spots around the mouth | Eczematous changes around the mouth | Inflamed yellow/red spots and pustules in beard area | Symmetrical inflammation, scaling in greasy areas of skin Recurrent and persistent |
| **Investigation** | Swab culture if infection suspected | Patch testing if allergy suspected | Swab pustules and nose for culture and sensitivities | Occasionally skin biopsy or fungal culture |
| **Treatment** | Stop topical steroids Apply topical metronidazole or erythromycin Apply oral tetracycline or erythromycin | Stop licking habit Apply emollients A mild topical steroid initially Wash with emollients Avoid allergen | Improve hygiene Grow the beard Oral flucloxacillin or erythromycin Topical mucopirocin Treat nasal carriers with chlorhexidin with neomycin cream | Topical anti-yeast creams Topical mild steroids Antibiotics for secondary infection If severe: an oral antifungal agent |

erythromycin or flucloxacillin, and topical antibiotics, e.g. mupirocin cream or ointment, may be prescribed (du Vivier, 2002).

Nasal carriers of the infection should be treated with a course of cream containing chlorhexidine and neomycin. This is applied to the nostrils four times daily for 10 days. Resistant cases may require mupirocin (Joint Formulary Committee, 2004: 545).

## Seborrhoeic dermatitis in adults

### Aetiology

Seborrhoeic dermatitis is extremely common. In its mildest form of simple dandruff, it is present in 15–20% of the population and is slightly more common in men (Selden, 2004). It develops after puberty and peaks at around the age of 40 years, but may also occur in the older age groups in greasy and hair-bearing areas of skin. It is associated with the yeast *Pityrosporum ovale* (*Malassezia*), but it is not contagious and appears to be aggravated by emotional stress, poor health and illness, in particular Parkinson's disease and immunological problems such as human immunodeficiency virus (HIV), in which case it tends to be more severe (DermNet NZ, 2004b). It may also be precipitated by certain drugs, e.g. chlorpromazine, cimetidine, gold, lithium and corticosteroids (Selden, 2004).

### Presentation

The patient complains of a symmetrical inflammation of areas of greasy skin. Seborrhoeic dermatitis occurs commonly on the face, in particular, in the nasolabial folds (*Figure 30.5*), on the forehead, eyebrows, behind the ears, in the beard area. There may also be a blepharitis of the eyelids (*Figure 30.6*).

Examination shows areas of greasy scaling that may burn and itch at times. Frequently the scalp is involved. Here symptoms may vary from simple dandruff to thick adherent crusts (*Figure 30.7*). Commonly there are similar changes in the presternal area (*Figure 30.8*) and between the shoulder blades where it is worth looking when seeking confirmation of the diagnosis.

Other sites that may be affected are the intertiginous regions of the axilla, groins and submammary regions. The severity of seborrhoeic dermatitis varies. At times it may be inactive, and then followed by intermittent flares, particularly in the winter months. Problems may persist or recur for years (Selden, 2004).

### Complications

Secondary infection may occur, particularly if the lesions are irritant and the patient scratches (Selden, 2004). *Figure 30.9* shows a patient with seborrhoeic dermatitis and itchy scalp which developed a spreading streptococcal infection (erysipelas) where this had occurred along the line.

### Investigation

Investigation is usually unnecessary. Examination and history of the intermittent symptoms are the usual clues. However, in severe cases a skin biopsy may be necessary or fungal culture should be taken to exclude a fungal infection of the scalp if this is suspected.

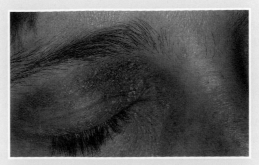

*Figure 30.6. Blepharitis in a patient with seborrhoeic dermatitis.*

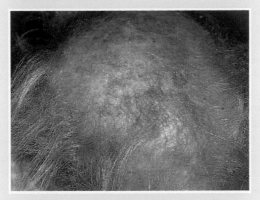

*Figure 30.7. Seborrhoeic dermatitis in the scalp of an adult.*

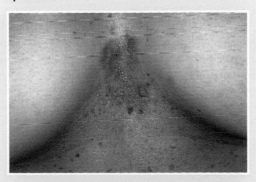

*Figure 30.8. Presternal lesion in a patient with seborrhoeic dermatitis.*

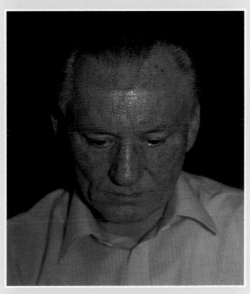

*Figure 30.9. Erysipelas (i.e. secondary infection) in a patient with seborrhoeic dermatitis.*

### Points to consider

It is important to consider that acute and severe seborrhoeic dermatitis may be suggestive of an underlying HIV infection.

Pre-pubertal children with dandruff are unlikely to have seborrhoeic dermatitis but the possibility of tinea capitis (unusual in adults) should be considered.

### Management

The patient should be warned that, although seborrhoeic dermatitis may respond to treatment, it may return when this is discontinued and that it is a condition that naturally comes and goes.

A topical anti-yeast cream or ointment, e.g. ketoconazole or imidazole rubbed into the skin 2–4 times daily for 2–4 weeks, usually settles the condition. For scalp and beard changes, shampoos containing ketoconazole and/or salicylic acid and coal tar are appropriate treatments. Some of these products are available to patients over the counter (Joint Formulary Committee, 2004: 567–72; 580–2).

Topical mild corticosteroids, combined with the use of topical ketoconazole, can be used with success but should be for short-term use only during acute flares. Patients should be warned to avoid the use of any potent steroids on the face (Selden, 2004). Secondary infection requires rapid control with oral antibiotics (Joint Formulary Committee, 2004: 263–305).

Phenoxymethylpenicillin is recommended for streptococcal infection. If a staphylococcal infection is suspected, flucloxacillin should be added. For those allergic to penicillin, erythromycin should be prescribed. In severe cases, an oral anti-fungal agent, e.g. ketoconazole or itraconazole may be used (Joint Formulary Committee, 2004: 305–10).

### References

DermNet NZ (2004a) Perioral dermatitis. www.dermnetnz.org/acne/perioral-dermatitis.html (accessed 9 February 2005)

DermNet NZ (2004b) Seborrhoeic dermatitis. www.dermnetnz.org/dermatitis/seborrhoeic-dermatitis.html (accessed 9 February 2005)

du Vivier A (2002) *Atlas of Clinical Dermatology*. 3rd edn. Churchill Livingstone, London

McMorran S, Prince C, YoungMin S, Pleat J, Wacogne I (2003) Sycosis barbae. In: GP Notebook. www.gpnotebook.com/cache/1449852957.htm (accessed 9 February 2005). Oxbridge Solutions Ltd

Joint Formulary Committee (2004) *British National Formulary 48*. September. British Medical Association and Royal Pharmaceutical Society of Great Britain, London

Kantor J (2004) Perioral dermatitis. In: Medline Plus Medical Encyclopedia. www.nlm.nih.gov/medlineplus/ency/article/001455.htm (accessed 9 February 2005)

Lawrence C, Cox N (2002) *Physical Signs in Dermatology*. 2nd edn. Mosby, London: 82–3

Mortimer J (2004) Facial eczema. National Eczema Society, London. www.eczema.org/Leaflets/facialeczema.PDF (accessed 9 Feb 2005)

Selden S (2004) Seborrhoeic dermatitis. *eMedicine*. www.emedicine.com/derm/topic396.htm (accessed 9 February 2005)

Sneddon IB (1976) The treatment of steroid induced rosacea and perioral dermatitis. *Dermatologica* **152**(Suppl 1): 231–7

Watkins J (2003) Dermatology clinic: *Practice Nursing* **14**(3): 121–6

Wells K, Brodell RT (1993) Topical steroid 'addiction': A cause of perioral dermatitis. *Postgrad Med* **93**(5): 225–30

## Test Your Knowledge

This man attended the surgery complaining of a rash on his chin. It had been present for some weeks and he felt that it was beginning to spread and getting worse. On examination there was a general inflammation of the area, among which were some reddish spots and pustules. He found that he was catching the spots with his razor when shaving and that it was getting sore. He had been applying an antiseptic cream to the area but without effect.

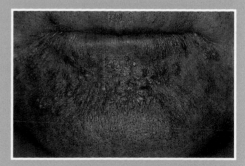

### Questions

1. What is the likely diagnosis and which features would help you come to this conclusion?
2. What investigations would you suggest?
3. What advice and treatment would you give to the patient?

# Acne vulgaris

Few of us find the teenage years easy. On the one hand, the growth from childhood to adult life is full of hopes, dreams and expectations, while on the other, doubts about our abilities and acceptance by those around us are constantly in the background. If we do not look the part and fit in with our peers we may feel rejected and lonely, both in the social world and on the job scene. Any spots and blemishes may leave us feeling conspicuous and embarrassed, particularly if they are on exposed areas such as the face.

Sadly acne most commonly strikes at this time of life. When a patient presents or asks for help, it is important that we take it seriously and listen to their concerns — even though the problem may appear to be a mild one.

The patient needs to know the likely course of the problem, the treatments available to control it and how to reduce the risks of subsequent scarring. If worrying reactions are ignored, in rare cases, the patient may resort to drastic measures. One study found that acne, without primary psychiatric illness, was the presenting symptom in 7 out of 16 cases of suicide (Cotterill and Cunliffe, 1997).

## Aetiology

The actual cause of acne vulgaris (AV) is unknown, but important factors in its development are an increased rate of secretion of sebum, obstruction and inflammation of the pilosebaceous duct and the bacteria *Proprionibacterium acnes* playing an important part. A trigger in acne would seem to be androgens. Often there is a family history of troublesome acne (Pearl et al, 1998).

AV occurs in 80% of teenagers between the ages of 13–18 years, and about a third of these sufferers require treatment because of its severity. In most cases, the condition will clear by the late teens or early 20s, but it will sometimes occur and/or persist in adult life. Sometimes this may be related to the intake of certain drugs or polycystic ovarian syndrome in women (Harper, 2007).

## Presentation

Symptoms of AV may be graded into mild, moderate or severe and should be assessed when deciding on management of each patient, as well as noting the effect that the condition is having in each individual case. Some people may not bother to mention their condition. However, if the nurse sees the signs when the patient is attending the surgery about something else, she/he may be able to offer advice that can improve appearance and perhaps avoid problems of permanent scars in later life.

### Mild acne

Comedones are the significant and early sign of acne vulgaris and may take the form of closed comedones (whiteheads), or open comedones (blackheads). Small inflamed papules and pustules may follow. Lesions occur most commonly on the face (*Figure 31.1*), but are also often seen on the upper chest, arms and back.

### Moderate acne

More lesions develop, with increased numbers of inflamed papules and pustules in the same areas (*Figure 31.2*).

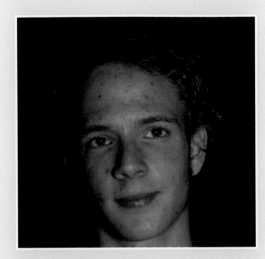

*Figure 31.1. Mild facial acne.*

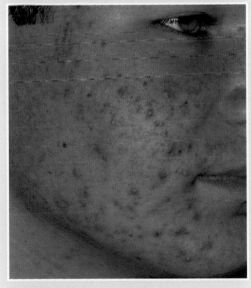

*Figure 31.2. Moderate, pustular acne.*

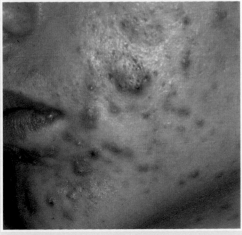

*Figure 31.3. Severe, nodulocystic acne.*

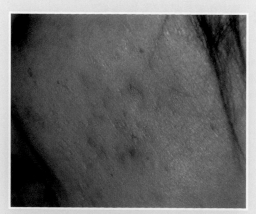

Figure 31.4. Ice pick scars.

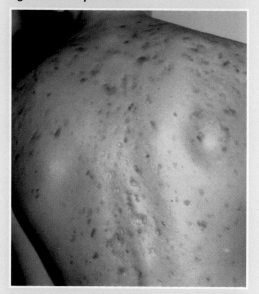

Figure 31.5. Scars resulting from severe
nodulocystic acne in a 17-year-old boy.

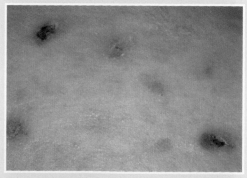

Figure 31.6. Acne excoriée: picked lesions on the
forehead.

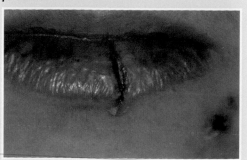

Figure 31.7. Dry, cracked lips in a patient on
systemic isotretinoin.

### Severe acne

Larger inflammatory lesions, nodules and cysts (*Figure 31.3*) develop, and these may well lead to permanent scarring in the form of small, deep pits (ice pick scars) (*Figure 31.4*) or larger deeper pits as can be seen on the back of this 17-year-old boy (*Figure 31.5*). Scars are more likely to arise if the lesions are 'picked' (*acne excoriée*) (*Figure 31.6*).

## Diagnosis

There is rarely any doubt about the diagnosis of AV. The lesions usually start in the teenage years and are typical in their appearance and distribution. Sometimes the condition may be associated with the taking of certain drugs such as steroids, lithium, progesterone, antiepileptics or iodides (Harper, 2007). The need for their use must be considered and alternatives substituted if this is possible.

### Polycystic ovarian syndrome

Polycystic ovarian syndrome may affect up to 10% of women. It is associated with enlarged cystic ovaries and a common cause is an excess of luteinizing hormone by the pituitary gland which, in turn, increases the production of androgens. A triad of symptoms of amenorrrhoea or oligomenorrhoea, hirsutism and acne will suggest the diagnosis. This can be confirmed by checks on the hormone profile and ultrasound examination of the ovaries. The specimen of blood is best collected on the 22nd day of the cycle and if raised levels of luteinising hormone (LH) and androgen are found, the patient will need further advice about this problem (Merck Manual, 2003).

## Management

The main consideration when treating acne is to help to avoid permanent scarring in the future. This must be coupled with the degree of concern that the patient has and how much it is affecting his/her life.

General advice may be given about twice daily antiseptic washes, the application of topical preparations over the whole of the acne area and not just on the individual spots, and a certain amount of sun exposure may be helpful (DermNet NZ, 2008a).

### Mild and moderate acne
### Topical treatment

Acne will often respond well to topical applications, of which benzoyl peroxide, clindamycin, erythromycin and tretinoin have been found to be beneficial. Other preparations such as adapalene, azelaic acid, erythromycin plus zinc or tetracycline (for inflammatory acne), isotretinoin (for comedonal, inflammatory and non-inflammatory acne) are likely to be beneficial but it is contra-indicated in pregnancy and women of child bearing age unless on contraception. If response to benzoyl peroxide is poor, a topical antibacterial should be considered. Some patients using these treatments will complain of skin irritation and scaling, but this may improve if the treatment is continued with lesser frequency (Joint Formulary Committee, 2010: 13.6.1).

### Oral antibiotics

For those with inflammatory lesions that fail to respond to

topical treatment alone, systemic antibiotics may be required. Erythromycin or tetracycline (500 mg twice daily) are most commonly used, but will need to be continued for at least 4–6 months, and in adequate dosage, to gain maximum improvement (Joint Formulary Committee 2008: 13.6.2)

### Hormonal treatment
Cyproterone with ethinylestrodiol is sometimes used in women with acne. It has no great advantages over other treatment, but may be useful for those who also require contraception, providing there are no other contraindications to the pill, such as increased risk of thrombo-embolism (Joint Formulary Committee, 2008: 13.6.2).

### Severe acne
In cases of severe acne or those that have failed to respond to adequate courses of topical and systemic treatments, oral isotretinoin is available, but only on a hospital prescription from a dermatologist. As the drug is teratogenic, careful supervision of the patient is necessary to ensure that the drug is not prescribed if there is any risk of pregnancy. Also, there are a number of possible side effects. In particular, dry mucous membranes and skin may lead to problems of dry, cracking lips (*Figure 31.7*) nose bleeds, and eczema.

As liver function and lipid levels may be affected, it is recommended that liver function and lipid levels should be checked before starting the drug and repeated 3 monthly, so that the drug can be discontinued if changes occur (Joint Formulary Committee, 2008: 13.6.2). There have also been concerns that mood changes with depression and possible suicide may occur.

Over the years there has been much debate about the part isotretinoin might play in this. A recent study has now shown that there is a potential for isotretinoin to reduce the availability of serotonin (5HT). These lower 5HT levels are thought to trigger aggressive behaviour and clinical depression (O'Reilly et al, 2007). Patients and their relatives must be told to be alert to any warning signs in this direction as it may be necessary to discontinue the drug. A course of isotretinoin is given for at least 16 weeks and in many cases the results are remarkable. Often the condition does not recur (DermNet NZ, 2008a). If it does, a further course of treatment may be required.

### Differential diagnosis
Although the diagnosis of AV is usually obvious, there are two other conditions that present with facial rashes with which it may occasionally be confused.

## Rosacea
### Aetiology
Rosacea tends to present later in life, between the ages of 30–50. The cause of rosacea has always been said to be unknown, but it does seem to be aggravated by the use of topical steroids, wind, UV light, certain facial creams, oils and spicy foods. However, studies in California, USA, suggests that the over-production of two interactive inflammatory proteins results in excessive levels of a third (Yamasaki et al, 2007).

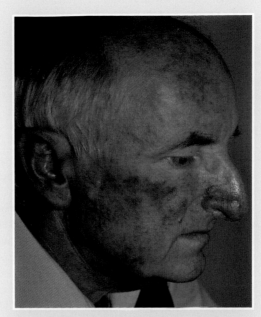

*Figure 31.8. Rosacea: red face, papules and telangiectasia*

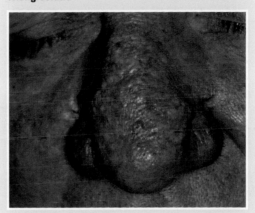

*Figure 31.9. Rhinophyma*

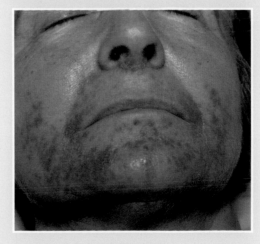

*Figure 31.10. Perioral dermatitis*

### Presentation
As in acne vulgaris, red papules and pustules develop on the nose, cheeks, chin and forehead, but unlike acne, there are no comedones or cystic changes and the chest is not involved. The face becomes persistently flushed and red and telangiectasia appear (*Figure 31.8*). In some, the nose becomes enlarged and thickened with prominent pores, a

state known as rhinophyma (*Figure 31.9*) and the eyes may become inflamed and feel gritty.

## Management

Topical steroids should not be offered to treat as they will aggravate rosacea. Although there may initially appear to be some improvement, it will gain new activity when the steroid is stopped, encouraging all the problems of a vicious circle as a further prescription is offered to control the flare:

- Any aggravating factors should, as far as possible, be avoided and sunscreens applied to the face when out of doors
- Systemic tetracycline antibiotics are most helpful in reducing the inflammation, papules and other symptoms. Tetracycline or erythromycin 500 mg twice daily, doxycycline 100 mg daily, lymecycline or minocycline are often used and should be continued for 6–12 weeks and repeated if recurrences occur. (Joint Formulary Committee, 2008: 13.6)
- Metronidazol cream or gel may be sufficient in mild cases, but more severe cases may require it to be combined with the oral antibiotic. Alternatively, azelaic acid cream or lotion may be useful (Joint Formulary Committee, 2008: 13.6)
- Isotretinoin may be offered by the dermatologist. It may be very effective in stubborn cases or in those who cannot tolerate other treatments. However, if used, it may need to be continued in low doses for a long time and the suitability and risks of side effects or pregnancy must be considered before prescribing

- Clonidine or a non-steroidal anti-inflammatory drug may sometimes be used if flushing is a problem.

*Persistent telangiectasia* can be improved with laser therapy or cautery, while *rhinophyma* may be helped by laser therapy or require referral to a plastic surgeon for surgical reshaping of the nose (Derment NZ, 2008).

## Perioral dermatitis

### Aetiology

The actual cause of perioral dermatitis is unknown, but recent work has suggested that it may be related to the proliferation of bacteria and yeasts in the hair follicles. It tends to occur on greasy skin and is more likely to occur in those who use make-up, moisturizers and sunscreens to the face. A common factor in its cause is the application of steroid creams or ointments to the face (DermNet NZ, 2008b). It nearly always occurs in women and is occasionally seen in children.

### Presentation

The patient develops small papules on the chin. These may spread to the upper lip and cheeks (*Figure 31.10*) and occasionally around the nose and eyes. The immediate area around the lips is spared.

### Management

The response to treatment is usually good and initially it is important to discontinue all topical make-up and moisturizers and in particular topical steroids.

If the steroids are suddenly withdrawn, the condition will flare, but the patient should be reminded that if they do

## Table 31.1. Differential diagnosis of acne vulgaris

| | Acne vulgaris | Polycystic ovaries | Rosacea | Perioral dermatitis |
|---|---|---|---|---|
| **Cause** | Unknown<br>Factors:<br>• increased sebum secretion<br>• Obstruction pilosebaceous duct<br>• Proprionibactrerium acnes<br>• Androgen<br>• Drug intake e.g. steroids, lithium, antiepileptics, progesterone, iodides | Enlarged cystic ovaries<br>Increased androgens | Unknown<br>Aggravated by topical steroids, wind, UV light, facial creams, spicy foods | Unknown<br>Possible proliferation of bacteria and yeasts in hair follicles<br>Associated with greasy skin, make-up, topical steroids |
| **Age** | 13–18 years and some into adulthood | Affects 10% of women | 30–50 year | Ususally women, occasionally children |
| **Presentation** | • Mild - comedones, small papules and pustules on face, upper chest, back and arms<br>• Moderate - More inflamed papules<br>• Severe-large nodules, cysts,scars | Amennorrhoea, oligomenorrhoea<br>Hirsutism<br>Acne | Papules, and pustules on cheeks, nose, forehead, chin<br>Flushed, red face<br>No comedones<br>Telangiectasia<br>Rhinophyma | Small papules chin—spread to upper lip and cheeks |
| **Investigation** | Unnecessary | Hormone profile—Day 22 cycle<br>Ultrasonography ovaries | Unnecessary | Unnecessary |
| **Management** | Mild - Topical, e.g. benzoyl benzoate, clinsamycin, erythromycin, tretinoin<br>Moderate-oral antibiotics - tetracycline,erythromycin 500 mg twice daily 4–6 months<br>Cyproterone with oestradiol if contraception required<br>Severe—isotretinoin (refer to hospital) | Refer for further advice | Stop aggravating factors<br>Oral tetracycline or erythromycin<br>Metronidazole cream<br>Clonidine (for flushing)<br>Telangiectasia—laser therapy<br>Rhinophyma—laser therapy or surgery | Stop all aggravating factors<br>Oral antibiotics–tetracycline 6–12 weeks<br>Topical-erythromycin, clindamycin or metronidazole<br>Azelaic acid—OK in pregnancy |

not stop it, the problem will be worse and more difficult to clear later. Occasionally it is necessary to apply the steroid less frequently and with less potent preparations so that the strength of the steroid is gradually reduced.

Rosacea normally responds well to a course of oral antibiotics for a 6–12 week period. Oxytetracycline, minocycline or lymecycline are normally used. If it recurs at a later date, a further course of treatment may be necessary. Topical antibiotics such as erythromycin, clindamycin of metronidazole are sometimes used, but tend to be less effective.

Azelaic acic has the advantage that it may be used in pregnancy (DermNet NZ, 2008b).

## Test Your Knowledge

James was 16. Life was tough. An ambitious boy, taking his GCSE that year, he was hoping for a good future. Recently he had had a few knocks. So-called friends were teasing him and had nicknamed him 'the pox'. Girls seemed to shun him and he had been turned down for a holiday job in the local newsagent as they thought his appearance might 'put people off'. He returned to the surgery begging for something to be done for his severe pustule/cystic acne vulgaris.

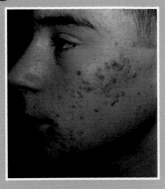

### Questions
1. What treatment would you be considering for his condition?
2. What advice would you have expected to give him before you proceeded to this step?
3. How would you discuss the pros and cons of the suggested new treatment?

## References

British Association of Dermatologists (2007) Acne: Patient information leaflet. BAD, London

Cotterill J, Cunliffe W (1997) Suicide in dermatological patients. *Br J Dermatol* **137**: 246–50

DermNet NZ (2008a) Acne management. http://dermnetnz.org/acne/acne-treatment.html (accessed 17 August 2008)

DermNet NZ (2008b) Perioral dermatitis. http://dermnetnz.org/acne/perioral-dermatitis.html (accessed 17 August 2008)

Harper J (2007) Acne vulgaris, emedicine. www.emedicine.com/DERM/topic2.htm (accessed 17 August 2008)

Joint Formulary Committee (2010) *British National Formulary 55*. March. BMJ Publishing Group Ltd and RPS Publishing, London

Merck Manual (2003) Polycystic ovarian syndrome (PCOS): menstrual disorders and abnormal vaginal bleeding. www.merck.com/mmhe/sec22/ch244/ch244g.html (accessed 17 August 2008)

O'Reilly KC, Trent S, Bailey SJ, Lane MA (2007) *Exp Biol Med* **232**(9): 1195–203. www.skintherapyletter.com/2007/12.10/3.html (accessed 17 August 2008)

Pearl A, ArrollB, Lello J et al (1998) The impact of acne: a study of adolescents' attitudes, perception and knowledge. *NZ Med J* **111**: 269–71

Yamasaki K, Di Nardo A, Bardan A, Murakami M, Ohtake T, Coda A, Dorschner RA, Bonnart C, Descargues P, Hovnanian A, Morhenn VB, Gallo RL (2007) Cause of skin condition rosacea discovered.*Science Daily* www.sciencedaily.com releases/2007/08/070805161110.htm (accessed 17 August 2008)

# Facial swelling

Since the introduction of the measles, mumps and rubella (MMR) vaccine in 1988, the incidence of mumps in young children has dropped dramatically. Notification of the disease in the UK became obligatory in the same year, and since then the numbers numbers reported have remained at only about 2000 a year. Between the years 2003–5 numbers increased to about 8000, mainly in young people over the age of 15 years, probably because this age group were too old to receive MMR when it was first introduced. As a result, this age group missed immunization, or received one dose only, and so lacked adequate protection from mumps (Department of Health (DH), 2005).

Mumps is still, therefore, only too likely to appear in surgeries making it important to be able to recognize the condition and be aware of other diagnoses that might mimic it (*Table 32.1*).

## Mumps
### Aetiology
Mumps is caused by the paromyxovirus and is transmitted by droplet infection. The incubation period is 15–24 days and exclusion from school for 5 days from the onset of mumps is recommended (Great Ormond Street Hospital for Children, 2007). In 20% of people the infection may be asymptomatic (Curtis and Sinert, 2006).

### Clinical presentation
The obvious signs of mumps may be preceded by low-grade fever, headache and muscle pains for up to a couple of days. This is followed by a high temperature and tender swelling of the parotid that may be unilateral or bilateral (*Figure 32.1*). Now that MMR is protecting the young, mumps is more likely to be seen in adults (*Figure 32.2*).

Opening the mouth, eating and swallowing may be painful and the patient may complain of earache and dry mouth. On examination the soft, tender swelling is seen and inflammation and swelling are noted around the orifices of the salivary ducts that drain the affected glands (Curtis and Sinert, 2006). Although it is usually the parotid glands that are affected, sometimes the submaxillary and sublingual salivary glands are involved.

### Diagnosis
The diagnosis can normally be made on clinical grounds, but if necessary, particularly in cases of meningitis without parotitis, a blood test will detect mumps-specific antibodies in the serum or a salivary swab with immunoglobin M (IgM) against mumps will detect it (Mentor authoring team, 2006).

Notification of mumps is required by the Central Public Health Laboratory, Colindale, London. On receipt of the information a salivary test kit will be sent to the surgery. The specimen is returned by post and allows accurate confirmation of the disease (Great Ormond Street Hospital for Children, 2005).

## Table 32.1. Differential diagnosis: facial swelling

|  | Mumps | Dental abscess | Salivary calculus | Tumours | Sarcoidosis |
|---|---|---|---|---|---|
| **Cause** | Paramyxovirus | Infection around tooth | Calculus - blockage of salivary duct | Benign or malignant | Unknown Autoimmune |
| **Presentation** | Prodromal headache low fever - leads to high fever, tender swelling of parotid gland(s) Duct orifices inflamed | Throbbing toothache Unilateral facial swelling Fever Tenderness of affected tooth | Usually >40 years Pain, swelling of gland when eating | Benign >40 years Malignant >60 years Painless lump in salivary gland Malignant: may have facial palsy | Parotid enlargement |
| **Diagnosis** | Serum for specific antibody or salivary swab | Clinical Swab of pus before starting antibiotics X-ray as needed | Clinic X-ray as needed | X-ray as needed, sialogram or ptylagram CT or MRI scan Biopsy | General examination ESR, ACE level Chest X-ray Biopsy |
| **Complications** | Orchitis Aseptic meningitis Deafness Pancreatitis Sontaneous abortion in first trimester | Dental extraction Cellulitis, osteomyelitis or abscess, e.g. brain | Secondary, infection abscess Dental sinus | Benign - good results Malignant - poor outcome if diagnosed late | Often spontaneous resolution Lung damage in 25% of cases chronic disease Fatal outcome occasionally |
| **Management** | Fluids, analgesics Notify Orchitis: scrotal support Admit to hospital if meningitis is suspected | Antibiotics -swab first if pus Refer to dentist Advise on dental hygiene | May pass spontaneously Surgical removal or lithotripsy | Refer any lump present for more than 3 weeks Surgery plus radiotherapy or chemotherapy if malignant | Refer to physician for full assessment Corticosteroids |

ACE = Angio converting enzyme; CT = Computed tomography; ESR Erthrocyte sedimentation rate; MRI = Magnetic resonance imaging

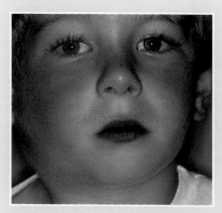

Figure 32.1. Mumps: Boy aged 4 years with parotid swelling.

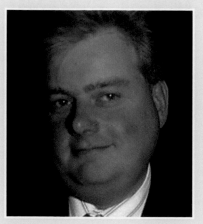

Figure 32.2. Mumps in an adult.

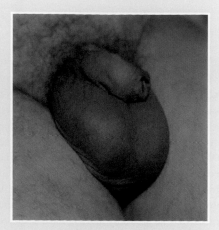

Figure 32.3. Orchitis.

## Complications

### Orchitis

After puberty, males may develop this problem in about 20% of cases. It usually develops about 5 days after the onset of the parotitis and will normally affect one testicle only. Occasionally it is bilateral. Testicular atrophy may follow, but sterility is unlikely. On examination the testicle is swollen, inflamed and tender (*Figure 32.3*). It is important to differentiate mumps orchitis from torsion of the testicle, in which there is no fever nor other symptoms of mumps.

### Aseptic meningitis or encephalitis

Meningitis may occur in 10% of cases of mumps between 3–10 days after the onset of the parotitis. It will normally settle without problems, although the risk of complication from mumps meningitis is greater in adults. Symptoms may include headache, vomiting and neck stiffness. Encephalitis is less common, but may occasionally lead to a fatal outcome or leave long-standing neurological problems. Symptoms may include high fever, fits and drowsiness.

### Deafness

Deafness may occur in about 4% of cases. This is usually unilateral and in most cases will clear spontaneously.

### Pancreatitis

Pancreatitis may occur in 5% of patients with mumps. The patient may complain of upper abdominal pain, nausea and vomiting. It may lead to a rise in the blood sugar level at the time, but as yet the condition has not been proven to result in diabetes mellitus (Curtis and Sinert, 2006).

### Pregnancy

Mumps does not pose any risk to the development of the fetus, but if a woman contracts contracts the disease in the first trimester, there is a risk of spontaneous abortion (Mentor authoring team, 2006).

### Management

Symptomatic treatment only is required for mumps, with paracetamol or ibuprofen to ease pain and a soft/fluid diet to be taken while eating is painful. In orchitis, scrotal support and ice packs may be helpful. If pancreatitis is severe, hospital admission may be necessary so that the patient can receive intravenous fluids; if meningitis or encephalitis is suspected, admission for further investigations to be carried out is necessary (Curtis and Sinert, 2006). Occasionally, if parotitis or orchitis is severe, prednisolone for a few days may help reduce symptoms (Mentor authoring team, 2006).

## Other causes of facial swelling

When a patient presents with a facial swelling, other possible conditions must be considered. The history of the problem, age of the patient and site of the presentation of the lesion must all be considered and differentiated. For example, parotid swelling must be distinguished from enlarged lymph glands.

## Dental abscess

### Aetiology

A dental abscess is associated with tooth decay and caries. Bacterial infection of the tooth may follow and extend to pus formation in the structures around the tooth. Dental caries may occur at any age, but is the most common cause of dental abscess in children. This child (*Figure 32.4*) was a candidate for such a problem. His teeth were affected when he was given a honey-filled dummy to suck as a baby. In the older age groups these problems may occur as the result of years of neglect (*Figure 32.5*). *Bacteroides*, *Fusobacterium*, *Peptostreptococcus* and *Streptococcus viridans* are usually involved (Schneider and Segal, 2007).

### Clinical presentation

The patient complains of toothache, which may be continuous or throbbing in nature, fever and unilateral facial swelling. This boy (*Figure 32.6*) had toothache and the left side of his face had become increasingly swollen in the previous 12 hours. His temperature registered 38.5°C. On examination there may be tenderness when pressure is exerted on the affected tooth. In more severe cases the patient may have difficulty in swallowing or fully opening the mouth.

## Diagnosis

The signs and symptoms of dental abscess usually make the diagnosis obvious and no further investigations are required. If the condition is associated with a cellulitis, a blood culture and a swab of localized pus should be taken for culture and sensitivities, before any antibiotic is administered. The dentist may require X-ray to further elucidate the problem.

## Complications

A patient with a dental abscess may need the tooth to be extracted. However, in many cases the dentist will be able to deal with the problem and preserve it. Other problems that may occur are related to the infection spreading to surrounding tissues, causing a cellulitis, osteomyelitis or more wide-spread infection to the brain (brain abscess), heart (endocarditis) or lungs. More chronic problems may occur if fistulae develop between the mouth and the skin, forming a dental sinus. The first sign of this may be a small 'dimple', pimple or ulcer that discharges from time to time.

These occur most commonly in the submandibular or submental region (*Figure 32.7*), but will sometimes be seen on the face. It is often the case that patients and professionals, fail to recognize the connection between such lesions and the teeth. Finally, recurrence of a dental abscess is likely if the initial infection is not adequately dealt with.

## Management

In the primary health care setting the professional, GP or nurse dealing with a dental abscess will offer antibiotics to settle the infection, and recommend the patient to contact the dentist straight away so that he/she can take over the management of the case. Warm, salt water mouth rinses may be helpful and analgesics are required to ease the pain. The dentist will be able to drain the abscess or extract the offending tooth as necessary. Sometimes, the tooth may be preserved by root canal therapy.

For the future, the patient must be advised regarding oral hygiene and dental care, including regular brushing of teeth with a fluoride toothpaste and the use of dental floss.

## Salivary calculi

### Aetiology

Stones may form in one of the ducts of a salivary gland causing an obstruction to the flow of saliva through the gland. The glands that may be affected are the parotid, sub-mandibular or sublingual glands. The problem is most common in men and those over the age of 40 years, but the reason for the formation of theses calculi, which usually consist of calcium, is unknown. They do not appear to be associated with any other medical condition and serum calcium levels are normal (Patient UK, 2008). A single stone may be present or as many as 8–10.

### Clinical presentation

The patient complains of pain and swelling of the affected gland associated with eating at a time when saliva is produced to lubricate and bind ingested food, assist taste and oral hygiene, and initiate starch digestion (Bowen, 2006). The pain and swelling then gradually subside.

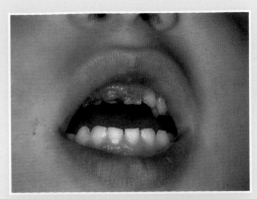

*Figure 32.4. Dental caries in a child.*

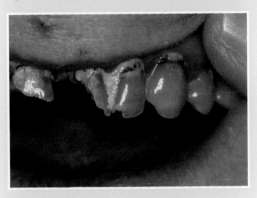

*Figure 32.5. Dental caries in an adult.*

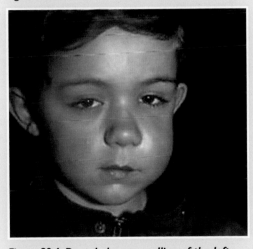

*Figure 32.6. Dental abscess: swelling of the left side of the face.*

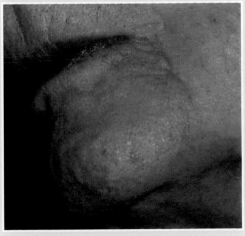

*Figure 32.7. Sub-mandibular dental sinus.*

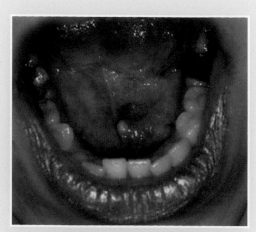

*Figure 32.8. Stone in the orifice of the submandibular gland.*

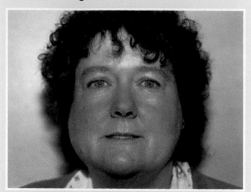

*Figure 32.9. Bilateral parotitis in a patient with sarcoidosis.*

Sometimes, if the blockage is not complete, these symptoms may be modified with variable pain and/or swelling of the gland. Occasionally, the patient will be symptomless and the stone only discovered when an X-ray of the area is performed for some other reason. On examination, a stone may sometimes be seen, and felt at the orifice of the duct (*Figure 32.8*).

### Diagnosis
Often there is no need to pursue any other investigations if the diagnosis is obvious. If necessary, X-ray or CT scan may be required to accurately locate the stone(s).

### Complications
Sometimes the gland becomes infected causing pain and inflammation. Occasionally, an abscess may form. The patient will then be unwell with a fever.

### Management
If a small stone is passed spontaneously, no other treatment will be necessary, but usually it will be necessary to remove it surgically or use lithotripsy to break up the stone

## Salivary gland tumours
### Aetiology
Tumours of the salivary glands are not common, affecting only about 1–2 out of 100 000 (Mentor Authoring Team, 2007). The tumours may be benign or malignant, with the former tending to present after the age of 40 years, while malignant tumours tend to occur later in life, after 60 years. Any of the salivary glands may be affected and there is an increased occurrence of malignant tumours in those who have previously received radiation to the neck.

### Clinical presentation
A tumours of the salivary glands presents as a discrete, painless lump in the gland, which grows slowly. If the swelling is associated with a facial palsy, the lesion is more likely to be malignant. Depending on the site of the tumour, some patients will suffer pain and occasionally there will be other symptoms such as difficulty in swallowing, hoarseness or nasal obstruction if the tumour extends to affect these parts. It is important that any lump involving a salivary gland or neck that persists for longer than 3 weeks is fully checked.

### Diagnosis
Once a salivary tumour is suspected, an X-ray of the gland (sialogram or ptylagram) should be carried out, and a CT or MRI scan done to locate the mass and exclude the possibility that it may have spread to lymph nodes. A fine needle biopsy of the lesion will confirm whether the lesion is benign or malignant.

### Complications
Spread of the malignancy to lymph nodes or other parts of the body is likely to occur where malignancy is diagnosed late. Caught early (Stage I), the 10-year survival rate is 83%, but later (Stage III) it is only 32% (Mentor authoring team, 2007). Facial palsy is not only associated with a malignant tumour, but may also result from surgery.

### Management
Where possible, surgery is the first approach to treat a benign tumour and should result in complete removal of the tumour and no recurrence. More extensive surgery is required for malignant tumours as well as radiotherapy. Chemotherapy may also be used although response is generally poor.

## Sarcoidosis
### Aetiology
The cause of sarcoidosis is as yet unknown, but it affects the immune system so that the patient is immunocompromised (Dermnet NZ, 2007; Perry. 2007). It tends to occur in young adults between the ages of 20–40 years and is more common in women than in men. It is a condition that may affect many organs of the body, including the skin, lungs and other major organs of the body. In 10% of cases, it affects the parotid gland (Mentor authoring team, 2007). In this multi-system, disease-scattered granulomatous lesions occur.

### Clinical presentation
The lungs are most commonly affected by sarcoidosis, and the changes that occur may pass unnoticed for years. If the head, neck or skin are affected, patients tend to present these more obvious symptoms early. This patient had bilateral swelling of the parotids and on further

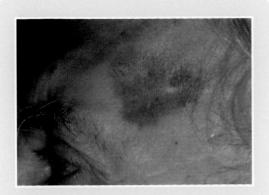

*Figure 32.10. Skin lesion in sarcoid.*

## Management

Referral to a physician will be necessary to investigate and confirm the diagnosis and assess the extent of the disease. Treatment with corticosteroids is the first line of approach. Topical steroids may suffice for skin lesions. Treatment may have to continue for many years as a relapse is likely if the drug is discontinued.

## References

Bowen R (2006) *Salivary glands and Saliva.* http://biology.about. com/library/organs/blpathodigest3.htm (accessed 9 April 2008)

Curtis K, Sinert R (2006) *Mumps - emedicine.* www.emedicine. com/emerg/topic324.htm (accessed 3 April 2008)

De Jong A (1995) *Otolaryngoligic Manifestations of Sarcoidosis.* Baylor College of Medicine. www.bcm.edu/oto/grand/3995.html (accessed 3 April 2008)

Department of Health (2005) Mumps - general information. http://194.74.226.162/infections/topics_az/mumps/gen_info.htm (accessed 3 April 2008)

Dermnet NZ (2007) *Sarcoidosis.* www.dermnetnz.org/dermal-infiltrative/sarcoidosis.html (accessed 3 April 2008)

Health Protection Agency (2005) *Mumps: Guidance for Healthcare Professionals.* www.fam-english.demon.co.uk/s/ NewsLetters/2005/MumpsGuidanceFinal.pdf (accessed 3 April 2008)

Great Ormond Street Hospital for Children (2007) *Nursery World. Quarantine (infectious diseases).* www.ich.ucl.ac.uk/gosh_families/advice_and_support/nursery_world/q/quarantine.html (accessed 9 April 2008)

Mentor authoring team (2007) Salivary gland disorders. Patient UK. http://www.patient.co.uk/showdoc/40000981/ (accessed 3 April 2008)

Mentor authoring team (2007) Salivary gland tumours. Patient UK. http://www.patient.co.uk/showdoc/40002085/ (accessed 3 April 2008)

Mentor authoring team (2006) *Mumps.* www.patient.co.uk/ showdoc/40024613/ (accessed 3 April 2008)

Patient UK (2008) Salivary stones (salivary calculi). www.patient. co.uk/showdoc/23069166/ (accessed 3 April 2008)

Schneider K, Segal G (2007) Dental Abscess, 2. *emedicine.* www. emedicine.com/ped/topic2675.htm (accessed 3 April 2008)

investigation was found to have sarcoidosis (De Jong, 1995) (*Figure 32.9*).

## Diagnosis

The diagnosis of sarcoidosis can be confirmed after full physical examination, erythrocyte sedimentation rate (ESR), angiotensin converting enzyme (ACE) level, serology and chest X-ray, and biopsy of lesions. A biopsy was taken from this persistent, thickened, darker patch on the forehead and sarcoidosis was confirmed (*Figure 32.10*).

## Complications

Many cases of sarcoidosis resolve spontaneously without further recurrence. However, in about 25% of cases the patient may be left with permanent damage to the lungs and/or a chronic form of the disease. In 5–10% of cases, if vital organs are involved, a fatal outcome may ensue.

## Test Your Knowledge

This elderly woman had been in pain for at least 2 days. In the last 24 hours, the right side of her face had become red and swollen. She was sitting in the chair, head in hands and moaning at the intensity of the severe, throbbing pain. She lived alone and seemed confused by her situation.

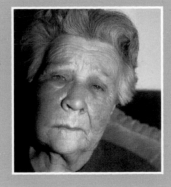

### Questions

1. What is the most likely diagnosis?
2. What signs would you look for that might confirm your suspicions?
3. How would you manage the case?

# Alopecia 1:
# Non-scarring forms

Our hair is said to be 'our crowning glory'. Whether we like it or not, it is there for all to see. Good comments may make us feel good, adverse remarks may cause embarrassment and upset. Changes in hair growth and alopecia may be hard to hide and so there may be considerable distress at the onset of any obvious hair loss. Even a small patch of alopecia may lead to anxieties not only about the current loss but fears that the condition may extend and/or never recover.

In the natural course of things, we continually lose hair. The majority of our hair is normally at the growing, anagen (growth) phase which may last from 2–3 years (*Table 33.1*). The catagen (transition) phase follows and lasts 2–3 weeks before entering the telogen (shedding) phase that, at any one time, affects 10–14% of the hair. During the telogen phase the hair is 'resting' and waiting to be shed. The normal rate of loss from the scalp is about 125 hairs a day and should have no appreciable effect on the general appearance. It is when there is excessive loss that baldness becomes obvious.

This chapter will consider non-scarring alopecia, which in some cases may be reversible, either spontaneously or with the help of medication. Non-scarring alopecia includes male pattern baldness, alopecia areata, some forms of trauma, ringworm, psoriasis and as a side effect of drugs or radiotherapy.

## Male pattern baldness: Androgenic alopecia
### Aetiology

Male pattern baldness (MPB) (androgenic alopecia) is due to a genetically inherited sensitivity to the effects of dihydrotestosterone (DHT), the production of which is regulated by the enzyme 5-alpha reductase. DHT is thought to shorten the anagen phase of the cycle and lead to the production of finer hairs. Hair follicles undergo a process of miniaturization. MPB is extremely common and affects about 50% of men at some time in their lives (Feinstein, 2009). Although this type of alopecia usually occurs in men, women may also be affected but generally to a lesser degree, with a generalized thinning of the hair (Feinstein, 2009) (*Figure 33.1*).

### Presentation

MPB may first be noticed in the mid-twenties with a receding hair line, particularly at the frontotemporal area. A further patch of receding hair may develop at the crown followed by more generalized spread (*Figure 33.2*) and complete baldness in 15% of cases (du Vivier, 2002).

### Management

Many accept baldness as a part of life and do not feel it necessary to seek advice. For some it may cause severe problems of poor self-esteem and depression. All patients

| Table 33.1. Cycle of hair growth | |
|---|---|
| **Anagen phase** | Stage of hair growth at rate of 0.4 mm/day<br>Lasts 2–3 years (occasionally much longer)<br>Affects up to 90% of the hair at any one time |
| **Catagen phase** | Transition stage<br>Affects 1–2% of the hair at any one time |
| **Telogen phase** | Stage at which hair is shed<br>Lasts approximately 3 months<br>Affects 10–14% of hair |

From: Alaiti, 2007.

should be reminded that alopecia leaves the scalp more vulnerable to sun damage and its possible consequences. Sunscreen and the wearing of a hat should reduce this risk.

### Minoxidil

Some time ago, patients taking minoxidil tablets for hypertension noticed regeneration of hair growth. Later it was found that applying topical minoxidil to the scalp had the same effect, after a period of 3–4 months (Feinstein, 2009). The disadvantage of minoxidil is that, if discontinued, the alopecia returns to its previous state within a few months. Also it may cause problems such as dermatitis or change of hair colour (Joint Formulary Committee, 2009: 13.9)

### Finasteride

Finasteride is now licensed for the treatment of MPB but beneficial changes are not felt for 3–6 months and alopecia reverts to its previous state within 6–12 months when discontinued (Joint Formulary Committee, 2009: 13.9).

### Hair transplantation

MPB may be managed with hair transplantation under local anaesthetic but may require several sessions. Surviving

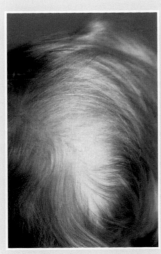

*Figure 33.1. Diffuse alopecia.*

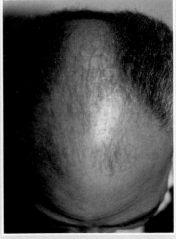

*Figure 33.2. Male pattern baldness.*

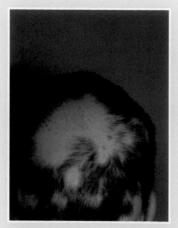

Figure 33.3. Alopecia areata.

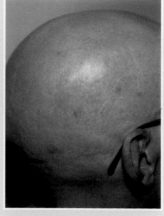

Figure 33.4. Alopecia totalis.

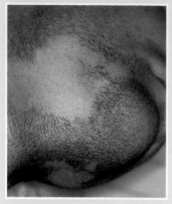

Figure 33.5. Alopecia areata (beard).

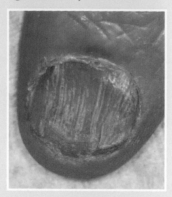

Figure 33.6. Alopecia areata
(nail with longitudinal ridging).

follicles are taken from the sides or back of the head and relocated to the bald area. Beneficial results are not immediate. Hair from the graft initially 'falls out' and regrowth does not follow for 1–3 months after the procedure. Complications such as infection, bleeding, paraesthesia or scarring at the donor site may occur. Also, the underlying balding process is likely to continue (Ngan, 2007). Some patients may be satisfied but the procedure is not available on the NHS. The use of wigs is a safe alternative, which may have good effect for the patient.

## Alopecia areata
### Aetiology
Alopecia areata (AA) affects between 0.1–0.2% of the population. It may occur at any age and either sex, including children (Safavi, 1992). It is thought to be an auto-immune disorder in which cytokines are released from lymphocytes around hair follicles. These cause the hair to be rejected. Patients with AA are more liable to develop other auto-immune problems such as pernicious anaemia, vitiligo or systemic lupus erythematosus (SLE). The fact that other members of the same family may have suffered AA or some other auto-immune disease suggests that there is a hereditary factor. Stress often seems to be a factor in the development of AA (Bolduc et al, 2008).

### Presentation
The extent and site of the alopecia may vary from a small, localized patch or patches (*Figure 33.3*) to complete loss of

hair on the scalp (alopecia totalis) (*Figure 33.4*) or loss of all body hair (alopecia universalis). Sometimes there is patchy loss in the beard area (*Figure 33.5*) or the eyebrows. The scalp appears normal on examination but 'exclamation-mark hairs' that are narrower near the base, can often be seen. There may be re-growth in some areas with hair still being lost in others. In 10–50% of cases, nail changes with pitting and longitudinal ridging may occur (*Figure 33.6*) and pterygium (Dermnet NZ, 2008).

### Management
There is usually little doubt about the diagnosis but if necessary dermoscopy may show the presence of yellow dots, that are a specific feature of AA. In about half of cases, hair will re-grow, without interference, within 1 year. In the majority of other cases there will eventually be re-growth but in about 10% of cases there will be no re-growth (Bolduc et al, 2008). A sign of recovery is the appearance of white or grey hair in the patches as the hair is re-growing, before it reverts to its previous colour. Poor prognostic features are the onset at a very young age, extensive hair loss or alopecia totalis, a previous episode of the condition or patients with asthma or atopic eczema (Dermnet NZ, 2008).

### Steroids
Intralesional steroids speed re-growth of the hair but are of limited value as they will only benefit the area injected and will not prevent further loss in other areas. Topical steroids may be particularly helpful in children. Minoxidil and some irritants such as dithranol may sometimes help but are likely to produce only temporary benefits (Bolduc et al, 2008). The greatest success may be achieved by stimulating an allergic contact dermatitis with an immunological agent such as diphencyprone (DPCP) but reactions may be quite severe and the health professional is at risk of also reacting to the preparation unless extreme care is taken (Bolduc et al, 2008).

## Trauma: Traction alopecia
### Aetiology
Culture or fashion may dictate hairstyles. For those that choose to use a style that persistently exerts a strong pulling force on the scalp hair, alopecia may develop at that site (Hantash and Schwartz, 2009) (*Figure 33.7*).

### Presentation
Regular braiding of hair leads to bald areas between the plaits. Pony-tails, both in men and women may also have the same effect.

### Management
Unless the problem is spotted early, traction hair loss will be permanent. Patients should, therefore, be advised to alter their hairstyle and warned of the likely results if they do not, and be informed that no treatment helps once the alopecia is fully developed.

## Trichotillomania
### Aetiology
Trichotillomania is a self-inflicted problem in which the

patient pulls or cuts the hair leaving bald patches. It is most common in women or teenage girls and may be associated with problems of anxiety, depression or psychosis (Chull-Wan, 2008).

### Presentation

Complaints are of hair loss and/or alopecia. Patients usually deny that they are the cause of their problem, and patients often say it happens in their sleep. Some will twiddle their hair while reading or watching the TV.

On examination, the patches tend to be small, single or multiple, with a geometric shape and no evidence of scarring. Broken and newly grown hairs may be seen within the area (Chull-Wan, 2008) (*Figure 33.8*).

### Management

Patients tend to be very resistant to any ideas of a psychological cause of their problem. The patient must be tactfully approached and the health professional must aim to establish a good relationship with the patient and help him/her to feel confident to discuss any problems he/she may have. Medication seems to offer little help, although a few patients may be helped by an antidepressant (e.g. selective serotonin reuptake inhibitor).

If and when the patient is ready, cognitive behavioural therapy seems to offer the best hope of success (Chull-Wan, 2008).

## Infection: Tinea capitis
### Aetiology

Tinea capitis (ringworm of the scalp) is caused by a dermatophyte fungus affecting the scalp (*Figure 33.9*). A number of different species may be involved, the most common being *Microsporum canis*, usually passed on from an infected cat or dog. It is seen most often in children but does occasionally occur in adults (DermNet NZ, 2007).

### Presentation

Patients notice hair loss. The scalp is either smooth or scaly with hairs broken off at the surface. In some there may be a dry scaling, while in others yellow crusts and matted hair will occur. Occasionally it may present with an abscess-like inflamed mass (DermNet NZ, 2007).

### Investigations

In cases caused by certain fungi, including *M. canis*, there is a green fluorescence under Wood's light. However, this is not positive for all, as some species do not fluoresce. Further confirmation can be made by microscopy and culture of skin scrapings or hair pulled out from the roots (DermNet NZ, 2007).

### Management

An oral antifungal agent such as terbinafine for 4 weeks is the preferred treatment for tinea capitis (DermNet NZ, 2007). Occasionally topical terbinafine cream may be sufficient for a small, localized patch or be added to the oral treatment for greater effect (Joint Formulary Committee, 2008: 5.2). It is also important to check any animals that may have been in contact with the individual and to get

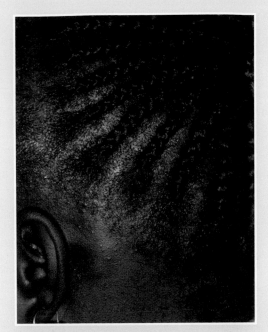

*Figure 33.7. Traction alopecia.*

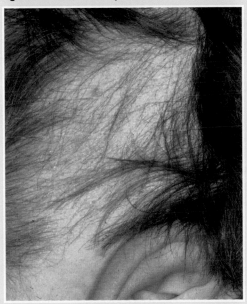

*Figure 33.8. Trichotillomania.*

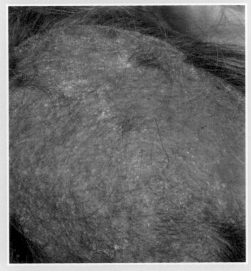

*Figure 33.9. Tinea capitis.*

## Table 33.2. A summary of non-scarring alopecia

| | Aetiology | Presentation | Management |
|---|---|---|---|
| **Androgenic alopecia** | Genetically inherited sensitivity to effects of dihydrotestosterone (DHT) Common in men | Receding hair line, bald patch at crown More generalized hair loss Total alopecia, scalp normal Women—usually just hair-thinning | Protect scalp from sun damage Minoxidil cream, finasteride Hair transplantation, wigs |
| **Alopecia areata** | Affects men and women. Occurs at all ages. Cytokines around hair follicles leads to rejection of hair Autoimmune disorder Possible hereditary factor | Small localized patch(es). Total alopecia, loss of all body hair. Patchy loss of beard, eyebrows. Exclamation mark hairs Nails—pitting, longitudinal ridging Grey/white hair heralds re-growth Scalp normal | 50% resolve in 1 year; 10% no re-growth. Poorer prognosis in the very young, extensive hair loss, recurrent cases or atopics. Intralesional steroids, topical steroids or minoxidil. Irritants, e.g. dithranol Immunological agents (DPCP). Wigs |
| **Trauma** | *Traction alopecia*: hair-style; *Trichotillomania*: hair-twiddling or psychological | Balding areas where hair is pulled or plaited | Advise about hairstyle, permanent if not changed. Counselling, Serotonin uptake drug occasionally |
| ***Tinea capitis*** | Dermatophyte fungal scalp infection Usually affects children | Hair loss, scalp smooth or scaly. Broken hairs, scaling, rusting, matted hair, occasional abscess-like mass | Woods light: green fluorescence if *microsporum canis*. Microscopy/culture skin-scraping. Oral antifungal agent. Topical if small area or added to oral treatment ung cocois co to lift scale |
| **Psoriasis** | One manifestation of psoriasis | Silvery/white scaly patches on reddish scalp. Dandruff, occasionally itchy, hair loss *Pityriasis amientacea*: thick yellow or white scales. Hair re-growth after treatment | Medicated or coal-tar shampoos plus antifungal agent. Topical: steroids, calcipotriol. Salicylic acid ung cocois co to lift scale |
| **Telogen effluvium** | Some drugs, especially chemotherapy, radiotherapy Severe stress, childbirth | Thinning—complete hair loss on scalp, whole body. Onset: few days–weeks after starting treatment | Re-growth 3–6 months after ceasing treatment. Short hair, mild shampoos, wigs, cold-cap treatment. Usually re-growth, takes up to 1 year |

them treated if they are affected. Hair can be expected to grow back normally after treatment (*Figure 33.10*).

## Psoriasis

### Aetiology
Psoriasis is a common problem and its management has previously been considered in depth in Chapter 13. The scalp may also be affected either in isolation or in association with any of the other forms of the condition.

### Presentation
Typically, patches of silvery-white scale on the background of reddened skin develop on the scalp and troublesome 'dandruff' occurs (*Figure 33.11*). It often has no symptoms but some patients complain of itching. Scalp psoriasis may be a persistent problem and in severe cases may be associated with hair loss (Stanway, 2008).

### Pityriasis amiantacea
In this type of scalp psoriasis, thick yellowish-white scales that coat the scalp and stick to the hair are seen (*Figure 33.12*). Although it often occurs in psoriasis it may also be seen in lichen simplex or seborrhoeic dermatitis. If hair loss occurs, re-growth follows (Stanway, 2008).

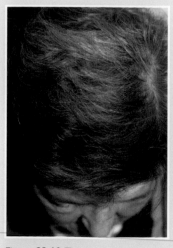

*Figure 33.10. Tinea capitis— re-growth.*

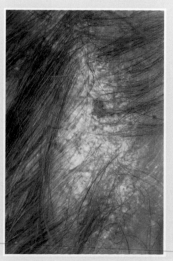

*Figure 33.11. Scalp psoriasis.*

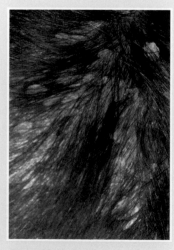

*Figure 33.12. Pityriasis. amientacia.*

## Management

Treatment of scalp psoriasis is often difficult, messy and psoriasis slow to respond to the treatment. Application is easier if the hair is kept short. Medicated or coal-tar shampoos, as well as shampoo with an anti-fungal component, e.g. ketoconazole may be helpful. Patience is required. The shampoo should be rubbed into the scalp and left for up to 10 minutes before rinsing. In more severe cases topical steroids, and calcipotriol may reduce inflammation but salicylic acid, coal-tar creams or Ung Cocois Co are better for lifting scale but should be left on for 1 hour or even overnight before rinsing. Dithranol may achieve some good results but this is messy, can stain and is even more difficult to use than the other treatments (Stanway, 2008).

## Telogen effluvium

### Aetiology

Hair loss may occur following childbirth, severe stress or certain drugs. Chemotherapy may lead to alopecia as it tends to attack the fast growing cells in the hair follicles. Not all the drugs used will cause alopecia and not all patients receiving treatment will suffer this effect. The effect of radiotherapy is different in that hair loss occurs only in the irradiated areas (Royal Marsden NHS Foundation Trust, 2008).

### Presentation

The extent of the loss related to chemotherapy may vary from just a thinning of the hair to complete loss of all body hair. Loss may begin within a few days or a few weeks of starting treatment but is not permanent. Initially there is re-growth of fine hair and after 3–6 months should be back to normal (Cancernet UK, 2009). Hair re-growth after radiotherapy may take longer, i.e. up to 1 year and in some cases may be patchy or fail to occur.

### Management

Some patients may wish to discuss the acquisition of a wig before starting treatment. Others may choose to try to prevent hair loss with 'cold cap' treatment. This involves putting on a cap to cool the scalp 15 minutes before chemotherapy and wearing it for 1–2 hours after, thus restricting blood flow to the hair follicles (Cancernet UK, 2009). Some patients find this approach difficult to tolerate and it may not work in all cases. More general advice when starting treatment is to adopt a short hairstyle, stick to mild shampoos and avoid hairdryers that may further damage brittle hair.

## References

Alaiti S (2007) Hair growth. Emedicine. http://emedicine.medscape.com/article/837994-overview (accessed 8 April 2009)

Bolduc C, Lui H, Shapiro J (2008) Alopecia areata. Emedicine 2008. www.emedicine.com/DERM/topic14.htm (accessed 8 April 2009)

Cancernet UK (2009) Hair loss and chemotherapy: Preventing and coping with hair loss. www.cancernet.co.uk/hairloss.htm (accessed 8 April 2009)

Chull-Wan I (2008) Trichotillomania. Emedicine. http://www.emedicine.com/derm/topic433.htm (accessed 8 April 2009)

DermNet NZ (2007) Tinea capitis. http://dermnetnz.org/fungal/tinea-capitis.html (accessed 8 April 2009)

DermNet NZ (2008) Alopecia areata. http://dermnetnz.org/hair-nails-sweat/alopecia-areata.html (accessed 8 April 2009)

du Vivier A (2002) *Atlas of Clinical Dermatology*. Churchill Livingstone, Philadelphia

Feinstein RP (2009) Androgenetic alopecia. Emedicine 2009. http://tinyurl.com/czfodn (accessed 8 April 2009)

Hantash B, Schwartz R (2009) Traction Alopecia. Emedicine. http://www.emedicine.com/DERM/topic895.htm (accessed 8 April 2009)

Joint Formulary Committee (2009) *British National Formulary 57*. March. BMJ and RPS Publishing, London

Ngan V (2007) Hair replacement surgery. DermNet NZ 2007. http://dermnetnz.org/procedures/hair-replacement.html (accessed 8 April 2009)

Royal Marsden NHS Foundation Trust (2008) Hair loss during treatment. http://tinyurl.com/cgagd6 (accessed 8 April 2009)

Safavi K (1992) Prevalence of alopecia areata in the first National Health and Nutrition Examination Survey. *Arch Dermatol* **128**(5): 702

Stanway A (2008) Scalp psoriasis. DermNet NZ 2008. http://dermnetnz.org/scaly/scalp-psoriasis.html (accessed 8 April 2009)

## Further resources

### The National Alopecia Foundation
US site with extensive information
www.alopeciaareata.com

### Help4Alopecia
Provides information and opportunities to share stories
www.help4alopecia.com

### Alopecia UK
Good links for further information on alopecia
www.alopeciaonline.org.uk

## Test Your Knowledge

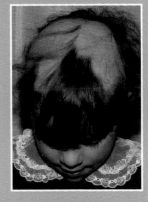

The mother of this 8 year-old child was really worried. The hair loss had started some weeks before and appeared to be extending rapidly. It was not the first time that the child had had such a problem but the previous episode had amounted to just a few small patches that could be hidden and the hair had re-grown normally within a few months. The mother had not been too concerned as she herself had once had a similar problem in the past. However, this time the child's hair-loss was more obvious and the child was being teased at school. On examination the scalp appeared smooth and a few exclamation-mark hairs could be seen but there were no encouraging signs of re-growth.

### Questions
1. What is the likely diagnosis?
2. How would you assess the likely prognosis in this case?
3. How would you advise the mother?

# Alopecia 2: Scarring forms

Whatever the cause, alopecia tends to be a concern for many people. In the previous chapter the possible causes of 'non-scarring' alopecia have been discussed. Many patients with this problem have some hope for recovery of a full head of hair, either spontaneously or with the help of some form of treatment. However, in cases of alopecia in which there is destruction of the hair follicles and the formation of scar tissue, permanent hair loss ensues. In some cases, destruction of the hair follicle may be preceded by inflammation in and around the follicles, known as primary cicatricial alopecia.

If recognized and treated early, it may be possible to halt the process before more permanent damage is done. In other cases the hair loss may be due to actual destruction of the hair follicles—a situation that cannot be improved by medication—known as secondary cicatricial alopecia. Some of the causes of scarring alopecia will be considered together with aids to diagnosis and ways in which the end result of alopecia any be reduced or averted (Cicatricial Alopecia Research Foundation (CARF), 2008).

## Primary cicatricial alopecia

In primary cicatricial alopecia condition, destruction of hair follicles occurs as the result of an inflammatory process. Patients may be symptomless, and if the hair loss is gradual, may initially be unaware of a problem. In others there may be rapid progression and the patient suffer itching and/or burning. As the follicles themselves lie below the skin surface, scalp may appear normal and without obvious scars. In other cases there may be signs

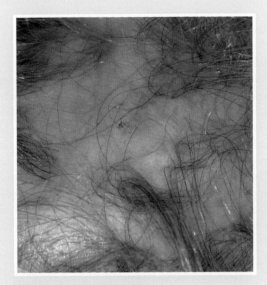

**Figure 34.1. Lichen pilopilaris.**

of inflammation, scales or pustules in the scalp (*Table 34.1*).

Diagnosis and management may be determined by the type of inflammatory cells involved. These may be lymphocytes, neutrophils or both. A scalp biopsy will, therefore, be required in order to confirm the diagnosis and ascertain the type of inflammation present. Treatment is best supervised by a dermatologist with a special interest in scalp problems (CARF, 2008). Cicatricial alopecia may be caused by a number of conditions which will be considered in this chapter.

## Table 34.1. Cause and presentation of cicatricial alopecia

| Type | Subtype | Cause | Presentation |
|---|---|---|---|
| Lymphocytic inflammation | *Lichen planopilaris* | • Unknown cause<br>• Precipitated by drugs | • Hair loss |
| | *Discoid lupus erythematosus* | • Autoimmune disease<br>• Precipitated by drugs | |
| Neutrophilic | *Folliculitis decalvans* | • Unsure, inflammation of hair follicles as reaction to micro-organisms, especially *Staphylococcus aureus*, yeasts or mites | • Inflammation and pustules round hair follicles<br>• Hair loss |
| Lymphocytic and neutrophilic inflammatio | *Erosive pustular dermatosis* | • Follows previous injury to scalp<br>• *Staphylococcus aureus*<br>• Crusting, pustular lesions | • Hair loss |
| | *Folliculitis keloidalis* | • Ingrown hair irritates hair follicles<br>• More common in Afro-Caribbeans<br>• Possibly a form of acne | • Itchy papules and pustules round hair follicles<br>• Keloid formation |
| | *Secondary alopecia* | • Injury<br>• Congenital<br>• Tumours<br>• Coup de sabre | • Hair loss |

### Cicatricial alopecia with mainly lymphocytic inflammation

Treatment of this type of problem is aimed at reducing the lymphocytic inflammatory cells that are attacking the hair follicles. Topical corticosteroids, tacrolimus or pimecrolimus, intralesional steroids or oral hydroxy-chloroquin, corticosteroids, doxycycline, the immuno-suppressant mycophenolate mofetil or ciclosporin may be tried depending on response and severity of the condition. If any drug is thought to have precipitated the condition it should be discontinued (CARF, 2008).

### *Lichen planopilaris*

Problems that fall into the category of cicatricial alopecia with mainly lymphocytic inflammation include lichen planopilaris (*Figure 34.1*). This patient had had problems with lichen planus of the scalp for many years. She had had to accept that hair loss was permanent but re-attended as she was experiencing trouble-some itching at the site. Examination found a few scaling areas and some white patches of old damage. In her case there were no other manifestations of lichen planus but the diagnosis had been confirmed by biopsy.

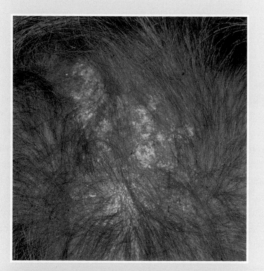

*Figure 34.2. Discoid lupus erythematosus.*

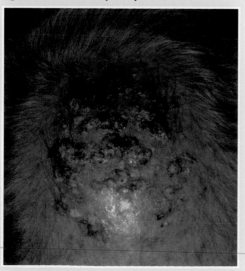

*Figure 34.3. Erosive pustular dermatosis.*

The cause of lichen planus is unknown but in some it may be precipitated by drugs such as beta-blockers, gold, penicillin or a non-steroidal anti-inflammatory drug (NSAID). This was a recurrence of the problem, some years after a previous episode had settled. Topical dermovate and hydroxychloroquin had been tried without success and eventually she decided to accept a hair piece to cover the area (Ross, 2007).

### *Lupus erythematosus*

Lupus erythematosus is an auto-immune disease which most commonly affects younger women. In some cases it may be precipitated by certain drugs such as carbamazepine, lithium, phenytoin or sulphonamides (Oakley, 2009). It may present in two forms, the first being systemic lupus erythematosus, which may have widespread effects on the skin and other major organs of the body. About 20% of these will have problems of diffuse, non-scarring alopecia. The second form is discoid lupus erythematosus, which may present with a thick, scaly rash that affects mainly sun-exposed areas such as the face, scalp or hands. Scarring and (if the scalp is affected) alopecia may follow (*Figure 34.2*). This woman had suffered some permanent hair loss starting a year previously; some signs of activity were still obvious.

### Management

Skin biopsy and direct immunofluorescence tests will confirm the diagnosis. Other tests may be normal in discoid lupus erythematosus but in systemic lupus erythematosus there will be high titres of antinuclear antibodies and other auto-antibodies. High titres are associated with more severe disease.

The patient should avoid sun exposure as much as possible and if the condition seems to be related to a drug, this should be discontinued (CARF, 2008). The patient should be offered treatments such as corticosteroids, oral hydroxychloroquin or ciclosporin.

### Cicatricial alopecia with mainly neutrophilic inflammation

Management of these problems are directed at the pathogenic organisms that are associated with the inflammation of the hair follicles. Antibiotics are therefore the most important approach to their treatment. Isotretinoin has also sometimes been found to be useful.

### Folliculitis decalvans

Forms of cicatricial alopecia with mainly neutrophilic inflammation include folliculitis decalvans (tufted folliculitis), where inflammation and pustules may be seen around the hair follicles. Although the scalp is often involved, it may affect hair at any part of the body and be followed by permanent hair loss. The true cause is not known but *Staphylococcus aureus*, *Propionibacterium acnes*, yeasts or mites can usually be isolated when a swab is taken from a pustule. Therefore antibiotics are the mainstay of treatment but in severe cases oral corticosteroids may be required (Ngan, 2008a).

### Cicatricial alopecia with lymphocytic and neutrophilic inflammation

This type of alopecia is associated with a mixture of inflammation of the hair follicles and infection. Treatment is, therefore, based on anti-inflammatory preparations and antibiotics. Isotretinoin is also used, especially in cases of folliculitis keloidalis.

### Erosive pustular dermatosis

Erosive pustular dermatosis is a form of alopecia with lymphocytic and neutrophilic inflammation. While the cause is unknown, it does appear to be more common on areas of the scalp that have suffered previous injury either through injury, skin malignancy, the sun or infection such as herpes zoster, or shingles. Sometimes it may be triggered by some minor injury or surgical procedure to the scalp.

The patient presents with pustular lesions on the scalp which crust over and which can frequently be shown to be associated with infection with *S. aureus* (*Figure 34.3*). The underlying skin is moist and red. Once settled, there is permanent scarring and alopecia.

### Management

A swab should be taken from the pustules for culture and sensitivities and the patient treated with a prolonged course (at least 6 weeks) of the appropriate antibiotic (usually flucloxacillin or erythromycin), together with a potent topical steroid (Duffill, 2009).

Biopsy may be necessary to confirm the diagnosis as the lesions may be difficult to distinguish from solar keratoses, basal cell carcinoma and squamous cell carcinoma. Recurrences commonly occur and would require further treatment. Crusts should be removed after soaking in potassium permanganate solution (Duffill, 2009).

### Folliculitis keloidalis

The cause of folliculitis keloidalis (acne keloidalis nuchae) is not known but it is usually associated with ingrown hairs that irritate the wall of the hair follicle.

It is most common in Afro-Caribbeans and may be a form of acne. Itchy papules and pustules form around the hair follicles in the region of the nape of the neck. In time, keloid-type scars form which are unsightly and more obvious as the areas becomes bald (*Figure 34.4*).

### Management

Response to treatment of this condition is often poor. Patients can be advised to avoid shirts that rub on the neck and if topical steroids and a prolonged course(s) of antibiotics such as tetracycline, clindamycin or rifampicin do not do the trick, intralesional steroids, oral isotretinoin, or surgical or laser excision of the affected area may improve the situation (Oakley, 2008).

## Secondary cicatricial alopecia

### Injury

If a portion of the skin of a hair-bearing area is destroyed, permanent hair loss will follow. Such damage may occur as the result of mechanical trauma, burns or radiation (Doctor's Doctor, 2008).

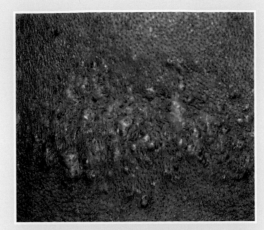

*Figure 34.4. Folliculitis keloidalis.*

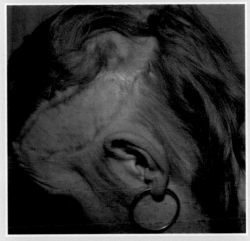

*Figure 34.5. Grafted area on scalp following road accident.*

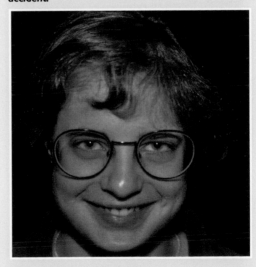

*Figure 34.6. Congenital alopecia.*

The girl in *Figure 34.5* was injured in a serious road traffic accident in which she was thrown headfirst through the windscreen and basically 'scalped'. The area had been grafted with skin taken from a non-hairy area of the thigh. Although it had healed well, hair could not be expected to grow.

She was to be provided with a wig and reviewed later for discussion regarding the possibilities of future hair transplantation.

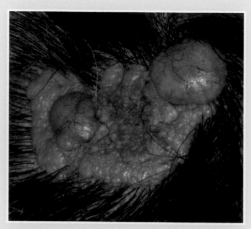

Figure 34.7. Sebaceous naevus with basal cell carcinoma.

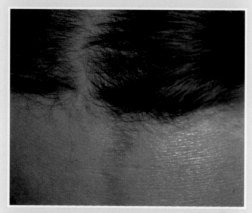

Figure 34.8. Coup de sabre.

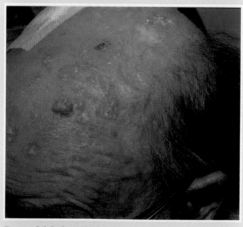

Figure 34.9. Actinic keratoses scalp.

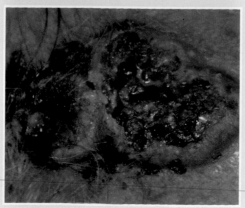

Figure 34.10. Squamous cell carcinoma scalp.

## Congenital alopecia
### Aetiology
Unlike other forms of alopecia in which there is hair loss from areas with previous hair growth, in congenital alopecia (hypotrichosis) the individual is born with areas on the scalp in which there are not, and will never be, actual hair growth. Congenital hypotrichosis is caused by genetic abnormalities or problems with embryonic development and may be associated with a number of rare syndromes.

### Presentation
The absence of hair dates from birth and in some cases tends to affect a triangular patch above the temples (triangular alopecia). In others there may be a developmental abnormality in which the skin fails to form, leading to an open area, like an ulcer, where hair fails to grow (WebMD, 2005).

### Management
This patient (*Figure 34.6*) managed to adapt her hairstyle to cover the bald areas; others may choose to have the 'barren area' excised and hair follicles transplanted (American Hair Loss Association, 2005).

### Scalp lesions that may be followed by alopecia
### Tumours
Both benign and malignant tumours as well as granulomatous lesion such as sarcoidosis or necrobiosis lipoidica may be associated with destruction of areas of skin and hair follicles thus leading to loss of hair at the site (Keratin.com). This patient (*Figure 34.7*) had a dual problem of a sebaceous naevus that had been present on her scalp since birth. As occasionally happens, she also developed a basal cell carcinoma in the naevus (Ngan, 2008b). Both these conditions will cause alopecia at the site of the lesions.

### Morphea (coup de sabre)
The cause of morphea is unknown. It is said to be a form of localized scleroderma which may affect the skin in a number of ways. One form of the condition is 'en coup de sabre' in which a linear lesion affects the skin and underlying tissue of the scalp and the temple (*Figure 34.8*). Hair in the affected area is lost for ever. Treatment, including intralesional steroids and some other medications such as methotrexate or phototherapy, although sometimes tried, are unlikely to achieve much benefit (DermNet NZ, 2008a).

## Complications of alopecia
Apart from the psychological effects of baldness, loss of hair leaves the scalp particularly vulnerable to skin damage and all its consequences. Patients with this problem frequently present with dry, wrinkled skin and rough, scaly patches which are a sure sign of solar keratoses (*Figure 34.9*). The fair-skinned, with blue eyes, who tend to burn easily in the sun are at the greatest risk of developing problems. These lesions, although unsightly, are in themselves harmless, but they are considered to be precancerous with a high risk of

developing basal cell carcinoma, squamous cell carcinoma (*Figure 34.10*), or sometimes malignant melanoma. It is said that patients with more than 10 solar keratoses have a 10–15% risk of change to squamous cell carcinoma (DermNetNZ, 2008b).

## Management

Prevention of solar damage is better than having to treat its effects. People should be advised to wear a hat or a wig when out, particularly in the summer months. Regular application of sunscreen also helps, even in patients who already have solar keratoses.

Treatment of solar keratoses includes cryotherapy, curettage and cautery or excision. If the abnormal skin is removed, the healed skin, formed from the deeper layers, is unaffected by sun damage (DermNetNZ, 2008b). Treatment can also entail topical application of 5-fluorouracil cream (once or twice a day for 3–4 weeks) (Joint Formulary Committee, 2009: 13.8.1) or imiquimod (3 times a week for 4 weeks) (Joint Formulary Committee, 2009: 13.7) or diclofenac gel (twice daily for 2–3 months) (NetDoctor, 2005) will help to clear the sun damaged skin.

## References

American Hair Loss Association (2005) Congenital hyopotrichosis. http://tinyurl.com/22hf9f (accessed 13 August 2009)

Cicatricial Alopecia Research Foundation (CARF) (2008) Frequently asked questions. www.carfintl.org/faq.html (accessed 13 August 2009)

DermNet NZ (2008a) Morphoea. http://tinyurl.com/nrqd5v (accessed 13 August 2009)

DermNetNZ (2008b) Solar keratoses. http://tinyurl.com/472yqh (accessed 13 August 2009)

Doctor's Doctor (2008) Scarring alopecia. http://tinyurl.com/m9ntrf (accessed 13 August 2009)

Duffill M (2009) Erosive pustular dermatosis of the scalp. http://tinyurl.com/ngwswq (accessed 13 August 2009)

Joint Formulary Committee (2009) *British National Formulary* 57. March. RPS and BMA Publishing

Keratin.com (2008) Secondary scarring alopecia from neoplastic disorders. www.keratin.com/at/at023.shtml (accessed 13 August 2009)

NetDoctor (2005) Solaraze gel. http://tinyurl.com/l2ytx8 (accessed 13 August 2009)

Ngan V (2008a) Folliculitis decalvans. http://tinyurl.com/ovlp7h (accessed 13 August 2009)

Ngan V (2008b) Sebaceous naevus. http://tinyurl.com/oqof6u (accessed 13 August 2009)

Oakley A (2008) Folliculitis keloidalis. http://tinyurl.com/lomyxp (accessed 13 August 2009)

Oakley A (2009) Cutaneous lupus erythematosus. www.dermnetnz.org/immune/cutaneous-lupus.html (accessed 26 August 2009)

Ross EK (2007) Primary cicatricial alopecia: clinical features and management. *Dermatol Nurs* **19**(2): 137–43

WebMD (2005) Congenital hypotrichosis. http://tinyurl.com/phde9f (accessed 13 August 2009)

| Type | Subtype | Management |
|---|---|---|
| Lymphocytic inflammation | *Lichen planopilaris and Discoid lupus erythematosus* | • Biopsy<br>• Stop any offending dru<br>• Topical /intralesonal/oral steroids or tacrolimus/picrolimus<br>• Doxycycline/mycophenolate/ cyclosporine<br>• Sun protection<br>• Wigs |
| Neutrophilic inflammation | *Folliculitis decalvans* | • Swab pustules for culture and sensitivities<br>• Antibiotics |
| Lymphocytic and neutrophilic inflammatio | *Erosive pustular dermatosis* | • Biopsy<br>• Swab pustules for culture and sensitivities<br>• Antibiotics for 6 weeks at least<br>• Soak crusts with potassium permanganate |
| | *Folliculitis keloidalis* | • Antibiotics: long course<br>• Topical steroids<br>• Intralesional steroids<br>• Isotretinoin<br>• Surgical/laser excision |
| | *Secondary alopecia* | • Hair transplantation<br>• Wigs |

Table 34.2. Management of cicatricial alopecia

## Test Your Knowledge

This 62-year-old woman had been complaining of an itchy scalp for some months. Topical sterioids seemed to have slightly eased the itching but problems continued and she was alarmed to notice hair loss in the affected areas. Her general health was good and she was not aware of any skin rash elsewhere on her body.

### Questions
1. How would you begin to try to make a diagnosis in this case?
2. How would you confirm the diagnosis?
3. How would you manage his case?

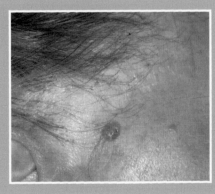

# Lip lesions

When a patient walks into the surgery, his/her lips are always on view. Patients may arrive with a specific complaint for which they are seeking advice or, if the nurse or doctor is observant, he/she may notice some abnormality themselves. Some of these problems may seem so trivial that the patient does not feel the need to discuss them but, from the medical point of view, it may be possible to offer advice that will at least render the patient more comfortable. Sometimes, however, action can be initiated that may save the patient more troublesome or serious consequences. Lacerations of the lip, infections, swollen and dry lips, non-healing lesions and vascular lesions are some examples of lip conditions which will be discussed in this chapter.

## Injury

### Cut lip

Lacerations of the lip are common following a fall or a punch in the mouth (*Figure 35.1*). Blood loss can be profuse but can usually be stopped by firm pressure on the wound (National Center for Emergency Medicine Informatics, 2006).

The wound will usually heal well without suturing but care should be taken to check for loose or missing teeth. In addition, it is important to check that there are no tooth fragments in the wound. If these are missed, the wound will, almost certainly, become infected. If the wound does subsequently become infected, it must be assumed that there is a remaining foreign body until proved otherwise (Roberts, 2002).

Some injuries can leave the patient with an unsightly deformity that may require reconstruction by a plastic surgeon.

## Mucocoele

This mucous retention cyst is sometimes seen on the inner side of the lip and stems from obstruction to the flow of saliva from the salivary gland as a result of trauma. It occurs most frequently in childhood and the teenage years. Mucocoeles present as painless, asymptomatic swellings that appear suddenly (*Figure 35.2*) and may fluctuate in size. Recent trauma may be recalled or the patient may be a persistent lip biter.

These lesions may rupture and clear spontaneously. If they are troublesome or persistent, they may be excised or treated with cryotherapy or laser therapy (Flaitz and Hicks, 2005).

## Infections

### Herpes simplex

Herpes simplex is one of the most common infections. It frequently presents with 'cold sores' on the lips. The patient first notices an itch and/or burning of the lip. This is soon followed by the development of clusters of small vesicles (*Figure 35.3*).

When it occurs on the lips (herpes labialis), it is usually caused by type 1 herpes simplex virus. Although it is occasionally transmitted sexually this is not usually the case.

Once the patient has suffered an initial infection, it is likely to recur at intervals at the same site. Recurrences

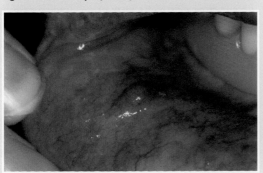

*Figure 35.1. Cut lip after a fall.*

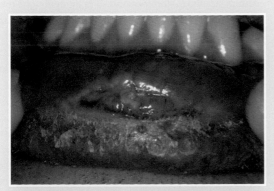

*Figure 35.2. Mucocoele.*

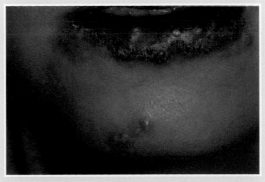

*Figure 35.3. Herpes simplex.*

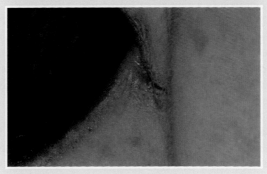

*Figure 35.4. Angular chelitis.*

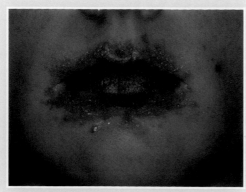

*Figure 35.5. Impetigo*

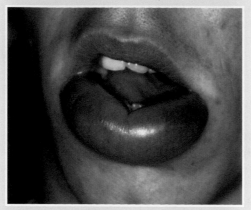

*Figure 35.6. Angio-oedema following wasp sting.*

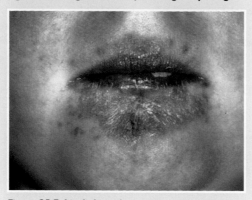

*Figure 35.7. Lip licking dermatitis.*

may be triggered by trauma, exposure to the sun, stress, hormones (e.g. premenstrual), or other infections such as coughs and colds.

High factor sunscreen protection may help avert attacks. If the lesions are left untreated, they resolve spontaneously within about 7–10 days.

Patients with recurrent problems may prefer to apply topical aciclovir five times daily at the first sign of trouble, in an attempt to halt progression of the problem. Oral antiviral treatment is required only in severe cases where complications such as eczema herpeticum or neurological problems may occur (DermNet, 2005).

### Candida

*Candida albicans* is a yeast infection that commonly affects the mouth. It is more likely to occur in the very young, the aged, smokers, the edentulous (i.e. those without teeth), those with ill-fitting dentures and those on inhaled corticosteroids or medications, such as antihistamines or diuretics that dry the mouth. Some patients will develop an angular chelitis in which red scaly areas and moist cracks form at the angles of the mouth (*Figure 35.4*).

*Candida* and/or *Staphylococcus aureus* (*Staph. aureus*) thrive in this situation (DermNet, 2005b). If necessary, a swab from the area will confirm the diagnosis.

An antifungal agent such as nystatin oral suspension or lozenge, or topical miconazole gel should clear the problem. Those with dentures should be advised to sterilize them thoroughly and not to wear them at night. If there is secondary infection with *S. aureus*, an antibiotic may also be required (Joint Formulary Committee, 2005: 12.3.2).

### Impetigo

Impetigo is a bacterial infection of the skin. It is usually caused by *Staph. aureus*. Occasionally a beta-haemolytic *Streptococcus* is involved. It frequently occurs on the face and often the lips are involved. It is contagious and easily passed around families and institutions, unless great care is taken to avoid contact with others.

The patient presents with yellow pus-filled blisters that rupture. The purulent exudates forms golden coloured crusts (*Figure 35.5*). Topical antibiotics such as fucidic acid or mupirocin will normally clear the condition but systemic flucloxacillin or erythromycin may be necessary in severe or widespread cases.

Patients should be advised to avoid close contact with others and not to share towels, bedding or clothes. Children should remain off school until they respond to treatment and no further lesions appear (British Association of Dermatologists, 2004).

Complications occasionally arise about 3 weeks later in the form of nephritis that may follow infection with certain strains of *Streptococcus*. It is thought to be related to an immune complex disorder, although the antigen-antibody reaction is still uncertain. Treatment of the infection with antibiotics does not prevent this complication (Geetha, 2005).

## Swollen lips
### Allergy

Angio-oedema may occur in association with an episode of urticaria or as a result of an allergic reaction. The patient shown in *Figure 35.6* presented with a grossly swollen lower lip after a wasp sting. The swelling occurs as a result of the release of histamine and other vasoactive agents from mast cells in the skin, leading to a diffuse swelling of the subcutaneous tissues. It often occurs during an attack of urticaria.

Antihistamines and corticosteroids may be needed to control an attack and antihistamines may be helpful given prophylactically in the hope of preventing further episodes.

If there is associated swelling of the tongue and laryngeal mucosa, the airway may be compromised and urgent action would also need to be taken using injected adrenaline and oxygen (Joint Formulary Committee, 2005: 3.4.30).

Any substance thought to have stimulated the attack should be avoided in future. A few patients may have occasional attacks of angio-oedema that is not explained. In these cases C1 inhibitor and C4 levels should be checked to exclude any hereditary factor or association with drugs such as captopril (du Vivier, 2002).

## Dry lips and erosions
### Chelitis
Patients may frequently complain of dry lips. There may be a number of different causes for this problem which can be relieved symptomatically by the frequent application of white soft paraffin as a regular moisturizer. This may be simple in patients with an obvious cause, such as those on the drug isotretinoin, where the problem of dry cracking lips is inevitable. The moisturizer will ease the symptoms that will resolve when the drug is discontinued.

Others may have lip problems associated with atopic eczema or develop a contact dermatitis as a result of using certain preparations such as lipstick, toothpaste or mouthwashes to which they have become allergic (Ashton and Leppard, 2005).

Those who repeatedly lick their lips may develop an eczematous rash mainly on the skin surrounding the lips (*Figure 35.7*). Emollients are helpful but somehow the patient must be encouraged to stop the habit. The application of topical hydrocortisone 1% ointment twice daily may also ease symptoms.

It is important to pick up those problems that may need another approach. If an allergy is suspected, skin tests can be done to identify the cause of the problem. (Ashton and Leppard, 2005).

### Actinic chelitis
Actinic chelitis is characterized by dry scaling of the lips, sometimes with white patches. It is most marked on the lower lip (*Figure 35.8*) because, owing to its greater prominence, it catches more sunlight over time.

Actinic chelitis is a premalignant condition that may progress to epidermal dysplasia and squamous cell carcinoma. In this situation squamous cell carcinoma is more likely to metastasize. It may therefore be advisable for a biopsy to be taken. The patient should be advised to avoid further exposure to the sun and to protect the lips with a high factor sunscreen in future.

Available treatments are cryotherapy, 5-fluouracil or surgery (du Vivier, 2002: 170).

### Other conditions
There are a number of other conditions that may involve the skin and changes on the lips. For example, some patients develop white, net-like lesions and/or erosions on the lips (*Figure 35.9*). Futher signs, such as a white lacey pattern on the mucous membranes of the mouth and/or an itchy rash of a violaceous colour on other parts of the body, will confirm suspicions of lichen planus (du Vivier, 2002: 95–105).

Patients with discoid lupus erythematosus, a condition exacerbated by sunlight, may also have a rash that affects or extends to the lips. The thick, scaly plaques that occur mainly in light-exposed areas leaves scars as the lesions heal (du Vivier, 2002: 490–502).

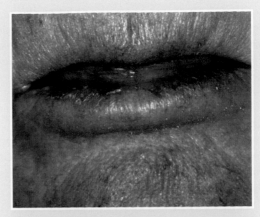
*Figure 35.8. Actinic chelitis.*

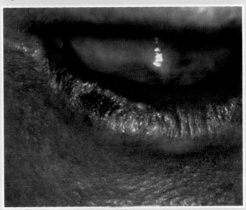
*Figure 35.9. Lichen planus with white streaking and erosions.*

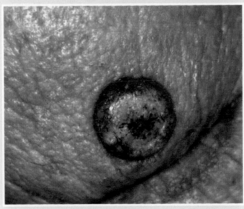
*Figure 35.10. Keratoacanthoma.*

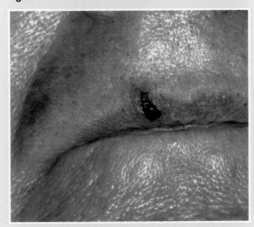
*Figure 35.11. Basal cell carcinoma on the lip: A persistent non-healing lesion.*

The diagnosis of such skin conditions should be investigated, confirmed and managed by the doctor or specialist but are likely to involve the use of topical steroids. Discoid lupus erythematosus is the one condition in which it may be necessary to use more potent steroids on the face to get the condition under control (Joint Formulary Committee, 2005: 13.4).

## Non-healing lesions

Any lesion on the lip that fails to heal should raise suspicion of malignant change. Basal cell carcinoma, squamous cell carcinoma and malignant melanoma may all develop on the lip.

### Keratoacanthoma

Keratoacanthoma may also occur in the sun-exposed region of the lips. It is a benign tumour that rapidly grows over a period of about 3 months. After this time there is slow regression over the ensuing months leaving a pitted scar. A well-defined papule grows to form a raised red or flesh-coloured papule that is filled with keratin (*Figure 35.10*). It may be confused with basal cell carcinoma or squamous cell carcinoma. Although resolution can eventually be expected, the lesion is best removed by curettage and cautery or excision; otherwise a malignancy could be missed (du Vivier, 2002: 176–7).

### Basal cell carcinoma

The patient shown in *Figure 35.11* had noticed this small ulcer on his upper lip which was confirmed as a basal cell

carcinoma on biopsy. He mentioned that it was gradually increasing in size, bled from time to time and then crusted over before breaking down again.

If left untreated, such lesions will slowly continue to grow and erode surrounding tissues. Metstases are unusual.

The treatment of choice in such cases is excision. Currettage and cautery is possible but carries a high risk of recurrence. Radiotherapy may be offered for large lesions or elderly patients who might prefer to avoid surgery (Ashton and Leppard, 2005: 243–4).

### Squamous cell carcinoma

The lip is vulnerable to the development of squamous cell carcinoma. It may present with a scaly or horny tumour that later ulcerates, bleeds, fails to heal and becomes covered in a crust. It tends to grow faster than basal cell carcinoma.

The treatment of choice is excision. Care must be taken to confirm histologically that the lesion has been completely removed. Radiotherapy is available for those with large lesions that might be difficult to excise, or for the very elderly (Ashton and Leppard, 2005: 288–9).

## Vascular lesions

### Venous lake

Venous lake is a benign vascular tumour that occurs on the lip in the elderly. It appears as soft purple papules that can be compressed (*Figure 35.12*). They are thought to follow long-term sun damage. A venous lake itself is harmless but must be distinguished from a malignant melanoma or pigmented basal cell carcinoma. Providing the doctor or nurse is confident of the diagnosis, no treatment is required.

If there is concern about the diagnosis or the patient is worried about cosmetic appearance, the lesion can be biopsied, excised or treated with laser therapy (Wang and Wang, 2005).

### Hereditary telangiectasia

Hereditary telangiectasia (Osler-Weber-Rendu syndrome) is an autosomal dominant disorder in which the patient may have multiple telangiectasia that have the potential to bleed. Patients have a family history of the condition. Recurrent nose bleeds are a common problem and some patients will have bleeding from lesions in the gastrointestinal tract. The blood loss may lead to problems of anaemia.

In this patient shown in *Figure 35.13*, who was found to be anaemic, the telltale telangiectasia that suggest the diagnosis could be seen on the lips. Once the condition is diagnosed, it is important to keep a watch on the patient's haemoglobin level and give the necessary supportive measure of iron and/or blood transfusion if or when necessary (du Vivier, 2002: 479).

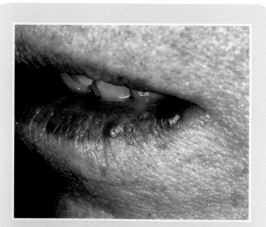

*Figure 35.12. Venous lake.*

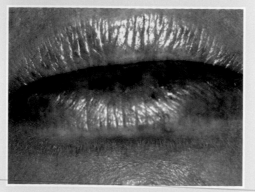

*Figure 35.13. Hereditary telangiectasia: petechiae on the lip in a woman with anaemia.*

## References

Ashton R, Leppard B (2005) *Differential Diagnosis in Dermatology.* 3rd edn. Radcliffe: 138–41

British Association of Dermatologists (2004) Impetigo. www.bad. org.uk/public/leaflets/impetigo.asp (accessed 10 April 2006)

DermNetNZ (2005a) Herpes simplex. http://dermnetnz.org/viral/ herpes-simplex.html (accessed 10 April 2006)

DermNetNZ (2005b) Oral candidiasis. www.dermnetnz.org/fungal/oral-candidiasis.html (accessed 10 April 2006)

du Vivier A (2002) Atlas of Dermatology. Churchill Livingstone

Flaitz C, Hicks J (2006) Mucoceoele and ranula. *eMedicine*. 24 January. www.emedicine.com/derm/topic648.htm (accessed 10 April 2006)

Geetha D (2004) Glomerulonephrittis, poststreptococcal. www.emedicine.com/med/topic889.htm (accessed 10 April 2006)

Joint Formulary Committee (2006) *British National Formulary 50*. September. Royal Pharmaceutical Society of Great Britain and British Medical Association, London

National Center for Emergency Medicine Informatics (2006) Lacerations of the mouth. Emergency Medicine on the Web. www.ncemi.org/cse/cse0403.htm (accessed 12 April 2006)

Roberts JRR (2002) Would you miss this diagnosis? *Emerg Med* **34**(2):61

Wang J, Wang K (2005) Venous lakes. *eMedicine*. 28 February. www.emedicine.com/DERM/topic451.htm (accessed 12 April 2006)

# Test Your Knowledge

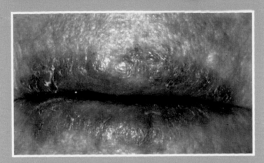

This elderly woman was troubled by persistent dry scaling of the lips. The problem had started some years before and was getting worse in spite of regularly applying a lip salve and emollient. The emollient seemed to soothe it at the time, but in effect did nothing to clear it. There were no complaints of skin rashes and her general health was good for her age. Apart from bendrofluazide and atenolol to control her blood pressure, she was on no other medication.

### Questions
1. What is the possible diagnosis in this case?
2. How would you help her to elucidate the problem?
3. What advise would you give to the patient?

# The tongue

A visit to a small traditional clinic in China, in a remote area of Yunan near to the Tibetan border, highlighted the fundamentals of medicine. In the demonstration of a routine examination of the patient, the areas of greatest importance in making the diagnosis were the pulse, the eyes and the tongue. Even with the wealth of technical advances available in modern western medicine, these basic checks remain important.

When examination is focused on the tongue, the practitioner should be aware of the patient's general condition and the presence of dehydration, localized problems that need treatment or further investigation and look for the sort of signs that may indicate or confirm problems of a more generalized disease. In this chapter some of the changes that may occur will be considered.

## Normal abnormalities
### Geographic tongue
Geographic tongue is so named because denuded, beefy red patches on the surface of the tongue cause it to resemble a map (*Figure 36.1*). The appearance may change rapidly. The condition may be symptomless but sometimes the patient may complain of soreness and a burning sensation.

### Management
No treatment is required. However, if it recurs repeatedly, some patients may find it helpful to avoid spicy food, alcohol or tobacco. Providing the professional is satisfied that there are no other problems, the patient can be reassured that it is not serious (Fung, 2005).

### Fissured (scrotal) tongue
Fissures on the tongue are common. They may occur in childhood but more often appear in adult life. Grooves of varying depths can be observed running along the dorsal and lateral aspects of the tongue (*Figure 36.2*). It is suspected it may be inherited (Kelsch, 2005). The patient is usually unaware of any problem.

### Management
No specific treatment is required. Fissured tongue does not affect general health unless it is associated with Down syndrome or Melkersson-Rosenthal syndrome (Eidelman et al, 1976). Patients with Melkersson-Rosenthal syndrome may complain of recurrent facial weakness and swelling of the lips. They will require specialist advice for this neurological disorder. (National Institute of Neurological Disorders and Stroke, 2006).

## Infections
### Candida
Oral thrush is caused by the yeast, *Candida albicans*. This organism is normally present in the mouth but as long as it is kept in check by the other organisms present, it will not cause problems. However, *Candida* may flourish and cause symptoms in a person who is immunosuppressed,

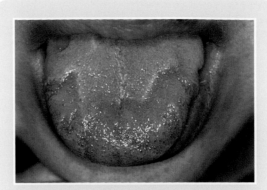
*Figure 36.1. Geographic tongue.*

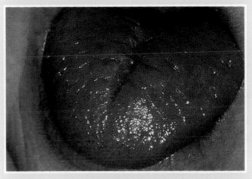
*Figure 36.2. Fissured (scrotal) tongue.*

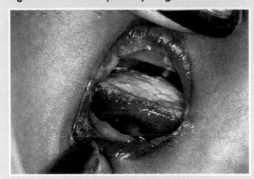
*Figure 36.3. Oral Candida in a young baby.*

diabetic, on chemotherapy or taking antibiotics or steroids, in poor health, or in the very young or very old.

### Presentation
The oral cavity and the tongue are inflamed and covered in white, velvety patches that gradually spread and merge. Oral *Candida* is common in a newborn baby (*Figure 36.3*) and should cause no particular worry as long as it does not persist for more than 2–3 weeks.

### Investigation
The diagnosis can usually be made by the appearance on examination but, if necessary, a swab taken from the area should confirm the presence of hyphae microscopically or *Candida* on culture in the laboratory. If there are no obvious causative factors, some patients may need further investigation to exclude an underlying cause (Medline Plus, 2005).

## Table 36.1. Altered appearance of the tongue

| | Cause | Features | Management |
|---|---|---|---|
| Geographic tongue | Unknown cause. Sometimes related to intake of certain foods, e.g. spicy food | Red, map-like red patches on the tongue | No treatment required |
| Fissured tongue | Possible genetic link | Usually symptomless | No treatment required unless associated with Melkersson-Rosenthal syndrome |
| Oral *Candida* | *Candida albicans* More common in the young, debilitated or immunosuppressed or after antibiotics | Spreading white velvety patches on the tongue | Swab as needed for microscopy and culture to confirm diagnosis Antifungal agents: topical or, if severe, systemic |
| Food affect | Dyes in foods | Discolouration | No treatment required unless symprtoms |
| Black hairy tongue | More common in tea or coffee drinkers, smokers HIV and intravenous drug users | Elongation of papillae on dorsum of tongue (black or brown) | Debride Dental advice Antifungal agent if complicated by *Candida* |
| Strawberry tongue | Group A beta-haemolytic *Streptococcus* (scarlet fever) | 1. Tongue coated white 2. Red strawberry appearance | Penicillin V for 10 days |
| Xerostomia | Medications, dehydration Smoking, diabetes mellitus, radiation to head and neck Sjögren's syndrome | Dry mouth, tongue smooth, cracked shiny | Attend to the cause Oral hygiene Sip water, ice cubes Saliva substitutes |

### Management

Oral *Candida* will usually respond well to topical antifungal preparations such as nystatin suspension or lozenges four times a day and continued for 2 days after resolution. In non-responsive or severe cases, systemic fluconazole or imidazole may be required (Joint Formulary Committee, 2006: 12.3.2).

### Discolouration

#### Food colouring

Sometimes, as a chance finding, a marked discolouration of the tongue, may be noticed, as in this child (*Figure 36.4*) who had been eating a red iced lolly. So long as there are nor other symptoms there should be no concern.

#### Black hairy tongue

Frequently black hairy tongue is asymptomatic but occasionally the patient may complain of a tickling sensation of the soft palate and throat, or gagging when swallowing. It usually occurs in those with poor oral hygiene or on a soft or liquid diet that fails to debride the tongue. It is said to be more common in men, those who drink a lot of coffee and tea, smokers, users of intravenous drugs or those who are HIV positive.

On examination, the filiform papillae on the dorsum of the tongue are elongated and may be discoloured black (*Figure 36.5*) or brown. In some cases there may be an associated *Candida* infection.

#### Investigations

If necessary, a swab can be taken from the surface of the tongue to exclude the presence of *Candida*. Any suspicion of HIV should be investigated.

#### Management

If the tongue is brushed with a toothbrush, scraped with a tongue scraper or dietary roughage is increased, it may help to remove the elongated papillae. A dental and/or dental hygienist's opinion may also be helpful. Otherwise interference is unnecessary unless complicated by *Candida*, in which case an antifungal agent such as nystatin, ketoconazole or fluconazole may be used (Mayo Clinic, 2005).

### Indicators of other disease

A number of other causes need to be considered when presented with an altered appearance of the tongue (*Table 36.1*).

### Scarlet fever

A patient presenting with scarlet fever is usually unwell with the sudden onset of high fever, sore throat, enlarged cervical glands, nausea, vomiting, abdominal pain and a rapidly developing rash that starts on the face and neck before spreading to the trunk and limbs. The rash consists of scarlet macules on an erythematous background. The cheeks are flushed but the area around the mouth remains pale (circumoral pallor).

Initially the tongue is coated white but then, as the inflamed papillae project through, it has the appearance of a 'white strawberry' (*Figure 36.6*). As the coating disappears, the tongue comes to look like a red strawberry.

Symptoms settle and the rash fades and peels after about the sixth day (DermNetNZ, 2006).

#### Investigations

A culture of a throat swab in the laboratory will confirm the presence of group A beta-haemolytic *Streptococcus*.

#### Management

Analgesics such as paracetamol are helpful for a fever, headache and sore throat. Penicillin V 250 mg four times a day for 10 days may also be taken. Erythromycin may be used in patients if they are allergic to penicillin.

## Xerostomia

Xerostomia (or dry mouth) is a common problem that is frequently caused by prescribed drugs such as diuretics, antihistamines, anti-spasmodics, antidepressants, some antipsychotics, and certain drugs used in the treatment of hypertension. It occurs when the production of saliva is reduced and may also be observed in cases of dehydration, in smokers, people with diabetes mellitus, following radiation to the head and neck, in neurological problems such as Parkinson's disease and in those who tend to breathe through the mouth. It is also seen in Sjörgen's syndrome, an autoimmune condition in which there is a reduction in the production of saliva and tears (Barker, 2006).

The patient becomes aware of dryness of the mouth, which may cause problems with halitosis, swallowing dry food or speaking for a long time. Dental decay may follow and *Candida* commonly occurs. On examination the tongue becomes smooth, cracked and shiny (*Figure 36.7*) (Betteroralhealth.info, 2006).

### Management

If the cause is recognized and treated, the condition may improve. Some useful ways of treating dry mouth are to ensure regular oral hygiene with mouthwash and brushing of teeth, frequent fluids, sips of cold water or sucking ice cubes (especially in cases of dehydration). Saliva substitutes in the form of a spray, lozenge or gel may also help. Luborant oral spray is recommended for dry mouth no matter what the cause, and pilocarpine tablets are licensed for use in cases following radiation of the head and neck or Sjörgren's syndrome, provided that they produce some response (Joint Formulary Committee, 2006: 12.3.5).

## Mouth ulcers

Patients often complain of pain or discomfort of the mouth or tongue (*Table 36.2*). On examination, one or more ulcers may be found that appear to be the cause. Such patients should be questioned to ascertain the reason for the ulceration. Important points to consider are:

- How long the lesion has been present
- The site of the ulceration
- The possibility of injury or localized trauma
- Any more generalized signs or symptoms that would suggest the correct diagnosis.

### Injury

Some patients may have a history of recent injury, dental work or problems with ill-fitting dentures or a broken tooth that irritate the tongue. One man had a painful ulcer after biting his tongue when he fell (*Figure 36.8*).

### Aphthous ulcers

Aphthous ulcers (or canker sores) are common on the oral or genital mucosa. It is thought that 20% of the population suffers from this problem from childhood onwards, often with recurrent episodes (Ngan, 2006).

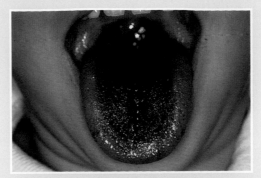

*Figure 36.4. Red tongue after eating a red iced lolly*

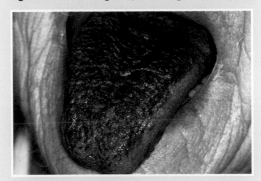

*Figure 36.5. Black hairy tongue*

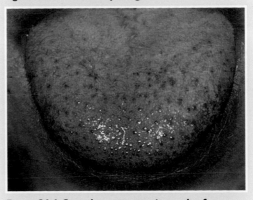

*Figure 36.6. Strawberry tongue in scarlet fever*

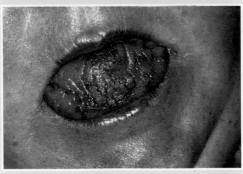

*Figure 36.7. Xerostomia*

The cause is uncertain but there have been links with stress, trauma, poor nutrition, certain foods or toothpastes and the menstrual cycle. There are also often family members who have had similar problems. Ulcers also occur more frequently in the immunosuppressed, in coeliac disease, Chron's disease and inflammatory bowel disease.

In the majority of cases the ulcers, which may be single or multiple, are usually less than 5 mm in diameter and heal within 1–2 weeks (*Figure 36.9*) (Ngan, 2006).

## Table 36.2. Ulcers on the tongue or oral cavity

| Type | Cause | Features | Management |
|---|---|---|---|
| Injury | Fall or blow to the mouth | History of injury | Cold, soft foods<br>Simple or antiseptic mouthwashes |
| Apthous | Uncertain: related to stress, trauma, poor nutrition, foods, toothpastes, immunosuppression | Single or multiple<br><5 mm in diameter<br>Heal within 1–2 weeks | Carmellose gelatine paste<br>Topical steroid paste or tablets to dissolve against the ulcer (as required)<br>Local analgesic ointment or lozenges |
| Herpes simplex | Herpes simplex virus | Associated with or history of cold sores | |
| Herpes zoster | Herpes zoster virus | Pain before ulceration occurs<br>Unilateral ulceration | Add a systemic antiviral, e.g. aciclovir |
| Hand foot and mouth disease | Coxackie virus | Rash on hands, feet and nappy area | Debride<br>Dental advice<br>Antifungal agent if complicated by Candida |
| Lichen planus | Unknown cause; autoimmune factors | Lacy, white reticulate pattern on the oral mucosa<br>White patches and/or ulcers on the tongue<br>Rash elsewhere on the body | Refer for medical opinion on any problem with associated generalized rash or other symptoms |
| Pemphigus | Autoimmune problem | Blisters and erosions in the mouth and this may also be on other parts of the body | Urgent referral for medical opinion |
| Cancer | Tobacco, heavy drinking | Non-healing ulceration<br>Lump or ulceration<br>Often painless initially | Refer any ulcer that does not heal in 3 weeks |

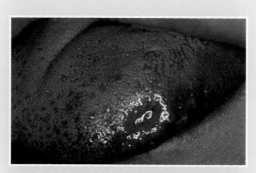

*Figure 36.8. Ulcer following bitten tongue in a fall.*

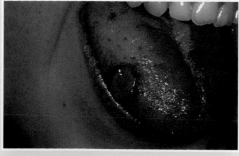

*Figure 36.9. Aphthous ulcer.*

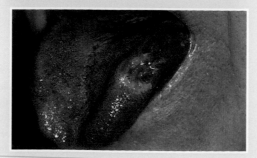

*Figure 36.10. Ulcer tongue associated with lichen planus.*

### Viral infections

#### Herpes simplex virus

Herpes simplex virus is often associated with other signs such as 'cold sores' on the lips.

#### Herpes zoster

Herpes zoster is where the cluster of vesicles and ulcers are limited to one side of the tongue and mouth. The ulceration is usually preceded by pain in the same area.

#### Hand foot and mouth disease

Hand foot and mouth disease is caused by the Coxsackie virus. A rash on the hands, feet and nappy area suggests the diagnosis. Typically there is a rash is on the palms of the hands and the soles of the feet.

## Contact dermatitis

Contact dermatitis may occur owing to contact with something such as dental amalgam.

## Lichen planus

The cause of lichen planus is unknown, but it is associated with some autoimmune conditions. The patient may present with the typical rash of flat-topped papules or hypertrophic lesions that tend to have a violaceous hue. There may also be oral signs of a white reticulate pattern on the buccal mucosa and/or white plaques or ulceration on the tongue (*Figure 36.10*). Sometimes the oral signs occur in isolation without the rash.

## Autoimmune disease

Tongue and mouth ulceration may occur in conditions such as lupus erythematosus or pemphigus. These patients are likely to have other signs of the condition such as a rash, malaise, fever and weight loss (du Vivier, 2002: 490–6). In pemphigus, the condition first presents in the

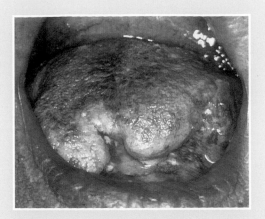

*Figure 36.11. Carcinoma of the tongue*

mouth in 50% of cases but there may be blistering elsewhere on the skin or other mucous membranes. The blisters rapidly break down to form erosions (du Vivier, 2002: 423–6).

## Cancer

Oral squamous cell carcinoma may occur anywhere on the buccal mucosa or tongue and is associated with tobacco smoking, chewing or snuff. It is more common in men, heavy drinkers and those with poor oral hygiene.

The patient presents with a lump or ulcer on the tongue or lip that is usually painless initially. As the lesion enlarges the ulceration spreads, bleeds and interferes with speech, chewing and swallowing (Medline Plus, 2006). The patient shown in *Figure 36.11* had allowed the condition to progress to a stage at which the ulcerated tongue was 'eaten away'.

## Management of oral ulceration

Early diagnosis of oral cancer is crucial. The cure rate in such cases is 75% but overall only 50% survive for more than 5 years because of delay and/or spread to the throat and cervical glands. Any oral ulcer that persists for more than 3 weeks should be biopsied to exclude malignancy (Medline Plus, 2006).

There is no specific cure for most oral ulcers so that the aim of any treatment is to reduce the pain while natural healing occurs. Cold, soft or pureed foods will be easier for the patient to take. Simple or antiseptic mouthwashes may help reduce the risk of secondary infection, while Carmellose gelatin paste may help protect the ulcer site.

Topical steroids such as oromucosal tablets dissolved next to the ulcer, the application of triamcinolone dental paste, or a beclometasone dipropionate inhaler sprayed twice daily (unlicensed for this pupose) may help ease symptoms. Local analgesics such as lidocaine ointment or lozenges may give temporary relief (Joint Formulary Committee, 2006: 12.3).

Systemic antiviral treatment such as aciclovir or famciclovir, should be given in cases of herpes zoster and in the immunocompromised with herpes simplex (Joint Formulary Committee, 2006: 5.3.2).

Any suspicion of more generalized disease should be referred to the doctor for further investigation and advice.

## References

Barker S (2006) Sjögren syndrome. DermNet, NZ. www.dermnetnz.org/immune/sjogren.html (accessed 24 October 2006)

Better Oral Health.info (2006) Dry mouth. www.betteroralhealth.info/Orbit/dry-mouth.html (accessed 24 October 2006)

Joint Formulary Committee (2006) *British National Formulary 52*. September. BMJ Publishing Group and Royal Pharmaceutical Society of Great Britain, London

DermNet NZ (2006) Scarlet fever. www.dermnetnz.org/bacterial/scarlet-fever.html (accessed 24 October 2006)

du Vivier A (2002) *Atlas of Clinical Dermatology*. 3rd edn. Elsevier

Eidelman E, Chosack A, Cohen T (1976) Scrotal tongue and geographic tongue: Polygenic and associated traits. *Oral Surg Oral Med Oral Pathol* 42(5): 591–6

Fung K (2005) Geographic tongue. *Medical Encyclopedia*. www.nlm.nih.gov/medlineplus/ency/article/001049.htm (accessed 24 October 2006)

Kelsch R (2005) Fissured tongue. *eMedicine*. 5 October. www.emedicine.com/DERM/topic665.htm (accessed 24 October 2006)

Medline Plus (2006) Oral cancer. *Medical Encyclopedia*. www.nlm.nih.gov/medlineplus/ency/article/001035.htm (accessed 24 October 2006)

MayoClinic (2005) Black, hairy tongue. www.mayoclinic.com/health/black-hairy-tongue/HQ003 25 (accessed 24 October 2006)

Medline Plus (2005) Thrush. *Medical Encyclopedia*. www.nlm.nih.gov/medlineplus/ency/article/000626.htm (accessed 24 October 2006)

Ngan V (2006) Aphthous ulcers, DermNet NZ. www.dermnetnz.org/site-age-specific/aphthae.html (accessed 24 October 2006)

National Institute of Neurological Disorders and Stroke (2006) Melkersson-Rosenthal syndrome information page. www.ninds.nih.gov/disorders/melkersson/melkersson.htm (accessed 24 October 2006)

## Test Your Knowledge

This 30-year-old woman was distressed. For several days she had been unable to eat solid food or take hot drinks because her mouth was so sore. The tongue was covered in a thick, white coating and there was some inflammation of the underlying mucosa. Any attempt to scrape off the coating showed the underlying mucosa

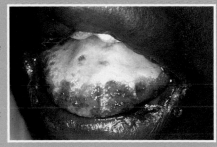

to be inflamed and friable. She complained that she had been feeling a bit 'off colour' recently and that this was the third episode of similar trouble that she had had in the last few months.

### Questions

1. What is the likely diagnosis?
2. What further questions and/or investigations might you consider?
3. What advice and treatment would you offer the patient?

# Abnormalities of the ear lobe

The ear lobe is obvious for all to see. The practice nurse may often be asked for advice about a particular lesion and is in a position to notice and comment on any unmentioned changes. Many lesions of the ear may be associated with years of exposure to the sun or created by desire for beauty and adornment. For others, more serious underlying problems may need to be considered, such as deafness in the presence of what might appear to be minor abnormalities of the earlobe.

## Congenital abnormalities

*'Bat' ears* (*Figure 37.1*) is a minor abnormality in which the ear lobes stick out prominently and/or are particularly large. This may cause problems for a child who is open to teasing and derision by his/her peers. Correction is possible at any time of life but is preferably done before starting school, at about 4–5 years of age. A general anaesthetic is usually required in the young. Complications of the operation are few unless an unsightly scar results. Haematoma and/or infection are possible but these are usually easily treated (American Society of Plastic Surgeons, 2004).

*Congenital deformity of the earlobe* (microtia) (*Figure 37.2*) is defined by an absent or rudimentary pinna. This is often associated with an absent ear canal and middle ear. The inner ear is usually normal. Very early hearing assessment is important so that hearing aids can be fitted as soon as possible. The opinions of facial plastic and ear surgeons should be sought because a bone-conducting hearing aid may need to be fitted. Reconstruction of the microtia and inner ear can be considered by the age of 4 years after an assessment by computed tomography (CT) scan (Levenson, 2003).

Accessory auricles, soft or cartilaginous skin-coloured tags or nodules are sometimes seen on the tragus or along the line from the tragus to the angle of the jaw. They are developmental abnormalities occasionally associated with deafness. They do not usually require any treatment (Logan Turner, 1988).

## Earrings

*Split ear* and *nickel dermatitis* (*Figure 37.3*) may both result from the wearing of earrings. In *split ear* the ear lobe may be torn if the earring is accidentally pulled or tugged at by a young child. Heavy earrings may also gradually elongate the hole and eventually tear the lobe.

Bleeding from a minor tear can be controlled by direct pressure. The area should be cleansed, and the earring removed until it has healed (Aurora Health Care, 2004). Once the wound has healed and any inflammation settled, the tear may be reconstructed surgically. Further use of earrings should be delayed for at least 6–8 weeks after such an operation. If the lobe needs to be pierced again, the patient should wait at least 6 months (Bermant, 2004).

*Nickel sensitivity* may be caused by nickel and cobalt (a contaminant of nickel), which are constituents of much

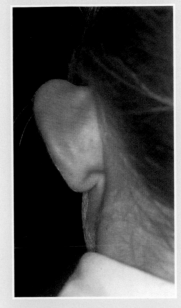

Figure 37.1. 'Bat' ears.

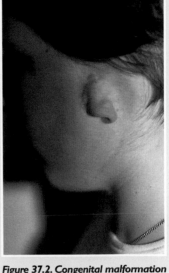

*Figure 37.2. Congenital malformation of the ear lobe.*

costume jewellery, including earrings. The patient develops an eczematous reaction at the site of contact. Symptoms should settle with the help of a mild topical steroid but any contact with nickel in the future will result in the same problem.

Patients should be advised to seek nickel-free adornments. Stainless steel, gold or plastic are possible alternatives. Patch testing confirms nickel sensitivity and highlights other substances that could cause similar problems (Du Vivier, 2002; Kunin, 2002).

## Infection

*Auricular perichondritis* (*Figure 37.4*) may follow trauma, surgery, ear piercing and infection of the ear lobe. The current fashion for high ear piercing may be more likely to be associated with this complication (Yahalom and Eliashar, 2003). If the perichondrium that surrounds the cartilage of the ear lobe becomes infected, the cartilage itself may become involved and necrose, causing a deformity and a shrivelling of the ear lobe that may be difficult to repair.

The patient presents with a painful, swollen, tender, red ear lobe and may be febrile. The infection is usually caused by *Pseudomonas pyocyanea* or *P. aeruginosa* or *Staphylococcus aureus*. Urgent treatment is required with an oral (or sometimes intravenous) antibiotic such as ticarcillin (Joint Formulary Committee, 2003: 274–5). If an abscess has formed, drainage will be required (Logan Turner, 1988; National Institutes of Health, 2002).

## Pressure

*Chondrodermatitis nodularis helicis* (*Figure 37.5*) is a common condition that presents with a painful nodule on

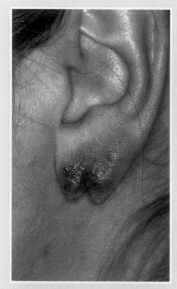

Figure 37.3. Earring complication: split lobe and nickel dermatitis.

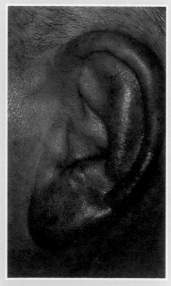

Figure 37.4. Auricular perichondritis.

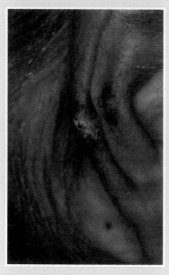

Figure 37.5. Chondrodermatitis nodularis helicis.

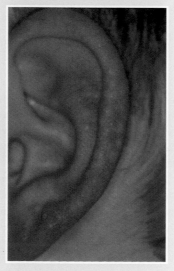

Figure 37.6. Juvenile spring eruption.

## Sun damage

*Juvenile spring eruption* (*Figure 37.6*) occurs most commonly in boys between the ages of 5 and 12 years. It is observed in spring at a time when the sun makes itself felt again. Often it recurs at the same time of year in the same patient but rarely continues into adult life. The child develops a papulo-vesicular rash on the earlobe that may become crusted and associated with a cervical adenitis. It usually settles spontaneously within a week and leaves no scars.

Lesions that irritate or are sore may be eased by the application of a mild topical steroid cream. Future episodes can sometimes be avoided if sunscreens are used or a hat worn at the appropriate time, or if the child can be encouraged to grow his/her hair to cover and protect the ears (Anonymous, 2004).

*Cutaneous horn* (*Figure 37.7*) occurs most commonly on sun-exposed skin. The ear is no exception. Both men and women can be affected and it is usually found in patients between the ages of 60 and 75 years. The hyperkeratotic lesion may increase rapidly in size and is usually symptomless. If traumatized, the base may become inflamed and painful. The lesion at the base of the horn is usually benign and associated with seborrhoeic keratosis, some naevi or premalignant actinic keratoses. However, in 16–20% of cases it is related to a squamous cell carcinoma or occasionally basal cell carcinoma (Silvis, 2001).

Treatment of a keratin horn depends on biopsy of the base of the lesion. A biopsy should be done to exclude an underlying malignant cause. Benign causes can usually be treated satisfactorily with cryotherapy (Silvis, 2001).

*Basal cell carcinoma* commonly develops on light exposed areas including the ear and is the most common cancer in people with white, fair skin who have enjoyed much exposure to ultra-violet light. Some of the other predisposing factors are immunosuppression, radiation and burns. It generally occurs after the age of 40 years and especially in old age. Any slowly progressive lesion that may bleed or ulcerate and fail to heal should be viewed with suspicion. It may present as a nodular, pigmented, superficial or scar-like lesion (morpheaform). Telangiectasia are often observed running across the lesion. The patient in *Figure 37.8* had noticed the lesion gradually increase in size in the previous 9 months.

The diagnosis is confirmed on biopsy and the treatment of choice is excision. Plastic surgery may be advised if the normal appearance of the lobe is to be maintained. Other approaches include radiation, curettage and cautery or cryotherapy but the recurrence rates after these procedures is higher. Metastases from basal cell carcinoma are rare but if the lesion is left untreated, gradual invasion and destruction of adjacent tissues will occur (Jiang, 2004; Leffel and Fitzgerald, 1999).

*Squamous cell carcinoma*, like basal cell carcinoma, is also related to sun exposure, immunosuppression and other injuries to the skin and is most common in people over the age of 65 years. It is common on the head and neck areas and is more common on the earlobe than basal cell carcinoma. It may present as a persistent, erythematous, ulcerated and crusting lesion (*Figure 37.9*) or a nodule without ulceration (*Figure 37.10*). Squamous

the most prominent part of the helix or antihelix. It is aggravated by pressure, cold or trauma. The pain often keeps the patient awake at night because he/she cannot stand the pressure of the pillow. It occurs more commonly in middle aged or elderly men and in those with fair, sun damaged skin, and may occur in people of all skin colours. The nodule may vary in size from 3–20 mm, is well demarcated, round or oval and may have a surface ulcer or crust. The cause is unknown but thought to be related to repeated trauma and/or pressure.

The patient should be encouraged to avoid further pressure by placing a foam pad, shaped with a hole in it, over the lesion at night. Other treatments available to 'cure' the problem include excision, curettage, electrocautery and carbon dioxide laser ablation. Unless the damaged cartilage is removed and the pressure relieved, the recurrence rate is high. If there is doubt about the diagnosis, a biopsy should be taken to exclude malignancy (Marks and Papa, 2002).

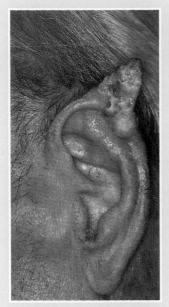

Figure 37.7. Cutaneous horn.

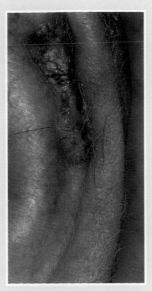

*Figure 37.8. Basal cell carcinoma.*

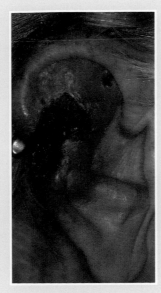

*Figure 37.9. Ulcerating squamous cell carcinoma.*

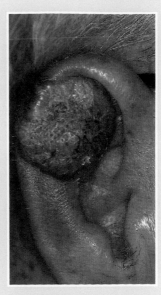

*Figure 37.10. Nodular squamous cell carcinoma.*

cell carcinoma may also be preceded by actinic keratosis or assocated with a cutaneous horn. It is defined as a 'malignant squamous neoplasm in which the cells have penetrated the epithelial basement membrane and invaded the dermis' (Benson, 2004). The diagnosis may be confirmed by punch biopsy, incisional biopsy or excisional biopsy.

The treatment of choice is excision with histological check to ensure complete removal. Occasionally, in patients unfit for surgery, radiotherapy or topical 5-fluorouracil may be used. There is always the potential for metastatic disease from squamous cell carcinoma and the risk of this may be increased in the case of the auricle where there is drainage to deep cervical nodes. As always with cancer, early diagnosis is critical to the long-term prognosis. (Shockley and Stucker, 1987).

Some lesions of the ear present minor health risks but others are more serious and may need to be referred to a specialist. It is important to ensure that the correct diagnosis is made so that the most effective treatment can be provided (*Table 37.1*).

## Table 37.1. Diagnosis of abnormalities of the ear lobe

|  | Cause | Presentation | Investigations | Management |
|---|---|---|---|---|
| 'Bat' ears | Congenital | Prominent large ears |  | • Surgical correction by 4–5 years of age |
| Microtia | Congenital | Absence or deformity of the ear lobe | • Early hearing check<br>• Specialist opinion<br>• CT scan | • Hearing aid as required<br>• Later surgical reconstruction after full assessment and specialist(s) |
| Split ear lobe | • Earrings<br>• Heavy earrings<br>• Trauma | Torn ear lobe |  | • Pressure to stop bleeding, cleansing<br>• Surgical reconstruction when healed<br>• Delay further earrings 6–8 weeks<br>• No further ear piercing for at least 6 months |
| Nickel sensitivity | Allergic reaction | Eczema at the site of contact | Patch test | • Mild topical steroid<br>• Never wear nickel again<br>• Use gold, stainless steel and plastic alternatives |
| Auricular perichondritis | • Trauma, surgery<br>• Ear piercing<br>• *Pseudomonas pyocyanea* or<br>• *P. aeruginosa*,<br>• *Staphyloccus aureus* | • Painful, red, swollen, tender ear lobe<br>• Sometimes fever |  | • Urgent antibiotics, e.g. ticarcillin<br>• Surgical drainage in cases of abcess |

## References

American Society of Plastic Surgeons (2004) Otoplasty, ear Surgery. www.plasticsurgery.org/public_education/procedures/Otoplasty. cfm (accessed 10 December 2004)

Anonymous (2004) Juvenile spring eruption. *GP Notebook*. Oxbridge Solutions, Ltd. www.gpnotebook.com/simplepage. cfm?ID=-2039807930 (accessed 10 December 2004)

Aurora Health Care (2004) Ear, pierced. www.aurorahealthcare. org/yourhealth/scd-adultcare/getcontent.asp?URLAdultCare= "EarPierced.htm" (accessed 10 December 2004)

Benson JF (2004) Squamous cell carcinoma of the skin. www. emedicine.com/ent/topic26.htm (accessed 10 December 2004)

Bermant M (2004) Torn ear lobe reconstruction and injury prevention. www.plasticsurgery4u.com/procedure_folder/split_earlobe.html (accessed 10 December 2004)

du Vivier A (2002) Allergic contact dermatitis. In: *Atlas of Clinical Dermatology*. 3rd edn. Churchill Livingstone: 59–65

Jiang SB (2004) Pathology: Basal cell carcinoma. www.emedicine. com/ent/topic672.htm (accessed 10 December 2004)

Joint Formulary Committee (2004) *British National Formulary 48.* September. Royal Pharmaceutical Society of Great Britain and British Medical Association, London

Kunin A (2002) Nickel contact dermatitis. AAA Skin Doctor. store. yahoo.com/skindoctor/nickel.html (accessed 10 December 2004)

Leffel D, Fitzgerald D (1999) Basal cell carcinoma. In: Freedberg IM, ed. *Fitzpatrick's Dermatology in General Medicine*. 5th edn. McGraw-Hill, New York: 857–64

Levenson MJ (2003) Congenital atresia and microtia of the ear. Eye Surgery Information Centre. www.earsurgery.org/atresia.html (accessed 10 December 2004)

Logan Turner A (1988) Diseases of the external ear. In: Maran ADG, ed. *Logan Turner's Diseases of the Nose, Throat and Ear*. 10th edn. John Wright: 263–4

Marks J, Papa C (2002) Chondrodermatitis nodularis helicis. www. emedicine.com/derm/topic76.htm (accessed 10 December 2004)

National Institutes of Health (2002) Perichondritis. In: Medline Plus Medical Encyclopedia. www.nlm.nih.gov/medlineplus/ency/ article/001253.htm (accessed 10 December 2004)

Shockley W, Stucker F Jr (1987) Squamous cell carcinoma of the external ear: A review of 75 cases. *Otolaryngol Head Neck Surg* **97**(3): 308–12

Silvis N (2001) Cutaneous horn. www.emedicine.com/derm/topic90.htm (accessed 10 December 2004)

Yahalom S, Eliashar R (2003) Perichondritis: A complication of piercing auricular cartilage. *Postgraduate Medical Journal* **79**: 29–30

## Test Your Knowledge

This 73-year old woman presented in the surgery with complaints of a very painful lesion on the antihelix of her left ear. It had become increasingly troublesome over the previous 6 months. She complained that it was tender to touch and that it kept her awake at night when she lay her head on the pillow. Examination showed a small, tender, slightly raised circular lesion with a small ulcer at its centre.

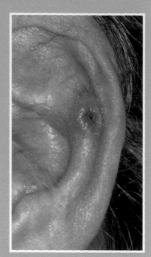

### Questions

1. What is the most likely diagnosis?
2. What treatment and/or investigations might you consider?
3. What other advice would you give the patient?

# Spots around the eyes

Patients sometimes worry about things that may seem trivial. A small blemish, particularly if it is on the face and visible for all to see, can be a real problem. The patient may be concerned that it is the start of cancer, that it may be a manifestation of an underlying disease, or that it will spread and he/she will be too embarrassed to go out in public.

Spots around the eyes raise these questions and it is helpful if general practice health professionals can recognize a problem, advise the patient of the diagnosis, reassure the person if possible and explain what, if any, action should be taken. This chapter will consider three problems that are commonly presented to, or noticed by, the practice nurse.

## Milia

Milia are benign, keratin-filled cysts that are thought to arise from the sebaceous glands. They are particularly common in newborn infants and it is thought that these primary milia arise in sebaceous glands that are not completely developed. However, primary milia may also occur in children and adults.

Secondary milia may develop in areas of skin that may have been damaged, thus affecting the sweat ducts. This may follow problems such as dermabrasion, a number of blistering disorders (e.g. bullous pemphigoid, sunburn or chronic solar damage), or in skin damaged by radiotherapy or the use of potent topical corticosteroids (Cooper and Ratnavel, 2001; du Vivier, 2002).

### Presentation

Milia present as symptomless, white or cream coloured papules. They may be single or multiple and are frequently seen on the eyelids and around the eyes (*Figure 38.1*) (Ratnavel et al, 1995), although no part of the body is exempt (*Figure 38.2*). Milia are particularly prevalent in newborn babies, where they are commonly seen on the face and nose (*Figure 38.3*). Occasionally they may be found on the mucosa or the palate (Epstein pearls).

### Diagnosis

The diagnosis of milia can easily be made by the appearance of the lesions. If there is doubt about this, a biopsy can be taken, but this is generally unnecessary. Sometimes it may be necessary to investigate the underlying cause in cases of secondary milia to exclude conditions such as pemphigoid (Cooper and Ratnavel, 2001).

### Management

No treatment is required for milia unless the patient is unhappy about his/her appearance. Milia occurring in infancy usually disappear spontaneously within a few weeks, but for patients in the older age groups, and those with secondary milia, it tends to persist longer. Milia can easily be dealt with if the cyst is pricked with a sterile needle or cold point cautery, and the contents of the cyst are squeezed out. However, those with multiple milia may decide not to undergo the discomforts of this treatment (Leppard and Ashton, 1998).

## Syringoma

Syringoma is a benign tumour of the sweat ducts. Syringomas occur more commonly in women, East Asians and African-Caribbeans. They usually first develop at puberty but new lesions may also develop later. The cause is uncertain, but in some patients there may be a family history of the problem. Syringomas are sometimes associated with Down's syndrome and diabetes mellitus (Horenstein and Shea, 2002).

### Presentation

Syringomas present as symptomless, skin-coloured or yellowish, round or flat-topped papules that are usually smaller than 3 mm in diameter (*Figure 38.4*). They are found most commonly on the upper part of the cheeks or lower eyelids where clusters of multiple, symmetrically placed lesions may be seen. However, they do occur elsewhere on the body, particularly the axilla, chest, abdomen, and genital areas (Horenstein and Shea, 2002).

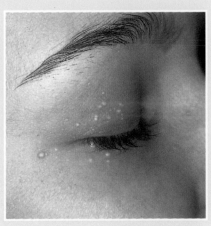
*Figure 38.1. Milia on the eyelid of a child.*

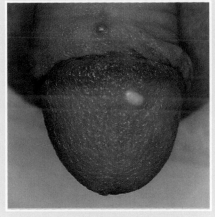
*Figure 38.2. Isolated milia on the penis.*

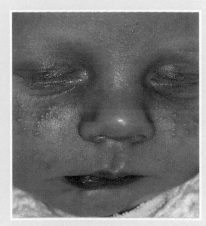
*Figure 38.3. Milia on a 5-week-old baby.*

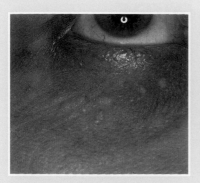

**Figure 38.4. Multiple syringomas.**

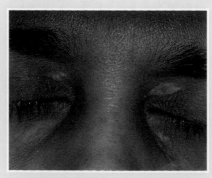

**Figure 38.5. Xanthelasma.**

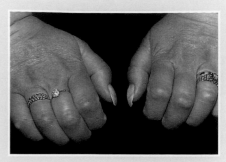

**Figure 38.6. Xanthelasma nodules on the knuckle of a woman with hyperlidaemia.**

### Differential diagnosis

Syringomas may appear similar to milia, basal cell carcinoma and trichoepithelioma (an inherited condition of tumours originating in the hair follicle) (Prieto and Shea, 2003). Therefore a careful differential diagnosis is required to enable decisions to be made about the correct treatment (*Table 38.1*).

### Investigations

A biopsy and histological examination may be taken, if necessary, to confirm the diagnosis and distinguish it from the other problems (Horenstein and Shea, 2002).

### Management

The patient can be reassured that syringomas are completely harmless and that no treatment or interference is necessary. If the patient is worried about the cosmetic effect they can be cleared by cautery under local anaesthetic if they are <2 mm in diameter, or removed by curettage and cautery if >2 mm in diameter (Leppard and Ashton, 1999).

## Xanthelasma

Xanthelasma occur as the result of deposition of lipid in the skin. Often they occur in patients with type II hyperlipidaemia and type IV phenotype. Approximately 50% of patients with xanthelasma have a raised plasma lipid level and some of these are likely to have low, high-density lipoprotein (HDL) levels (Schumucker and Hampton, 2001). This may be caused by a primary genetic defect or abnormal metabolism (du Vivier, 2002).

### Presentation

Xanthelasma may occur at any stage from puberty to old age but usually appear between the ages of 40–60 years. They are more common in women than in men.

Soft, yellow plaques develop around the eyes and mainly affect the medial sides of the upper eyelids. However, they are also found on the lower lids and are often bilateral (*Figure 38.5*). Xanthelasma rarely causes the patient any problems other than the fact that they are unsightly and cause embarrassment. Once established,

## Table 38.1. Differential diagnosis

|  | Milia | Syringoma | Xanthelasma |
|---|---|---|---|
| **Cause** | • Keratin-filled cysts arising from sebaceous gland | • Benign tumour of sweat ducts | • Deposits of lipid in the skin |
| **Age** | • Newborn<br>• Others in later life | • Puberty onwards | • Commonest age 40–60 years |
| **Associated problems** | • Skin damage<br>• Blistering problems | • Occasionally family | • Hyperlipidaemia (50%)<br>• Xanthomas<br>• Down's syndrome<br>• Diabetes mellitus |
| **Presentation** | • White or cream coloured papules (single or multiple)<br>• Often around the eyes but may occur anywhere | • Skin coloured or yellowish papules <3 mm in diameter<br>• Multiple lesions<br>• Usually upper cheeks and eyelids but can occur anywhere | • Soft, yellow plaque<br>• Usually around the eyes |
| **Investigations** | • Clinical diagnosis<br>• Biopsy if in doubt<br>• Check for underlying problems in secondary milia, e.g. pemphigoid | • Clinical diagnosis<br>• Biopsy if in doubt | • Clinical diagnosis<br>• Fasting lipids and high-density lipoprotein (HDL) and low-density lipoprotein (LDL) |
| **Management** | • Nil necessary<br>• If patient requests, prick lesion and squeeze out contents | • Nil necessary<br>• Cautery under local anaesthetic if needed | Nil necessary or:<br>• Surgical excision<br>• Carbon dioxide and argon laser<br>• Chemical cautery<br>• Cryotherapy and management of hyperlipidaemia if detected |

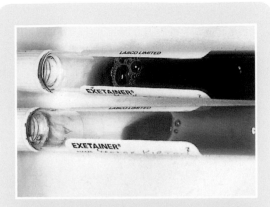

*Figure 38.7. Fasting lipid test. Top-normal blood. Lower-hyperlipidaemia.*

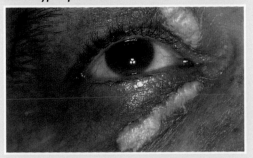

*Figure 38.8. Xanthelasma immediately after treatment with trichloracetic acid.*

they may continue to increase in size or remain static (Schumucker and Hampton, 2001).

## Investigations

The patient should be examined for any other obvious signs of hyperlipidaemia, e.g. xanthomas. These lobulated, yellowish nodules can sometimes be found over the knees, elbows, Achilles tendon and backs of the hands (*Figure 38.6*) (du Vivier, 2002: 523–4).

In order to recognize patients who have xanthelasma that is associated with a hyperlipidaemia, HDL and low-density lipoprotein (LDL) levels should also be requested (*Figure 38.7*).

## Management

*Xanthelasma*

If the patient is not concerned, no treatment is required. If treatment is requested, the following choices are available:

- Surgical excision may be satisfactory for small lesions, but there is a 40% risk of later recurrence of the lesion
- Carbon dioxide and argon laser ablation may be successful, but there may be subsequent scarring and pigmentation of the treated area
- Chemical cauterization using carefully applied trichloracetic acid may achieve good results with minimal scarring (*Figure 38.8*). More than one treatment may be required
- Superficial xanthelasma may respond to cryotherapy but scarring and pigmentation of the area my follow and several treatments may be required (Schumucker and Hampton, 2001).

*Hyperlipidaemia*

The patient with xanthelasma should always be checked to see if hyperlipidaemia is present. The patient should then be given advice about following a low-fat diet and making life-style changes if appropriate, e.g. weight loss and smoking cessation. Lipid-lowering agents should also be considered (Joint Formulary Committee, 2004).

## References

Cooper S, Ratnavel R(2001) *Milia*. www.emedicine.com/derm/topic 265.htm (accessed 28 May 2004)

du Vivier A (2002) Benign tumours of the skin. In: *Atlas of dermatology*. 3rd edn. Churchill Livingstone, London: 126–7

Horenstein M, Shea C (2002) *Syringioma*. www.emedicine.com/ DERM/topic414.htm (accessed 28 May 2004)

Joint Formulary Committee (2004) *British National Formulary 47*. March. British Medical Association and Royal Pharmaceutical Society of Great Britain, London: 124–9

Leppard B, Ashton R (1998) *Treatment in Dermatology*. Radcliffe Medical Press, Oxford: 117

Prieto V, Shea C (2003) *Tricho-epithelioma*. www.emedicine. com/derm/topic429.htm (accessed 28 May 2004)

Ratnavel R, Handfield Jones S, Norris P (1995) Milia restricted to the eyelids. *Clin Exp Dermatol* **20**(2): 285–6

Schumucker T, Hampton R (2001) *Xanthelasma*. www.emedicine. com/oph/topic10.htm (accessed 28 May 2004)

## Test Your Knowledge

This 78-year-old woman had always loved the sun. Whenever she had the opportunity she was out there, soaking it up. On occasions, when abroad she had suffered sunburn to her face and neck. She now complains that for the last 13 years she had noticed increasing numbers of small, white papules spreading over her forehead, round her eyes and down onto her neck.

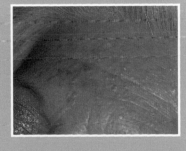

### Questions

1. What is the likely diagnosis and what investigations would you feel might be necessary?
2. What explanation would you give to the patient?
3. What treatment and further advice would you give the patient?

# Adverse reactions to topical steroids

Ingested drugs are not the only ones to cause adverse effects. Topical preparations such as the many creams, ointments, gels, lotions, eye and nasal drops, and sprays that are prescribed or acquired over the counter may also cause adverse reactions. These may result in allergic reactions, localized irritant reactions to the substance, or exacerbation of underlying infections. Often preparations are used inappropriately by a patient who happens to have a tube of ointment in the cupboard or buys a tube in ignorance from the local pharmacy (Davies, 2001).

Topical corticosteroids are a valuable tool in many cases but care must always be taken when recommending their use for patients. In general, the moderately and mildly potent preparations such as hydrocortisone 1% or clobetasone butyrate 0.05% rarely cause adverse reactions, but more potent forms such as betamethasone and clobetasol propionate may cause problems, particularly if they are used for long periods or over large or raw areas where absorption may occur (Joint Formulary Committee, 2005:13 4) *(Table 39.1)*.

## Systemic effects

More potent topical steroids may cause pituitary-adrenal suppression and Cushing's syndrome in rare cases if the steroid is absorbed (Joint Formulary Committee, 2005: 13.4). Absorption may be increased if the preparation is used under occlusion or over thin, macerated skin and the intertriginous areas. Occasionally, patients have developed a Cushingoid appearance (moon face, erythema and hirsutism), or osteoporosis, and there has been stunted growth in some children (Tang and Su, 2003).

## Local effects

### Contact dermatitis

Contact dermatitis is not common but should be considered in a patient with a dermatitis that responds well to steroids and then begins to deteriorate, despite still using the application. The problem may lie with the base of the ointment or cream, which may contain a variety of ingredients including a preservative or stabilizer, an antimicrobial such as neomycin, or it may be caused by the steroid molecule itself (Tang and Su, 2003). Patch testing can confirm the problem. Often it is sensible to patch test the patient with the application before starting treatment (du Vivier, 2002a).

### Infected skin

If topical steroids are applied to infected skin, the infection is likely to get worse. In particular, *Staphylococcus aureus* is often an exacerbating factor in eczema *(Figure 39.1)*. Streptococcal infections may also occur. Infection is suspected where there is crusting, weeping and surrounding cellulitis. Such an infection may need to be treated with an appropriate systemic antibiotic. If the infection is localized, a topical antibiotic might be considered (Primary Care Dermatology Society and British Association of Dermatologists, 2003).

## Fungal infections

### *Tinea incognito*

If the rash of tinea is treated in error with a topical steroid, it may spread and become difficult for a nurse or doctor to recognize. The typical rash will become larger, less scaly and the margins will be flatter and less obvious. Also pustules develop within the area *(Figure 39.2)*.

Skin scrapings should be taken from the lesion and be examined for fungal elements. However, if the patient has recently used the steroid cream, the results may be negative. It may then be necessary to wait a few days until the lesion has flared and become more inflamed, before a positive result can be obtained.

To treat the tinea incognito, the steroid preparation should be discontinued and an antifungal preparation with terbinafine or itraconazole given (du Vivier, 2002b).

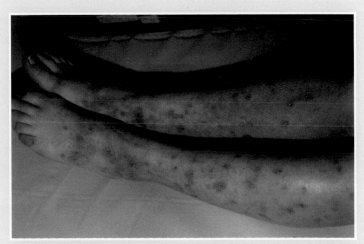

*Figure 39.1. Infected eczema – Antibiotic treatment necessary.*

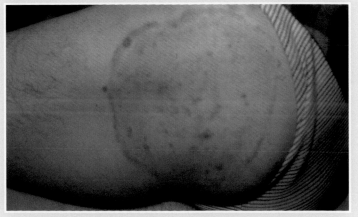

*Figure 39.2. Tinea incognito treated incorrectly with topical steroids.*

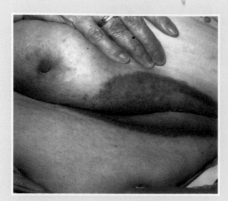

Figure 39.3. Candida intertrigo: the patient had tried to ease the soreness with topical steroids.

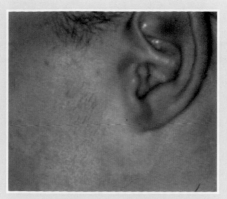

Figure 39.4. Pityriasis alba - topical steroids had been used on the face.

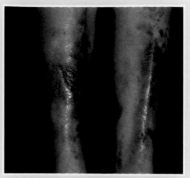

Figure 39.6. Skin fragility and bruising after the use of systemic and potent topical steroids.

### Candida

*Candida* may be altered and exacerbated by the use of topical steroids in the same way as tinea. This may be observed particularly in the warm, intertriginous areas of the groin, nappy and submammary area *(Figure 39.3)*. *Candida* may also become a problem for those using inhalers that contain steroids such as beclometasone. In such cases, the patient may complain of a sore mouth or hoarseness. A spacer may be recommended when using the inhaler, and rinsing the mouth out with water after inhalation may reduce this risk (Joint Formulary Committee, 2005: 3.2). Antifungal lozenges or oral suspension should help control the problem. It is important, when starting a new treatment, to ensure that the patient is well instructed in its use and can recognize any side effects if they occur.

### Skin damage

#### Pigmentary changes

Repeated use of topical steroids may cause changes in skin pigmentation. This is more likely in association with potent steroids or in infants and young children (Tang and Su, 2003). Some patients develop hypopigmented areas of the skin following the use of topical steroids. This problem is most common on the face and is more noticeable in dark or tanned skin. The changes may be reversible (Joint Formulary Committee, 2005: 13.4). The patient in *Figure 39.4* had a mild eczematous rash on his face. He had used some betamethasone cream that he had in the cupboard in an attempt to clear it. The pale patches lasted long after stopping the cream. His colour gradually returned to normal.

### Striae and telangiectasia

Striae and telangiectasia will remain a permanent disfigurement. The patient in *Figure 39.5* had been using a potent topical corticosteroid (betamethasone) for 2 years to control an eczematous rash on her inner thighs. If such treatment is required for the face, only a weak corticosteroid (e.g. hydrocortisone 1% may be used, and then only for as short a time as possible (Joint Formulary Committee, 2005: 13.4).

### Bruising and skin fragility

In some cases skin damage caused by the use of steroids may be such that the patient finds that the skin is very fragile, tears and bruises extremely easily (DermNet NZ, 2005c) *(Figure 39.6)*. This patient was a severe asthmatic and had taken oral steroids for some time but also had a persistent eczematous problem on her legs for which she had used a potent topical steroid. It may be hoped that there will be some improvement of the skin once the steroids are stopped, but complete resolution is unlikely (Joint Formulary Committee, 2005: 13.4).

### Perioral dermatitis

Perioral dermatitis *(Figure 39.7)* is characterized by itchy, tender red spots around the mouth, chin and upper lips. It is associated with the use of moisturizers, make-up, sunscreens and topical steroids around the mouth. It may be caused by proliferating bacteria in the hair follicles (DermNet NZ, 2005a), which is encouraged by steroids. This patient had developed a few spots under her nose. Mometasone cream seemed to clear it but the condition flared every time she tried to discontinue it. She was advised to stop the steroid (despite the flare up) and was prescribed a course of minocycline to treat it. The condition cleared within a few weeks.

## Table 39.1. Common topical steroids by strength

| Strength | Steroid | Examples |
|---|---|---|
| **Mild** | Hydrocortisone | Efcortelan<br>Canesten HC*<br>Daktacort*<br>Fucidin H*<br>Vioform<br>Hydrocortisone* |
| **Moderate** | Clobetasone butyrate 0.05% | Eumovate<br>Trimovate* |
| **Potent** | Betamethasone dipropionate 0.05%<br>Betamethasone valerate 0.1%<br>Diflucortolone valerate 0.1%<br>Fluocinolone acetonide 0.025%<br>Fluocinonide 0.05% | Diprosone<br>Betnovate<br>Nerisone<br>Synalar<br>Metosyn |
| **Very potent** | Clobetasol propionate 0.05% | Dermovate |

\* Steriords combined with antibiotics and/or antifungal agents
From: Joint Formulary Committee, 2005

## Acne

Acne vulgaris may develop or become worse at the site of application of topical steroids (Joint Formulary Committee, 2005: 13.4). Acne rosacea is aggravated by topical steroids, which should never be prescribed for this condition. If steroids are used in error for the red face, papules, pustules and telangiectasia of rosacea, there is improvement, but when the steroids are withdrawn, symptoms return *(Figure 39.8)*. The patient must be persuaded to stop the steroids. Oral tetracycline or topical metronidazole cream or gel can then be introduced (DermNet NZ, 2005b).

## Psoriasis

Topical steroids are often used in psoriasis to good effect but may provoke complications, some of which have serious outcomes. For example, there is a risk of tachyphylaxis, in which continued use of the cream or ointment leads to decreased efficacy and may result in an acute flare up or severe pustular psoriasis when the treatment is discontinued. If potent topical steroids are used in widespread psoriasis, any of the local or systemic side effects may occur. It is recommended that a short course of a weak steroid may be used in flexural or facial psoriasis, so long as nothing stronger than hydrocortisone 1% is used on the face. A more potent steroid is needed for the scalp (Joint Formulary Committee, 2005: 13.4). Patient education on management is crucial.

## Eyes

Topical steroids (drops or ointments) should be used only under supervision to treat the eye. 'Red eye' may be the result of a bacterial or viral infection; treating it with a steroid would risk aggravation, corneal ulceration, impaired vision, or even loss of the eye. Steroid glaucoma or steroid cataract can also occur. If topical steroids are used to treat blepharitis, eczema or other conditions of the eyelid or periorbital area there is a risk that any steroid cream might contaminate the eye itself and cause these problems (Joint Formulary Committee, 2005: 11.4.1)

## Nose

Corticosteroid nasal drops and sprays may be used for hay fever and allergic rhinitis, sometimes in combination with an antihistamine or cromoglicate. If such a patient has an untreated nasal infection, the infection may be aggravated. Steroid nasal drops and sprays should not be used in cases of pulmonary tuberculosis or until healing is complete after nasal surgery.

Locally, the patient may complain of a dry nose or nose bleeds and occasionally ulceration of the mucous membrane. Systemic effects are also possible in long-term users, particularly if they are using nasal drops rather than a spray (Joint Formulary Committee, 2005: 12.2).

## Conclusions

Topical steroids are safe in the short term for symptomatic relief, so long as a number of important safety precautions are considered *(Table 39.2)*.

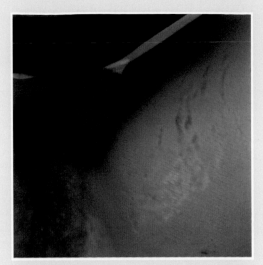

*Figure 39.5. Striae after prolonged use of potent steroids to the area.*

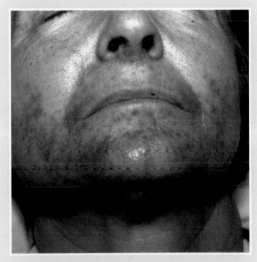

*Figure 39.7. Perioral dermatitis that flared after use of topical steroids.*

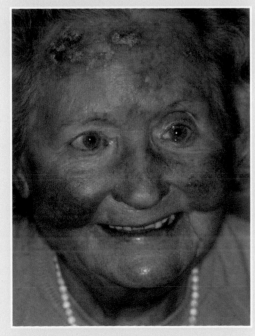

*Figure 39.8. Acne Rosacea that flared after the use of topical steroids.*

## Table 39.2. Important considerations when prescribing topical steroids

**Do:**

Match the potency of the steroid to the severity of the problem

Choose the weakest steroid that will control the condition

Use steroids for a few days in acute eczema

Use steroids for up to 4–6 weeks in chronic eczema

Review all steroid use regularly

Apply emollients 30 minutes after a topical steroid

**Do not:**

Use very potent steroids in children without specialist advice

Use topical steroids to provide emollient effect

**Beware:**

Treating infected areas with topical steroids

Using topical steroids near the eyes

Using topical steroids on the face— use only a mild topical steroid (hydrocortisone 1%) for as short a time as possible

**Consider:**

New immunomodulatory agents, e.g, tacrolimus or pimecrolimus, in those who may be intolerant to topical steroids or where conventional therapy has failed

**Ensure:**

When treatment is started, that the patient understands the purpose and use of each preparation and how to recognize any side effects

From: Primary Care Dermatology Society and British Association of Dermatologists, 2003.

## Test Your Knowledge

This middle aged woman presented in the surgery complaining of a sore mouth and throat and that her friends had noticed her to be rather hoarse recently. She did not attend the surgery very often but she was a known asthmatic who coped well with her condition. Repeat prescriptions for her inhalers were given from time to time. She mentioned that she had had a little more trouble than

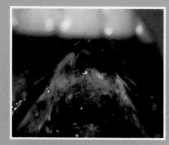

usual since the hot weather began. On examination, there were some smooth red patches on the tongue and a white coating at the back of her tongue. A diagnosis of Candida was made.

**Questions:**

1. What do you think may be the cause of the candidal infection?
2. What further investigations might you wish to pursue?
3. What advice would you give to the patient?

## References

Davies C (2001) Paradoxical reactions to commonly used drugs. *Adverse Drug Reaction Bulletin* 211: 807–10

DermNet NZ (2005a) Perioral dermatitis. May. http://dermnetnz.org/acne/perioral-dermatitis.html (accessed 18 August 2005)

DermNet NZ (2005b) Rosacea. May. http://dermnetnz.org/acne/rosacea.html (accessed 18 August 2005)

DermNet NZ (2005c) Topical steroids. July. http://dermnetnz. org/treatments/topical-steroids.html (accessed 18 August 2005)

du Vivier A (2002a) Contact dermatitis. In: *Atlas of Clinical Dermatology*. 3rd edn. Churchill Livingstone, London: 59–64

du Vivier A (2002b) Superficial fungal disorders of the skin. In: *Atlas of Clinical Dermatology*. Churchill Livingstone, London: 326–7

Joint Formulary Committee (2005) *British National Formulary 49*. March. Royal Pharmaceutical Society of Great Britain, London

Primary Care Dermatology Society, British Association of Dermatologists (2003) Guidelines for the management of atopic eczema. www.bad.org.uk/healthcare/service/Eczema_11.03.03.pdf (accessed 26 August 2005)

Tang YM, Su R (2003) Principles of prescribing topical preparations and topical steroids. In: Sá Cabral

P, Leite L, Pinto J, eds. *Handbook of Dermatology and Venereology*. Social Hygiene Handbook, 2nd edn. Department of Dermatology, Hospital Pulido Valente, Lisbon. www.hkmj.org.hk/skin/steroids.htm (accessed 19 August 2005)

# Drug induced reactions of the skin

Skin rashes are often associated with prescription and over-the-counter medications. Drugs should be considered as a possible cause of any cutaneous eruption. At least 1% of rashes seen in general practice and 3% in the hospital setting will be related to the use of medications, particularly in older people and the immunocompromised (Ehrlich et al, 2004). A nurse's ability to recognize a drug-induced rash and discontinue treatment quickly can help relieve suffering and reduce the potentially toxic effects of the drug. Although such reactions are usually mild, sometimes they can be serious or even life threatening (Lee and Thomson, 1999).

Reasons for the development of drug-induced eruptions may be toxic or allergic. Some eruptions may be normal but will have unwanted problems, such as alopecia (hair loss) during chemotherapy. Others may be the result of an excess dose of a drug or a drug intolerance owing to altered metabolism. Some people may have an allergic response to a drug, or the skin may become photosensitive to ultraviolet light.

Almost any drug may be responsible for a skin reaction but common offenders are antibiotics, non-steroidal antiinflammatory drugs (NSAIDs) and aspirin, diuretics, drugs for treating cardiovascular disease, medicines which act on the central nervous system such as antidepressants or the phenothiazines, drugs used for the management of rheumatic problems, and sulphonamide preparations (du Vivier, 2002) (Table 40.1).

Drug-induced rashes may mimic almost any of the inflammatory dermatoses, and drug reactions may be

## Table 40.1. Characteristics of drug-induced skin reactions

| Type of rash | Presentation | Distribution | Onset | Differential diagnoses |
|---|---|---|---|---|
| Erythematous, morbilliform rashes | Erythematous Macules/papules | Widespread Palms/soles spared | 2–3 weeks | Infections |
| Photosensitivity | Erythema Blisters | Sun-exposed areas | <24 hours | Sunburn Idiopathic Porphyria |
| Pigmentation | Brown pigment | Sun-exposed areas | Gradual | |
| | Slate grey | Generalized - phenothiazines | | Amodiderone Minocycline |
| Vasculitis and purpura | Palpable purpura Does not blanch on pressure\ From pinpoint size to a few centimetres Haemorrhagic blisters ulceration | Legs Systemic: fever, joint pains | 1–3 weeks | Infection Immunological problems |
| Urticaria and angioedema | Itchy, oedematous weals | Any site | <36 hours | Allergies, e.g. to foods such as fish, nuts, or strawberries Infections |
| Erythema multiforme | Asyptomatic red/purple rash Various shapes Target lesions Blisters | Symmetrical Limbs/palms/trunk Soles feet Mucous membranes | Usually within 4 weeks | Infections Collagen disease Bacterial Malignancy Herpes simplex Sarcoid |
| Stevens Johnson syndrome | Ill patient, fever Blisters, erosions | Generalized Mucous membranes | | As erythema multiforme |
| Erythema nodosum | Tender, red nodules 1–5 cm Last 4–8 weeks | Shins – extensor surfaces | | Streptococcal Infections Tuberculosis Sarcoidosis |
| Fixed-drug eruption | Erythematous; dusky round/ oval, brown/purple | Recurs at same site whenever the drug is taken | <8 hours | |
| Psoriasis | Psoriatic lesions | Whole body/scalp | | |
| Lichenoid eruptions | Shiny papules Violaceous colour | Localized or widespread | Weeks or months | Lichen planus |
| Acne | Papular/pustules | Face, chest, back, may extend | | |
| Eczema | Dry itchy skin Dry lips | Any site | | |

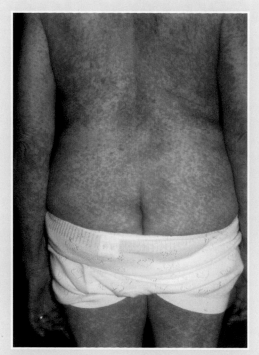

*Figure 40.1. Erythematous morbilliform rash in a patient treated for a urinary infection with trimethoprim.*

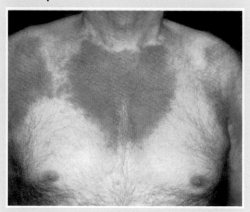

*Figure 40.2. Photosensitivity rash in a patient recently treated with trimethoprim for urinary infection after a day in the sun.*

difficult to distinguish from a disease that is associated with a similar rash *(Table 40.2)*. As with any rash, drug intake must remain a part of the differential diagnosis. Unless the drug is discontinued, symptoms will deteriorate. Patients who experience a reaction to a drug must not receive the same drug again because the reaction will recur and may be worse. Medicines administered both topically and systemically can cause problems but the following discussion considers only those used systemically.

## Types of skin reaction

### Erythematous morbilliform rashes

Erythematous morbilliform reactions *(Figure 40.1)* are the most common type of skin eruption that occurs in reaction to drugs. They account for 30–50% of cutaneous drug eruptions (Erlich, 2004). The patient develops a widespread rash made up of erythematous macules and papules. The whole body may be covered by the rash but the palms and soles are normally spared. The rash usually appears about 2–3 weeks after treatment has begun (Lee and Thomson, 1999).

Ampicillin, amoxycillin and sulphonamides cause this type of reaction most commonly, but may other preparations can have the same effect.

### Photosensitivity rashes

Some drugs lead to rashes in areas that have been exposed to light. A photosensitivity reaction usually develops within 24 hours of exposure (Bergamo and Elmets, 2004). It may take a variety of forms. Some appear like bad sunburn with erythema *(Figure 40.2)*, which may proceed to blistering. In others the rash may be lichenoid or eczematous in appearance. Hyperpigmentation may be a feature after the rash has subsided. Other patients develop annular, scaling and psoriasiform, or rashes of the type associated with lupus erythematosus. The areas commonly affected are the 'V' area of the neck, and the backs of the arms and hands, but in some cases the rash may extend beyond these limits. Amiodarone and chlorpromazine are frequent causes, but are not alone in causing this type of rash (Bergamo and Elmets, 2004).

### Pigmentation

Pigmentation occurs as a phototoxic skin reaction in which pigmentary changes develop, particularly in sun exposed areas, as the result of taking certain drugs. A slate grey colour may be caused by a number of drugs among which chlorpromazine, amiodarone and minocycline are the most frequent offenders *(Figure 40.3)*. Patients should be warned to discuss the problem with their doctor as the medication should be stopped and an alternative found if necessary. Oestrogens in the contraceptive pill or hormone replacement therapy (HRT) may lead to patchy brown pigmentation on the face (chloasma). It becomes more marked after exposure to the sun and may not fade completely when the drugs are discontinued (Bergamo and Elmets, 2005).

### Vasculitis and purpura

Acute cutaneous vasculitis may be difficult to distinguish from thrombocytopenic or Henoch Schonlein purpura, but the problem is probably drug related in 10% of cases (Lee and Thomson, 1999). Vasculitis leads to inflammation and necrosis of the walls of the blood vessels. Initially the patient develops erythematous macules that blanch on pressure. These are followed by purple lesions of palpable purpura that do not blanch *(Figure 40.4)*. The size of the lesions may vary from pinpoint to several centimetres. Some may form haemorrhagic blisters or ulcerate. As other organs become involved other symptoms may occur, e.g. fever and joint, muscle and abdominal pain. The rash lasts for up to about 4 weeks and gradually resolves leaving yellow or brown patches. It usually develops between 1–3 weeks after the patient has started the offending drug. The drugs most often associated with simple vascular purpura are NSAIDs, sulphonamides and anticonvulsants. Other causes of vasculitis include infections and immunological problems (du Vivier, 2002).

## Table 40.2. Types of rashes and more common associated drug causes

**Erythematous morbilliform rashes**

Antibiotics: penicillins (e.g. ampicillin, amoxycillin), cephalosporins, erythromycin, gentamycin
Diuretics: frusemide, thiazides
Sulphonamides, nitrofurantoin
Antituberculous drugs
Barbiturates
Carbamazepine
Phenothiazines
Phenytoin
Gold

**Photosensitivity rashes**

Amiodarone
NSAIDs
Phenothiazines
Retinoids, including isotretinoin
Sulphonamides
Tetracycline
Thiazides
Occasionally: antidepressants, carbamazepine, griseofulvin, sulphonylureas (e.g. glicazide, tolbutamide), quinolones (e.g. ciprofloxacin)

**Pigmentation**

Amiodarone
Chlorpromazine
Minocycline
Oestrogens

**Vasculitis**

Penicillin
Phenothiazine
NSAIDs, aspirin
Sulphonamides
Phenytoin
Allopurinol
Cimetidine
Diuretics: thiazides, frusemide

Hydralazine
Propylthiouracil

**Urticaria and angioedema**

ACE inhibitors
Antibiotics, especially penicillin
Salicylates
Hydrallazine
Insulin
NSAIDs
Muscle relaxants
Opiods: morphine, codeine

**Erythema multiforme and Stevens Johnson syndrome**

Antibiotics: penicillins, tetracyclines
Sulphonamides
Rifampicin
Diuretics: thiazides
NSAIDs
Barbiturates
Phenothiazines
Phenytoin, lamotrigine
Chlorpropamide
Gold

**Erythema nodosum**

Barbiturates
Sulphonamides
Oral contraceptive pill
Salicylates
Bromides and iodides
Gold

**Fixed-drug eruptions**

Analgesics, NSAIDs, aspirin
Barbiturates
Hyoscine
Dapsone
Phenolphthalein
Sulphonamides
Quinine

Tetracycline
Griseofulvin
Oral contraceptives

**Psoriasis and psoriasiform eruptions**

Lithium
ACE inhibitors
Beta-blockers
Chloroquin and hydroxychloroquin
Gold
Interferon
NSAIDs
Tetracycline
Nicotine
Alcohol

**Lichenoid eruptions**

Antimalarials
Beta-blockers
Gold
Antituberculous drugs: streptomycin, isoniazid
Carbamazepine
ACE inhibitors: captopril, enalapril
Thiazides
Penicillamine
Chlorpromazine

**Acne**

Corticosteroids: topical and systemic
Oral contraceptives
Androgens in women
Isoniazid
Lithium
Anticonvulsants

**Eczema**

Isotretinoin
Methyldopa
Gol

From: Primary Care Dermatology Society and British Association of Dermatologists, 2003.

### Urticaria and angioedema

Urticaria presents with itchy, raised, oedematous blotches or weals *(Figure 40.5)* that may come and go within a few hours before disappearing without trace (du Vivier, 2002: 375). In cases of angioedema, fluid leakage leads to oedema of the deeper layers of the skin or mucosa.

Such swelling of the tongue or upper respiratory tract may cause obstruction of the airway and require urgent treatment with adrenalin, injectable antihistamines and systemic steroids du Vivier, 2002: 337–8). In acute urticaria, oral or injected antihistamines are usually sufficient. The rash may occur anywhere on the body within about 36 hours of exposure to an offending drug. Other causes may be related to certain foods, infections or rubber. Angiotensin converting enzyme (ACE) inhibitors, antibiotics, salicylates and NSAIDs are commonly associated with these problems (du Vivier 2002: 374–8; Lee and Thomson, 1999).

### Erythema multiforme

Erythema multiforme may present in a number of different ways but should be thought of as a diagnosis in the case of any asymptomatic, symmetrical, red or purple rash that takes on a variety of shapes. Its classic presentation is as the so-called annular, 'target' lesions in which there is a raised, cyanotic central area *(Figure 40.6)*. The lesions occur particularly on the limbs, palms of the hands and soles of the feet but may be more widespread. Blisters may occur. Infections, in particular herpes simplex, are the most frequent cause of erythema multiforme but it may sometimes be related to drugs (du Vivier, 2002: 369–71).

### Stevens Johnson syndrome

Stevens Johnson syndrome is a much more serious condition in which there is a fatality rate of 5% (Lee and Thomson, 1999). The patient is ill with fever, joint and muscle pains and a widespread rash of the erythema

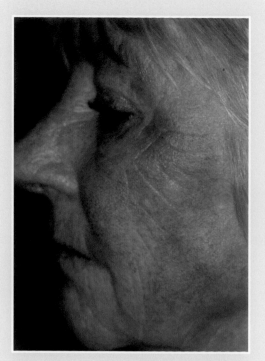

*Figure 40.3. Slate-grey staining of the cheek in a patient on minocycline.*

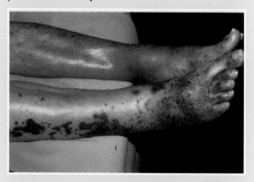

*Figure 40.4. Vasculitic purpura.*

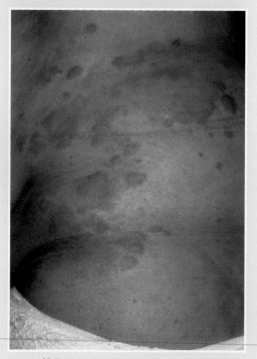

*Figure 40.5. Urticaria in a patient on trimethoprim.*

multiforme type over the whole body. Blisters and painful erosions develop *(Figure 40.7)*. Other organs such as the joints, bronchi, gastrointestinal tract and kidneys may be affected (du Vivier, 2002: 371–2). It may be associated with a number of drugs in particular penicillins, tetracyclines, sulphonamides and NSAIDs (Lee and Thomson, 1999).

### Erythema nodosum

Erythema nodsum is most common in young women. The patient presents with tender, red nodules that are usually on the extensor surfaces of the shins *(Figure 40.8)*. The patient may feel unwell and have a slight fever. Symptoms gradually subside over 3–6 weeks. This hypersensitivity reaction may be associated with a number of causes. Sarcoidosis or infections (e.g. streptococcal bacteria or tuberculosis) are often at the root of the problem, but drugs such as barbiturates, sulphonamides or the oral contraceptive may also be the cause (DermNet NZ, 2004).

### Fixed-drug eruptions

A patient with a fixed-drug eruption develops single or multiple, round or oval, erythematous lesions that may be 'dusky purple' or brown, anywhere on the skin or mucous membranes *(Figure 40.9)*. Vesicles or blisters sometimes occur. This is the only skin reaction that is related solely to the intake of a drug. It will occur at the same site within 8 hours, every time the patient takes the specific drug. The most common cause of this reaction is phenolphthalein, which is present in some laxatives, but other drugs may also cause the problem (Lee and Thomson, 1999).

### Psoriasis and psoriasiform eruptions

Psoriasis is a very common condition that affects 1–2% of the population (du Vivier, 2002). The scaly lesions of plaque psoriasis are unmistakable *(Figure 40.10)*. Many patients have a family history of psoriasis and it may be triggered by infection or injury. In patients with known psoriasis, exacerbations may occur in association with certain drugs, and drugs may trigger psoriasis for the first time. Lithium exacerbates psoriasis but other drugs may also be implicated. In the case of steroids, rapid withdrawal can exacerbate psoriasis (du Vivier, 2002; Lee and Thomson, 1999).

### Lichenoid eruptions

Some drugs may cause a rash to develop that is very similar to lichen planus. Very itchy, small, shiny papules appear that are violaceous in colour *(Figure 40.11)*. The lesions may be localized or widespread and severe. Sometimes the rash has a photosensitive component. A lacy, white pattern may be seen on the buccal mucosa. Lichenoid rashes may present weeks or months after the medication has been started, but the rash usually clears within a few weeks of discontining the drug.

A topical steroid may help ease the rash but severe cases may require systemic steroids. A number of drugs have been associated with this problem, in particular, anti-malarials, beta-blockers and gold.

### Acne

Acne is a common problem in the teenage years. Some will continue to have problems into adult life. Acne or skin reactions that mimic acne vulgaris may be induced or exacerbated by certain drugs. Papules and pustules can be seen on the face *(Figure 40.12)* and chest and sometimes spread to the abdomen, lower back, upper arms and thighs. Comedones tend not to be a feature of drug-induced acne.

The drugs most commonly associated with acne are corticosteroids, androgens,oral contraceptives, isoniazid and lithium (Lee and Thomson, 1999).

### Eczema

Ingested drugs do not often cause problems with eczema but in a few cases patients will complain of the problem of dry, itchy skin. In particular, isotretinoin, used in the treatment of severe acne, reduces sebum secretion, which dries the skin causing greater susceptibility to eczema (Joint Formulary Committee, 2004: 574–5). Dry lips and cheilitis (inflammation and cracking of the lips) *(Figure 40.13)* must be expected, providing the patient is taking the medication correctly. Frequent applications of Vaseline and plenty of emollients for the eczema should help. Nose bleeds, muscle and joint pains are the the most common problems (du Vivier, 2002: 407).

Patients taking isotretinoin should be advised to stop treatment if they develop a problem with depression.They should also be warned that isotretinoin is teratogenic and that they should avoid pregnancy while on it or for at least 3 months after stopping (Joint Formulary Committee, 2004: 749). (There is some debate about whether the gap should be longer.) Such women should also be offered contraception.

## Investigations

A combination of knowledge about drug intake and the type of rash are usually sufficient to be confident about the diagnosis of drug allergy. In cases where a rash persists or recurs, a full blood count will detect problems of leucopenia and thrombocytopenia (Ehrlich et al, 2004). Serum amylase and lipase may be elevated and autoimmune antibodies may be altered in drug-induced lupus erythematosus (du Vivier, 2002: 408). Skin tests are not particularly helpful and may prove dangerous to the patient (Ehrlich et al, 2004).

## Management

As soon as the problem is recognized, the offending drug should be discontinued. Most patients require symptomatic treatment only. Oral antihistamines help address itchy rashes and emollients are useful for dry and eczematous skin problems. Sometimes topical steroids are helpful and, occasionally, prednisolone may be needed for more severe problems (Lee and Thomson, 1999). The patient should be warned never to take the offending drug again.

### Severe cases

Topical applications, tetracyclines or, in severe cases, isotretinoin, may help the acne. For girls on the combined oral contraceptive pill, the preparation that contains the

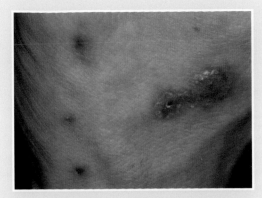

*Figure 40.6. Erythema multiforme with target lesions.*

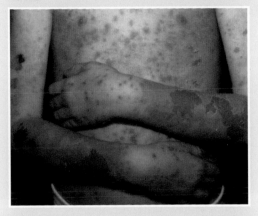

*Figure 40.7. Steven's Johnson syndrome: recovering after 3 weeks.*

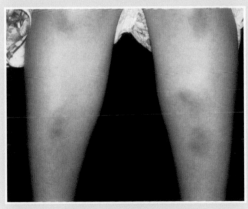

*Figure 40.8. Erythema nodosum.*

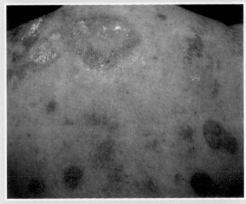

*Figure 40.9. Fixed-drug eruption, which recurred in the same place when patient took trimethoprim for recurrent urinary infections.*

anti-androgen cyproterone with ethinylestradiol can be a useful alternative. (Joint Formulary Committee, 2004: 576; Lee and Thomson, 1999; du Vivier, 2002: 406).

Severe problems such as Steven's Johnson syndrome require immediate hospital admission for administration of systemic corticosteroids, intravenous fluids and antibiotics (Ehrlich et al, 2004).

## Conclusions

The presentation of drug induced skin reactions are varied. A knowledge of drug intake and the types of rash associated with particular drugs are important to making the correct diagnosis.

## References

Bergamo B, Elmets CA (2005) Drug induced photosensitivity. *eMedicine*. http://www.emedicine. com/derm/topic108.html (accessed 16 June 2005)

DermNet NZ (2004) Erythema nodosum. http://dermnetnz.org/ vascular/ erythema-nodosum.html (accessed 16 June 2005)

DermNet NZ (2005) Fixed drug eruption. http://dermnetnz.org/ reactions/ fixed-drug-eruption. html (accessed 30 June 2005)

du Vivier A (2002) Reactive disorders of the skin and adverse drug reactions. In: *Atlas of Clinical Dermatology*. 3rd edn. Churchill

Livingstone, London: 400–16 Ehrlich M, Helm TN, Camisa C (2004) Drug eruptions. *eMedicine*. www.emedicine.com/derm/topic 104.htm (accessed 16 June 2005)

Joint Formulary Committee (2004) *British National Formulary 48*. September. Royal Pharmaceutical Society of Great Britain, London

Lee A, Thomson J (1999) Drug induced skin reactions. *The Pharmaceutical Journal* **262**:357–62. www.pharmj.com/Editorial/ 19990313/education/ skinreactions.html (accessed 16 June 2005)

## Test Your Knowledge

This elderly woman presented in the surgery with a florid rash that had started on her legs and arms and was now spreading to the trunk. She was alarmed by the extent of it but surprised that it caused her no irritation or other symptoms. She had been on medication for hypertension for some time but it was only since she had been in hospital, for a minor operation under general anaesthetic that the rash had occurred.

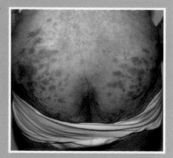

### Questions

1. What is the likely diagnosis?
2. In this case, what is the most likely cause of the patient's rash?
3. What advice would you give to the patient?

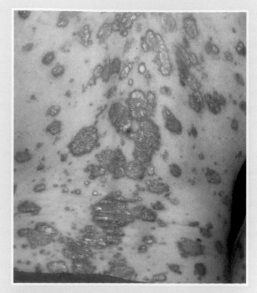

*Figure 40.10. Plaque psoriasis.*

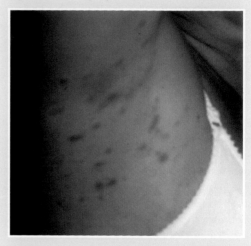

*Figure 40.11. A lichenoid reaction to gold.*

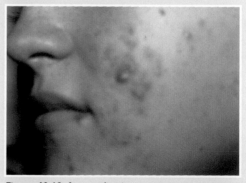

*Figure 40.12. Acne vulgaris.*

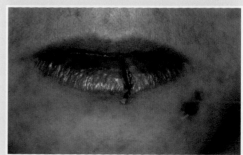

*Figure 40.13. Dry, cracked lips, reaction to isotretinoin.*

# Test your knowledge answers

## Chapter 1: Malignant melanoma

1. As this lesion was increasing in size, had irregular borders, was itching and more than 7mm in diameter, the likelihood of malignant melanoma is very high. The lower leg of women is a common site for MM, if they have been used to wearing skirts.

2. Any patient with a lesion suspicious of MM should have a full examination to exclude other pigmented lesions and there should be a check on the regional lymph glands and liver, in case of metastatic spread. BAD guidelines recommend that any potential MM should be seen by the specialist (Dermatologist/Surgeon/Plastic Surgeon) within 2 weeks of receipt of the referral letter from the GP. If the lesion is excised by the GP and reported as MM, the patient should be seen immediately by the specialist. In view of the area excised anD the site of the lesion, the patient required a skin graft in order to achieve healing.

3. In this case the histology report confirmed the diagnosis of superficial, spreading melanoma and stated that the lesion had been excised with 2cm margin but that the Breslow thickness was 3.7mm. There as no evidence of spread to the lymphatics or liver. The prognosis for a 5 year survival rate was 60-75% and the patient would require regular follow up, 3 monthly for 3 years and 6 monthly for a further 2 years. She should also be advised to avoid further sun exposure, to wear a hat and cover-up clothes when out doors and to apply sun lotion (at least factor 30), to any exposed parts.

## Chapter 2: Malignant melanomas and seborrhoeic wart

1. A lesion such as this in a young man would inevitably raise concerns about the diagnosis of malignant melanoma. The fact that it had recently increased in size, had irregular borders and irregular pigmentation would all point to this.

2. The following actions should be taken:
- Urgent referral to a dermatologist or surgeon
- Full advice about future sun protection with hats, clothing and use of high factor sun cream to exposed parts
- Full examination to excludes any other lesions elsewhere on his body that would have been at risk of sun exposure and check of the lymph glands and liver to ensure that there were not already signs of spread.

## Chapter 3: Mimickers of malignant melanoma

1. There are a number of features about this lesion that might lead you to suspect a superficial, spreading malignant melanoma. In particular the lesion was said to have recently increased in size and become darker. On examination, the 'mole' showed an irregular outline and colour pattern.

2. The patient should be urgently referred to a dermatologist or surgeon for excision and histology of the lesion.

3. In this case, the concerns about this patient were unfounded. The lesion was excised and in the histology it was reported to be a 'warty, compound naevus and simple lentigo with no evidence of malignancy'. This example shows that you cannot always be sure. It is always better to play safe and seek a second opinion if the history and appearance of the lesion suggest that there is any room for doubt. In this case the lesion was benign, but had a malignant melanoma been missed, the patient would have suffered and the health professional might well have ended up in court. Advice for the future was to encourage the woman to continue to watch for change in other moles and not to be afraid to seek an opinion if necessary. She was also reminded to observe good sun protection when out of doors, either by avoidance, or applying sunscreen.

## Chapter 4: Keratoacanthoma /Basal cell caricinoma/Squamous cell carcinoma

1. Basal cell carcinoma (BCC). This patient with a long history of sun exposure, is a high risk candidate for skin malignancy. The history of slow development of the non-healing lesion that started as a small spot is typical of BCC, together with the raised, rolled rim that can be seen around its edge.

2. The treatment of choice for BCC is complete excision, followed by histological examination to confirm complete removal of the lesion. An alternative treatment is radiotherapy, but this would require a biopsy of the lesion first to confirm the diagnosis as well as several visits to the hospital for treatment. .For the elderly, infirm or housebound, curettage and cautery or cryotherapy are an option but recurrences after these procedures tend to be high. The patient should be advised to avoid sun exposure in the future by covering with clothing and a hat, when out of doors, and to use sunscreen on areas that cannot be covered.

3. Full examination of other areas of the body that may have suffered sun damage should include the head, neck, limbs, back and chest in case other lesions have occurred. Metatstases from BCC are rare.

## Chapter 5: Cutaneous T-cell lymphoma

1. The recent history of a sore throat followed the sudden onset of 'drop like' rash would strongly suggest the diagnosis of guttate psoriasis. Guttate psoriasis may settle spontaneously or with the help of ultraviolet light, but can progress to the plaque stage. The plaques of chronic psoriasis are usually covered in a silvery scale. This patient had presented during the acute phase where inflammation was the main feature. Unlike the plaques of mycosis fungoides, these plaques are all of similar size, shape and colour.

2. Other signs to look for in mycosis fungoides would be follicular mucinosis or in a black skinned patient, hyper- or hypopigmentation. Check for any enlargement of the lymph glands.

3. Skin biopsy would be necessary to confirm the diagnosis of mycosis fungoides and full blood count, so check the lymphocyte count or Sézary cells. If the test suggest MF the doctor should be asked to review the patient, with the expectation that referral to a dermatologist would be made for further care.

## Chapter 6: Skin manifestations of breast cancer

1. The most likely diagnosis in this case is carcinoma of the breast. A full history, including family history, should be taken regarding the changes and the patient's health and discuss with her, her thoughts, feelings, fears and expectations are about the problem. A general examination should include check of the respiratory system, abdominal examination to exclude enlargement of the liver and for any lymphadenopathy, particularly in the axilla and supra-clavicular glands.

2. The patient should be referred urgently to a Breast Clinic. The patient did actually attend the clinic but when a biopsy of the lump was suggested, she refused point blank to proceed and quickly left the department.

3. She did return to see the nurse in the surgery where possible treatments with surgery, (lumpectomy or mastectomy and axillary clearance), radiotherapy &/or chemotherapy were discussed and the patient asked to contact them again if and when she had decided how she would like to proceed. She was asked to return, with a relative, for a further discussion. Eventually, she was encouraged to return to the hospital where she decided to try a course of treatment with tamoxifen, with some success: at the last hearing, the lump had shrunk and she was beginning to gain in confidence once more. She was also given the contact number for the Breast Cancer Support Group where she could talk with a trained volunteer who has been through the same problem and gained much insight and personal experience. Phone 0845 077 1893 or email ukpeersupport@ breastcancercare.org.uk

## Chapter 7: The nipple

1. Eczema of the nipple. The bilateral nature of the problem, the long history of recurrences of the condition and the fact that it cleared completely at times, with the help of treatment, would make this diagnosis more likely.

2. The patient gave a history of problems with eczema and asthma as a child. Also on examination the changes affected the areola only, the nipple was normal. No other breast abnormality or lump could be found.

3. As the time of delivery was near, it was important to try to settle the problem as quickly as possible. She was prescribed topical hydrocortisone ointment 1% to apply regularly three times a day and reviewed a week later. When she returned, the eczema had cleared,. A biopsy of the lesion was, therefore, felt to be unnecessary.

## Chapter 8: Brown pigmented lesions

1. Post-inflammatory hyperpigmentation. The lesion is completely symptomless with no irritation or skin changes other than the discolouration.

2. It was necessary to go carefully into the history in order to ascertain the cause. She certainly could not remember any injury or bruise to the area in the preceding weeks. Eventually she recalled that she had developed a blistery rash at the site "It was strange" she said "because it took the form of streaky lines". It had settled after about a week. It had occurred after she had been out in the garden cutting back the chysanthemums on a lovely sunny day. It seemed likley that she had developed phytophotodermatitis which, typically, produces such a rash after contact with plants containing furocoumarin, when the skin is exposed to sunlight. This was a post-inflammatory problem.

3. There is no treatment for this condition that should gradually tend to fade over the weeks and months. There seemed no need for cover up with cosmetic camouflage. The patient left reassured.

## Chapter 9: Telangiectasia

1. Close inspection of the 'spots' would find a group of small vessels radiating from a central arteriole. If the central arteriole is compressed, the whole lesion would blanch.

2. In a young, fit woman such as this patient, the sudden development of these telangiectases would be most likely to be stimulated by hormones. This patient was not pregnant but had recently started taking the combined oral contraceptive pill. When further questioned about her drinking habits, they were found to be moderate only and, therefore, in view of her generally good health, it seemed unnecessary to pursue liver function tests.

3. The patient was advised that the telangiectasia were probably related to the oestrogen in her contraceptive pill and that the lesions might resolve within 9 months if she changed her method. A contraception alternative method were discussed.

## Chapter 10: Viral warts

1. This lesion is, almost certainly a verruca (plantar wart). The clearly demarcated, keratotic lesion, within which can be seen a few small haemorrhages, is typical of the problem that so often occurs on the sole of the foot. Should it be carefully pared with a scalpel, the appearance of small bleeding points would distinguish it from a corn.

2. Although warts will frequently clear without treatment, in this case, because the pain was interfering with her life, some treatment would seem to be required. She had already tried "wart paint", although it was uncertain as to whether she had applied it correctly, after soaking in warm water for five minutes, and whether she had rubbed off the dead skin with a pumice stone or emery board about twice a week. In any case, it would be expected to take at least 12 weeks to respond and her need was more urgent. Instead, she elected to try cryotherapy at the surgery, but understood that it might be painful and that she might need to attend up to three sessions with gaps of 2-3 weeks between. She hoped that this might avoid the need for curettage to get rid of the wart.

3. As regards spread of warts in the swimming pool, the viral wart may spread by direct contact, particularly in damp places such as bathrooms, showers and pools. However, if simple precautions are observed, towels, shoes and socks are not shared and plastic verruca socks or waterproof plasters worn in these situations, the risk of spread is minimal.

## Chapter 11: Genital warts

1. Genital warts are usually associated with HPV type 6 or 11 and as such are not likely to lead to malignant change. However, other types of HPV may coexist with these, so his condition should be kept under review.

2. As these warts were inflamed and in a situation where healing was impaired by intertriginous situation, it was recommended that he should have the warts treated with cautery, under a local or general anaesthetic. He was also prescribed a topical cream containing hydrocortisone, nystatin, benzalkonium and dimeticone to try to settle the inflammation. He was also advised to attend a GU clinic to exclude any other STIs.

3. Although genital warts often appear within about 3 months of contact with a partner with HPV, there may sometimes be a delay of several years before symptoms develop. He should not, therefore, assume that his girlfriend has been unfaithful. Nevertheless, she should be advised to attend a doctor or GU clinic to be checked for STI and would need to have a cervical smear taken if one had not been performed recently.

## Chapter 12: Diagnosing spots and vesicles

1. From the history and findings on examination, there seemed little doubt the patient had chickenpox and there were no other findings to suggest any complications. The signs and symptoms were such that there was no need to pursue further investigations. General advice about paracetamol and topical calamine lotion should be given.

2. Chickenpox is potentially a more serious problem in adults, especially in a pregnant woman: the risks are both to herself and the child. Serious complications such as pneumonia, hepatitis and encephalitis may affect the woman, and there is a small risk of fetal varicella syndrome in those who get chickenpox in the first 28 weeks of pregnancy. These potential problems should be discussed with the woman so that she knows when to seek help and what action she might consider for the pregnancy.

3. The advent of antiviral treatment has reduced morbidity and mortality rates considerably, but should be given within 24 hours of the onset of the rash. By the 3rd day it seemed too late to offer this, and in any case, its use is not advised in pregnancy before 20 weeks. Detailed ultrasound, in a specialist unit, might confrrm abnormalities such as limb deformity, microcephaly, hydrocephalus if done at least 5 weeks after the primary infection. This would still give time to discuss with the patient, the option of a termination, if serious abnormalities were detected. If any symptoms of chest

involvement, neurological symptoms, haemorrhagic rash or bleeding or if the woman is immunosuppressed, she should be referred immediately to hospital. She should be advised to avoid contact with others until 5 days after the onset of the rash, if she has been in contact with a non-immune, pregnant woman, that contact should be advised to seek VZIG within 96 hours of contact.

## Chapter 13: Plaque psoriasis

1. Plaque psoriasis. Psoriasis often presents for the first time at this age. The well define scaly plaque with its silvery scale is typical of a psoriatic plaque.

2. On inspection of the extensor surfaces of his knees and elbows there were some small plaques on both elbow and some of the finger nails showed some pitting and early onycholysis. It also transpired that his grandmother and an aunt had also suffered with psoriasis. All these signs added to the likelihood of psoriasis.in his case. His scalp was actually clear. It was not necessary to pursue any further investigations.

3. One could discuss with him the fact that the cause of psoriasis is still unknown but that frequently there does seem to be a genetic link to the problem. He was on no drugs that could have aggravated the problem but reminded that should he be travelling to an area where malaria occurred, some antimalarials could trigger an exacerbation. The fact that the condition tends to run a natural course of exacerbations and remissions was mentioned and that there is no specific cure for the condition. However, sunlight is often helpful and the holiday might be just what the doctor ordered! In the meantime he should apply an emollient to soften the scale, and initially a topical coal tar preparation such as coal tar and salicylic acid ointment could be applied to the plaque once or twice a day. Should this not be successful or he find it unpleasant to use, he should return to get advice regarding moving on to dithranol, a topical steroid (as it was a small area), or calcipotriol &/or UVL. He was given the contact address and telephone number of the Psoriasis Association.

## Chapter 14: Lichen planus

1. Hypertrophic lichen planus (LP). LP often presents with lesions on the flexor surfaces of the wrists, does tend to spread and is very itchy. Hypertrophic lesions often occur on the legs and the purple colour of the lesions is characteristic of LP.

2. On further examination of the mouth, a symptomless, white, lacy pattern was noticed on the buccal mucous membrane and a small bald, scaly bald patch of papules was found in her hair all suggesting the diagnosis of LP. Her nails were normal.

3. The diagnosis seemed obvious and therefore biopsy was not recommended. She was reassured that the condition usually clears spontaneously within about 18 months but, as she was so troubled by the rash, an antihistamine and a potent topical corticosteroid was prescribed, to be applied also to the scalp. However, a few weeks later there was still no improvement and the rash was so widespread that it was virtually impossible to apply the

cream to all areas. She was therefore referred to a dermatologist who started her on systemic steroids. The rash gradually subsided, the itch improved and she was weaned off her steroids.

## Chapter 15: Intertrigo

1. Erythrasma. This presentation of a symmetrical rash in the flexures or between the toes, in this case the axillae, with the brown scaly wrinkled surface is typical of this condition. He noticed the irritation but no other symptoms.
2. Erythrasma is caused by corynebacterium minutissium and confirmation of the diagnosis may be made in the laboratory if skin scrapings are taken and cultured. A diagnosis may be confidently made in the surgery if Wood's Lamp is shone onto the area (in the dark). The lesion will fluoresce a coral pink
3. No local treatment is required but the patient will need a prescription of Erythromycin tablets 250mg qds for two weeks. The condition should then be "cured".

## Chapter 16: Scaly feet/Keraroderma

1. Pustular psoriasis. The appearance of the rash and the pustules is typical of this condition. Some cases with pustular psoriasis will have a family history of psoriasis or previous or current manifestations of the problem. Many, however, will have none of these.
2. The patient should be examined for other signs of psoriasis. The elbow, knees and nails will commonly be affected. The patient should be asked if she is a smoker and checked to ensure that there are no other indications of associated problems such as diabetes or thyroid disease.
3. The patient may be encouraged by the fact that many cases of pustular psoriasis resolve spontaneously.
   - Smoking must be discontinued
   - Topical salicylic acid preparations may help to remove scale
   - Topical coal tar or dithranol – nursing help may be require if the patient has problems managing the treatment.
   - Specialist advice may be required for stubborn cases.

## Chapter 17: Hand dermatitis/ Tinea manuum

1. The most likely diagnosis in this case is dermatitis. The distribution of the rash, with the well defined margin suggested contact with some irritant substance. Close questioning it was discovered that the problem first occurred at the time when, in his job as a carpenter, and using the wood preservative, capronil, his gloves had leaked. Repeated skin contact with cuprinol is known to lead to a dermatitis with dryness and cracking of the skin.
2. If there was any doubt as to the cause, an allergic cause could be excluded by patch testing and/or if tinea is thought to be involved, skin scraping for microscopy and culture may be undertaken
3. Anyone using cuprinol should be advised to avoid direct contact with the substance with protective overalls/ coveralls and gloves. Should contact occur, any

contaminated clothing should be removed and the skin thoroughly washed with soap and water or cleansed with a proprietary skin cleanser. Treatment of the dermatitis requires the frequent use of moisturisers and a topical corticosteroid preparation. The 1% hydrocortisone cream that the patient had been using did not seem to be having any effect. He was therefore prescribed a potent corticosteroid ointment to use until the condition was under control. The potency could be reduced as progress continued. He was reminded that an ointment for this dry scaling condition was likely to be more effective tan an ointment. It was suggested that he would be well advised to stop work until the condition had resolved,

## Chapter 18 Insect bites/Bullous pemphigoid/

1. The most likely diagnosis in this case would be bullous pemphigoid. The history of itching, urticarial type of rash followed by crops of large, tense and often haemorrhagic blisters, is typical of the presentation in this condition. Other factors in favour of the diagnosis are his age, and the fact that he had been on frusemide for his hypertension, a drug which has been found to sometimes precipitate the condition.
2. As Bullous pemphigoid is going to require systemic steroids for a considerable length of time, it is always important to confirm the diagnosis before starting on the medication. This can be done by taking a biopsy from a fresh lesion and sending a specimen of fluid from a blister to be checked for immunofluorescence.
3. In view of the extent and severity of the rash and blisters, the patient was offered hospital admission for full nursing care until the condition was under control, and to watch for, and deal with any problems of secondary infection that might occur. Initially, he was started on a high dose of prednisolone (30-60mg daily) and advised that the dose could later be reduced by 5 mg every 5 days down to a lower maintenance dose, sufficient to prevent further exacerbation of the condition. Also, it was hoped that the dose could be reduced if topical steroids were applied and also by the addition of the steroid sparing agent, azathioprine.

   As he was likely to be on systemic steroids for longer than 3 months, he should be started on a prophylactic biphosphonate such as alendronate, etidronate or risedronate, in order to reduce the risk of the development of osteoporosis and fractures.

## Chapter19: Urticaria

1. Urticaria occurring as the result of an acquired aller gy to a sulphonamide. The fact that she had never previously reacted to the drug is explained by the fact that this is an allergic immunoglobulin E (IgE) mediated reaction that requires previous dose(s) to sensitize the patient to the drug.
2. This patient was prescribed a non-sedating antihistamine (fexofenadine 180 mg daily) to take until the condition subsided, and a mild topical steroid cream to apply to the rash if it was troublesome. The patient was advised to discontinue the trimethoprim

and was prescribed an alternative antibiotic to treat the urinary infection.

3. The patient was warned that she should not take any sulphonamide drug in the future as she would almost certainly suffer the same reaction. A suitable warning was added to her medical records. Further investigations were felt to be unnecessary as the association between the drug and the relatively quick reaction seemed clear.

## Chapter 20: Erythema multiforme

1. Erythema multiforme.
2. Factors suggesting the diagnosis are:
   - The sudden onset of a widespread, non-irritant macular rash of varied size and shape.
   - The rash did not itch
   - The rash was symmetrically distributed
   - The child was not ill.
   - The probable trigger for the problem was the course of trimethoprim that she had been given for her urinary infection 2 weeks before.
3. The mother should be;
   - told the diagnosis
   - reassured that it was not a serious condition
   - the condition should resolve without treatment within the next three weeks
   - The condition was not infectious and it would be safe for her to mix with her friends if she felt well enough
   - The probable trigger factor for the rash was probably the trimethoprim and she should therefore avoid treatment with any sulphonamide preparation in future.
   - Once better there should be no unpleasant after effects.

## Chapter 21: Atopic eczema

1. A sudden flare such as this would suggest that the eczema had become infected. In view of the cirumstances and the stress of exams, it is likely that the boy had neglected to continue with adequate moisturization of his skin (as the picture also indicates), which would tend to increase the eczema and itching. This, together with the increased temptation to scratch, would account for infection and the sudden flare.
2. A swab taken from a weepy part of the rash would be necessary. If swab results confirm the presence of Staphylococcus aureus, which is sensitive to flucloxacillin, a course of oral flucloxacillin could then be commenced. Fusidic acid ointment with betamethasone could be prescribed to apply to the rash.
3. The boy should be advised to find time to continue regular application of emollients and, as the condition improves, to move 'down' to 1% hydrocortisone ointment before discontinuing it. He should be reminded that, given his age, with proper care the eczema should remit.

## Chapter 22: Compulsive itch

1. The most likely diagnosis in this case is lichen simplex. It may well have started all those years ago with a bit of eczema, possibly initiated by the wearing of his

watch. He had never worn a watch since. However, repeated scratching had worsened the condition and led to more itching and thickened scaly plaque. Scratch marks were there for all to see.
2. In his case there did not seem to be much point in pursuing investigations of this localized, itchy rash. The diagnosis seemed pretty obvious. The story of initial eczema could suggest that he did have some atopic tendencies that would be backed if a blood test demonstrated a raised immunoglobulin E (IgE) level. Also, the suggestion that maybe it had developed in association with the wearing of a watch could lead to patch testing to detect any specific allergy to the metal (such as nickel) or other substances.
3. The patient was reminded that it was crucial that he stopped scratching. He should keep his nails short and wear gloves at night to reduce trauma to the area. A sedating or an antihistamine, promethazine, was also prescribed at night to help him sleep and ease the itch. He was also supplied with a potent topical cor ticosteroid ointment, clobetasol, to apply twice a day. When this did not help sufficiently, he was advised to apply it under occlusion for 2 weeks. Eventually the condition settled and he continued with regular emollients and for a time a milder corticosteroid ointment and managed to stop scratching.

## Chapter 23: Scabies

1. Eczematised scabies.
2. Search should be made for burrows so that a scraping can be taken and viewed under the microscope, mixed with potassium hydroxide, in the surgery or the pathology laboratory. The finding of the scabies mite or eggs should definitely confirm the diagnosis.
3. The patient should be prescribed 5% perimethrin cream or malathion lotion to apply at night to the whole body apart from the face and scalp, (not just the rash), including the areas between the fingers, toes and genitalia. The application should be washed off 24 hours later and the treatment repeated a week later. Bed linen and clothing should be washed and ironed. The eczematous reaction would need the application of a topical steroid to settle it down, together with a sedative antihistamine if the itching was troublesome. The patient had probably not responded to the first prescription of perimethrin because:
   - He applied the cream to the areas of the rash only
   - He did not repeat the treatment a week later
   - He did not launder his bedding or clothing
   - Close contacts were not treated which left the patient at risk of reinfestation

## Chapter 24: Infestations

1. The most likely diagnosis in this case, especially as both she and her husband were affected, was that, in their involvement with the dogs, that they had the problem of flea bites
2. They were advised to apply 1% hydrocortisone cream to the spots to ease the irritation and to take an oral antihistamine, such as desloratidine or fexofenadine if the itching was not sufficiently relieved. They had no

other pets in the home; however, they were advised to launder their bedding and clothes, and to vacuum carpets and upholstered chairs. This was to be followed up with a spray of insect growth regulator and repeated over the next 2 weeks in order to catch any emerging fleas

3. They were advised to contact the bed and breakfast owners to alert them to the problems and suggest they get advice from the vet as to how to deal with the infestation in the home and 'deflea' the dogs with an adulticide and insect growth regulator. He would also advise on the question of de-worming the dogs.

## Chapter 25: Genital

1. The most likely diagnosis in this case is Lichen sclerosus atrophicus. The smooth white appearance of the skin and troublesome itching are typical of the condition. Although it often affects the vulva, it is not uncommon in the perianal region and the appearance of a "figure of eight" pattern in this area.

2. In her case the diagnosis was clear, but if in doubt or there is concern about malignant change that could present with a lump or persistent ulceration, a skin biopsy can be taken to confirm the condition. Sometimes there can be confusion between LS&A and eczema. As thyroid disease is frequently associated with LS&A, the thyroid function should also be checked.

3. Initially a potent topical steroid was prescribed to get the condition under control and then changed to a weaker preparation. There are times when it is preferable to refer the patient to a specialist in vulval disease to establish the diagnosis and advise on treatment. In the meantime the patient should use emollients instead of soaps and just a moderate potency topical steroid. Warning should be given that she should report the event of the development of any lump or ulcer. She could also be put in touch with the National Lichen Sclerosis website at www.lichensclerosus.org

## Chapter 26: Tinea corporis

1. Tinea corporis – the lesion seen here in this picture is typical of the condition. Particular features are the well defined, itchy annular rash that is rapidly increasing in size. The margin is made up of papules that are breaking down and crusting, while the central area appears to be clearing. The rash is spreading to other areas of her body and it would appear to be infectious, as her granddaughter has developed a similar problem on one arm.

2. Skin scraping – if microscopy is available in the surgery, the scrapings should be mixed with potassium hydroxide. Branching hyphae would be seen under the microscope. If the scrapings are sent to the laboratory, this can be confirmed and fungal culture will identify the fungus.

3. Treatment for a fungal infection should be initiated, in this case, before receiving a lab report as the diagnosis seems certain and the problem rapidly deteriorating. She would seem to have passed it on to the granddaughter who should also be treated and kept away from school until treatment appeared to be working. A topical antifungal agent would probably suffice in the case of

the granddaughter as she had developed just one lesion. However, with the widespread distribution in the case of the grandmother, a 4 week course of terbinafine, 250mg daily was given, as well as the topical imidazole or terbinafine cream. Alternative oral treatments include fluconazole or itraconazole. In fact this patient rapidly improved. Four weeks later the condition had completely cleared

## Chapter 27: Nails 1- A pointer to disease

1. The most likely cause of these changes is psoriasis. The classic features of pitting and onycholysis are present.

2. Although nail changes may occur in isolation, it is always worth checking to see if there are any signs of psoriasis or another skin condition. In particular, thickening and silvery scale over the elbows are common and often ignored by the patient, as well as 'dandruff' and scaly patches in the scalp. When challenged, the patient will often be aware of others in the family with psoriasis or may have had a previous episode him/herself that may have been forgotten. The fact of recent pain and stiffness in the fingers could raise the possibility of an early psoriatic arthritis that might need advice and treatment from a doctor or rheumatologist. As the patient's employer was concerned about infection, nail clippings could be taken to exclude a fungal infection. A biopsy of the nail could be done but is probably unnecessary.

3. The patient should be advised that the most likely diagnosis is psoriasis and that should not in any way preclude her from doing her job. Treatment could be discussed but she should be discouraged from following this path as the risks of side effects from the various medications could well be troublesome. The nails might improve spontaneously but there is always the risk of recurrence - both with and without treatment.

## Chapter 28: Nails 2 - The traumatized nail

1. Chronic paronychia associated with Candida albicans. The changes in the nail folds, together with the history of slow development over a period of months are typical of this condition. One would expect the nail to be affected by the problem. In fact, her own nail was ridged and discoloured but she had resorted to false nails in order to improve the appearance, in the hope that none of her customers would be aware of the problem.

2. A swab taken from the nail fold for culture should confirm the presence of Candida albicans and also demonstrate any other associated infection.

3. As a hairdresser and housewife this woman was constantly immersing her hands in water. She should be advised to always wear cotton-lined rubber gloves when working and at home when there was a risk of contact with water, and reminded that she should try to keep her hands dry as much as possible. Providing she could wear gloves there should be no problems of 'contaminating' her clients. Additionally, she could coat the nail folds with flexible collodion that would act as a barrier to water and infection. She could apply topical antifungal imidazole lotion, to the nail folds twice daily. However, further damage to the cuticles by trimming or

the use of cuticle removers will only potentiate the problem. If response is poor, an oral antifungal agent such as itraconazole, terbinafine or fluconazole may be given but treatment would need to continue for up to 3 months. Response to treatment is slow and relapse common so that it is important to continue to avoid contact with water even when the problem has cleared.

## Chapter 29: Red faces

1. Vague rashes like this are common in children. Often an accurate diagnosis is not reached and one has to assume that the rash is caused by some viral infection.

2. This child was not 'ill'. He was bright and cheerful, and on examination had no signs of a throat infection. He did, however, have firm, enlarged occipital and posterior cervical glands, making the diagnosis of rubella most likely.

3. In view of the mother's pregnancy, it was important to be sure about the diagnosis and, if it was rubella, to know the mother's rubella status. If her rubella titre has already been done and she has been shown to be immune to rubella, the worry is over. However, if this result is not available it would be necessary to take blood for a check on her rubella status. If this test demonstrated that she is non-immune, a further test should be repeated after 10 days to see if there has been a rise in the rubella titre that would indicate that she had developed the disease. A mother who has suffered rubella in the first 3 months of pregnancy is at considerable risk of producing a child with serious abnormalities. After the 4th month these risks are less. She should be counselled about the risks to the baby and allowed the opportunity, discuss her feelings about a termination and offer referral if she feels that would be her choice.

## Chapter 30: Red and spotty faces

1. Sycosis barbae. A rash of this kind in the beard area of a man is most likely to be due to this problem. Perioral dermatitis is unusual in men and he had not, at any stage, been using topical steroids on the face.

2. A swab should be taken from the pustules as well as a swab from the nose to see if there is a problem of being a nasal carrier of staphylococcus aureus.

3. The patient should be advised to observe good hygiene and, if he is agreeable, to allow the beard to grow. An antibiotic, preferably flucloxacillin, should be prescribed to clear the underlying infection. If the patient is allergic to penicillin then erythromycin is an alternative. Should nasal carriage of S.Aureus be proven than he should use a cream containing chlorhexidine with neomycin to the nostrils 4 times daily for 10 days.

## Chapter 31: Acne vulgaris/ rosacea

1. Isotretinoin would undoubtedly be helpful in improving his severe acne and would be recommended in his case, if ignored as there was great risk of permanent scarring.

2. James had been attending the surgery with his acne for about 18 months. Initially he had been started on topical benzoylperoxide which he had religiously applied twice a day to the whole of his face twice daily after washing with an antiseptic wash. When this did not help he was changed to topical clindamycin and the moved on to oral oxytetracycline which he had taken 500mg twice daily for at least 9 months.

3. At this stage the treatment of choice would be isotretinoin but first it was important to explain to him that although this should produce dramatic improvement in his condition, the drug was not without its side effects and risks. As a male, there was no concern about a possible pregnancy, although he must remember that he should never pass the tablets on to any female friend or donate blood until a month after stopping the drug. He was given a sheet outlining all the possible side effects but advised that serious problems were very unlikely to occur, other that it unavoidable problem of dry, cracking lips that would be helped by frequent application of Vaseline: other problems might be nose bleeds, dry eyes and eczema. He and his mother were warned to alert the doctor should there be problems with depression. As he was desperate he decided to start the medication and so liver function and serum lipids were checked prior to starting the treatment and advised that this should be repeated 3 monthly. His progress was carefully watched and 6 months later he stated that he was delighted with the improvement.

## Chapter 32: Facial swelling

1. This is almost certainly owing to a dental abscess. The typical symptoms and nature of the toothache, together with the swelling, inflammation, fever and signs of caries are all present.

2. On examination it looked as if dental care had been ignored for a very long time. Three stumps of teeth could be seen in the right upper jaw, pus could be seen oozing from around one of them and was extremely tender on pressure.

3. The patient required penicillin and rapid referral to a dentist. Before starting the antibiotic, a swab was taken of the oozing pus and sent to the laboratory for culture and sensitivities. In her confused state it was doubtful that she would comply adequately with the taking of pills on her own, so a starting dose of intramuscular penicillin was to be followed up by full course of penicillin V tablets. A supply of analgesics (paracetamol or ibuprofen) was also prescribed. Her daughter was alerted to the problem and it was arranged that she should supervise the taking of further medication and make the arrangements with a dentist for her to be seen as soon as possible.

## Chapter 33: Alopecia 1- Non-scarring

1. The history and presentation of this case was typical of alopecia areata (AA). The normal looking scalp exclamation mark hairs, previous and family history all suggested AA to be the most likely cause. Dermoscopy might have also indicated the diagnosis if the typical yellow dots could be seen in the bald areas.

2. The prognosis in this child might not be good. The alopecia was extensive, there was a family history of AA, she was young and had already had a previous episode of the problem. In her favour was the fact that she had no history of asthma or eczema.

3. At her age and with the extent of the alopecia, intralesional steroids were not a practical suggestion but topical steroids could be tried as the alopecia was of recent onset and they tend to be more successful in children under 10 years. However, one could not expect improvement of at least 3 months. The question of a wig could be discussed with the mother who could also be put in touch with the National Alopecia Foundation for support and advice.

## Chapter 34: Alopecia 2 - Scarring

1. A careful history of the problem should be taken and the patient should be fully examined. There was no previous or family history of skin problems. The scalp showed definite areas of scarring alopecia and in her case a symptomless lacy white pattern could be seen on the buccal mucous membrane, which was highly suggestive of lichen planus. She was not on any drug that might be suspected of precipitating the condition.

2. Skin biopsy of an affected area confirmed the diagnosis of lichen planus.

3. The patient should be referred to a dermatologist who is experienced in dealing with problems affecting the scalp. It was recommended that she continue the use of a topical steroid, possibly a more potent one to get the condition under control. Also, as the problem was spreading and she was started on a course of oral hydroxychloroquin. She was reminded that she should receive a regular ocular examination to pick up any possible changes that might suggest the side effect of retinopathy.

## Chapter 35: Lip lesions

1. The most likely causes of the chelitis in this woman are a contact dermatitis as the result of the use of some substance that could provoke this reaction. Actinic chelitis is less likely as both lips are affected, rather than just the bottom lip. If it were related to another skin condition one would expect to find signs of such a disease elsewhere.

2. Questions should be asked about which lipstick, toothpaste or mouthwash that the patient might use. The patient could be offered patch skin testing to ascertain whether she was allergic to any of these preparations or other substances that can be routinely tested for. In fact she was found to have a positive reaction to lanolin and when enquiries were made this was found to be present in the lip salve that she was using.

3. The patient should be advised to stop the use of the lip salve and any other preparation, such as lipstick, that could contain this wool alcohol. This ban would apply not only at the time but also for the future, as the allergy will not go away. Instead she should apply white soft paraffin frequently as a moisturiser

## Chapter 36: The tongue

1. This appearance of the white coating on the tongue is typical of candida (Thrush).

2. A swab could be taken from the tongue for microscopy and culture but with such a typical presentation this is probably unnecessary in her case but it would be worth enquiring whether she also had any symptoms suggestive of vaginal thrush. One would wish to pursue the fact that she had had recurrent episodes and been feeling less well of late. It appeared that she had not been "ill enough" to seek medical advice and had not therefore been prescribed any antibiotics, steroid inhalers or systemic steroids recently. It would be well worth while to check a urine specimen for glucose and follow this up, if positive, with a fasting blood sugar in case she proved to be diabetic. She was not on steroids or any other immunosuppressive drugs but the severity of the condition might also suggest immuno-suppression for which further medical opinion and investigation, including a full blood count to exclude leukaemia and HIV testing might be required.

3. The patient should be advised to take cold fluids by mouth and rinse the mouth with an antifungal mouthwash such as nuystatin oral suspension, 5-10ml four times a day. In view of the severity of the condition, oral fluconazole 50-100mg daily for 7-14 days might be more helpful.

## Chapter 37: Abnormalities of the ear lobe

1. The most likely diagnosis is Chondrodermatitis nodularis Helicis. Her story of pain and loss of sleep when her head rests on the pillow at night is typical and the appearance of the lesion suggestive. One should always consider the possibility of a basal cell carcinoma but generally these are less tender and telangiectasia can frequently be seen running across the lesion. In this case there are none.

2. One must always be sure that such a lesion is not a BCC and biopsy is therefore sensible. If excision of the lesion is recommended or curettage performed the lesion should be sent to the laboratory for histological examination and the problem solved in one operation.

3. It can be explained to the patient that this problem has developed as the result of pressure on the ear. The patient can be advised whilst awaiting removal of the lesion, by helping her to find ways of relieving the pressure on the ear lobe, especially at night. A foam pad strapped to the ear is helpful. If a central "hole" is made in the foam so that it overlies the lesion. Sometimes analgesics may be necessary.

## Chapter 38: Spots around the eyes

1. Multiple milia. The diagnosis is obvious and the patient would not require a biopsy to confirm it.

2. One could explain to the patient that this is a common but harmless problem in which small cysts develop in the sebaceous glands. She should understand that more could develop but that there is no risk of any serious consequence such as malignancy, other than her affecting appearance. One could explain that milia often develop on sun-damaged skin and that her earlier sunbathing had contributed to the problem

3. She should be reassured that treatment is unnecessary but that if she feels that she would like to be rid of them, the only approach would be to prick each one individually

with a sterile needle or cold point cautery and to squeeze out the content. A mammoth task in a lady with so many. In fact, she chose the cold point cautery option and was advised to apply EMLA cream ( a local anaesthetic cream) to the area to be tackled, 2 hours before attending, in order to numb it. (BNF 2003 – sect 15.2 – p616).

She should also be advised to avoid exposing herself to the sun in the future. She should wear a hat and apply sunscreen – at least factor 30 – whenever out of door in the spring and summer months.

## Chapter 39: Adverse reactions to topical steroids

1. Oral candida is a common problem but may be precipitated by the use of inhaled steroids. It is also common in those with dentures, HIV, infancy and old age, xerostomia, diabetes mellitus or poor nutrition. In this case, the patient admitted to the recent greater use of her inhalers, so this was the most likely reason for her to be affected.

2. a) A swab can be taken from the mouth and sent to the laboratory for confirmation of the diagnosis. However, this is probably unnecessary unless one is concerned that there may also be some other bacterial infection present.
   b) A full asthma check should be done to try to ascertain the reason for the recent deterioration in her condition. Her peak flow level was low at 350 l/min and she had particular problems with hay fever in the hot weather, which she thought was related to the worsening of the asthma. Her chest was clear and there were no signs of other infection.

3. a) The question of antifungal oral suspension or lozenges to treat the candida was discussed but as the infection seemed to be spreading down her throat she was prescribed oral fluconazole 50mg daily for 7-14 days. (BNF Sect 5.2).
   b) The patient was reminded of how and when to use her inhalers most effectively and reminded that if the dose was gradually reduced when the asthma was controlled that there would be less risk of the candida returning.
   c) A prescription for an oral antihistamine and nasal spray was provided. With the suggestion that a steroid nasal spray might be more effective once the candida was better.
   d) She was offered a spacer to use with her inhaler and it was suggested that she rinse her mouth out with water after each inhalation in order to reduce the risk of candida.

## Chapter 40: Drug induced reactions of the skin

1. Erythema multiforme. This florid symptomless rash, of many shapes is most likely to be EM. Closer inspection found evidence of target lesions on her legs and arms.

2. It is probable that the anaesthetic – thiopental sodium – a barbiturate had caused the problem as this was the only new medication that she had received in the last month. She was also on bendrofluazide, a thiazide diuretic, which can also cause EM. However, she had been on it for many years, so this seemed less likely. An infective cause for the rash was ruled out as the patient had been well and there had been no problems with herpes simplex.

3. The patient could be reassured that the rash would probably settle, without treatment, over the ensuing 3 weeks. She was provided with aequeous cream and hydroxyzine tablets to use if there were any problems with skin irritation or dryness. She was also advised to avoid barbiturates and to be sure to alert any anaesthetist should she require their attention in the future. At the same time the medication for her hypertension was reviewed and, as it appeared to be well controlled with atenol, the bendrofluazide was discontinued.

# Index

acne rosacea   34, 183
acne vulgaris   137–41, 183, 185, 189, 197
  aetiology   137
  diagnosis   138
  differential diagnosis   140
  management   138–9
  presentation   137–8
actinic chelitis   163
allergic reactions   68–70, 162–3
alopecia   62
  androgenic   149–50, 152
  areata   150, 152, 197–8
  complications   158–9
  congenital   157–8
  injury-related   157
  non-scarring   149–53, 197–8
  primary cicatricial   155–7
  scarring   155–9, 198
  secondary cicatricial   157–8
  totalis   150
  traction   150, 152
angioedema   81–2, 85, 162, 185, 187
angioneurotic oedema   79
angular chelitis   161
antidepressants   97
antihistamines   97
anxiety   119
athlete's foot see interdigital tinea pedis
atopic facies   89
atrophic disorders   35
auricular perichondritis   173–5
autoimmune disease   170–1
bacterial infections   68–70
basal cell carcinoma   13–14, 36–7, 163, 191
  ear   174–5
basal cell papilloma   8, 10
'bat' ears   173, 175
BCC see basal cell carcinoma
bed bugs   106
black heel syndrome   9, 10
blisters   77
blue naevus   7, 10
body lice   107–8
Bowen's disease   57–8
Bowenoid papulosis   43–4
breast abscess   27
breast cancer   21–4, 192
  acute puerperal mastitis   22
  aetiology   21
  inflammatory   22
  inverted nipple   22–3
  management   23–4
  peau d'orange   21–2
  physical signs   22–3
  ulceration of skin   23
breast examination   21–2
brown pigmented lesions   29–32, 192
bullous pemphigoid   77–8, 80, 194
callosities   73–4
Campbell de Morgan spots   33–4, 36
Candida albicans   162, 167–8, 67, 69–70
Candida intertrigo   182
cavernous lakes   9
cervical cancer   43
chelitis   163
chickenpox (varicella)   49–51, 193
chondrodermatitis nodularis helicis   173–4, 198
chronic vasodilation   34
ciscoid lupus erythematosus   16

compulsive itch   95–9
corns   73–4
coup de sabre   158
cryotherapy   40
CTCL see cutaneous T-cell lymphoma
cutaneous horn   174–5
cutaneous T-cell lymphoma   17–20, 191–2
dental abscess   143–5
dental caries   145
dermatitis
  contact   181
  artefacta   96, 98
  genital   110–11
  hand   75–6, 194
  lip licking   93–4, 133–4, 162
  nickel   173, 175
  perioral   133–4, 140–1, 182
  seborrhoeic   68–70, 135–6
dermatofibroma   8–10, 79
dermatomyositis   35–7
dermatophyte infections   69
Dhobi itch   67
discoid lupus erythematosus   35–6, 57–8
drug induced reactions   185–90, 199
duct ecstasia   25
ear lobe   173–6, 198
  congenital malformation   173
  infection   173
  juvenile spring eruption   174
  pressure   173–4
  sun damage   174–5
earrings   173
eczema   185, 189
  allergic contact   93
  atopic   89–94
    complications   91
    diagnosis   90–1
    differential diagnosis   92–3
    management   91–2
    presentation   89–90
  chronic superfical   18
  contact   93–4
  discoid   57–8, 113, 116–17
  hand   75
  irritant contact   93–4
  nails   120–1
  nipple   23, 26–7
  pompholyx   71–3
  seborrhoeic   68
erosive pustular dermatosis   157
erythema multiforme   87–8, 185, 187, 189, 195, 199
  aetiology   87
  differential diagnosis   88
  major   87
  presentation   87
erythema nodosum   185, 188–9
erythematosus   185
erythematous morbilliform rashes   186
erythrasma   68–70
eyes   177–9, 183, 198–9
facial swelling   143–7, 197
fifth disease   129–30
fixed-drug cruption   188–9
fleas   105–6, 195–6
folliculitis   109–10
folliculitis decalvans   156
folliculitis keloidalis   157
galactorrhoea   25
gene rearrangements studies   19

genital conditions 109–12
genital naevi 46
genital warts 39–40, 43–7, 193
  aetiology 43
  Bowenoid papulosis 43–4
  complications 44
  diagnosis 44–5
  differential diagnosis 45–7
  malignancy 44
  management 45–6
  pregnancy and 44
  presentation 43–4
  prevention 46
  psychological effects 44
  transmission 44
  vaccination 43, 46
German measles (rubella) 128–9, 197
granuloma annulare 113, 115–16
guttate psoriasis 63–4
haemosiderin pigmentation 30, 32
halo naevus 7, 10
hand-foot-and-mouth disease 51–3, 170
head lice 106–8
herpes simplex 161–2, 170
herpes zoster 49–51, 170
HPV see human papilloma virus
human papilloma virus 39, 43
  see also viral warts
hyperlipidaemia 179
hyperpigmentation owing to drugs 30, 32
immunophenotyping 19
impetigo 68, 162
infestations 105–8, 195–6
ingrowing toenails 123–5
insect bites 78–80
interdigital tinea pedis 67–8, 70, 73–4, 115
intertrigo 67–70, 194
  aetiology 67
  complications 67–8
  differential diagnosis 68–9
juvenile plantar dermatosis 72–3
juvenile spring eruption 174
Kaposi's sarcoma 10
keratoacanthoma 13–14, 163–4, 191
keratoderma
  climactericum 71, 73
  differential diagnosis 73
  feet 71–4, 194
Koebner phenomenon 55–6
laser therapy 40
lentigo maligna melanoma 3
leuconychia 123, 125
lice 106–8
lichen planopilaris 62, 156
lichen planus 61–5, 73, 170, 193–4
  aetiology 61
  differential diagnosis 63–4
  management 62–3
  nails 120–1
  presentation 61–2
lichen sclerosus et atrophus 35–6, 109–10, 196
lichen simplex 63–4, 95–6, 98, 110–11
lichenoid eruptions 185, 188
lichenoid reaction 63
lip lesions 161–5, 198
lip licking dermatitis 93–4, 133–4, 162
lupus erythematosus 156
male pattern baldness 149–50
malignant melanoma 1–6, 191

aetiology 1–2
diagnosis 1–2
incidence 1
mimickers 7–11, 191
prognosis 3
seborrhoeic warts and 5–6
symptoms 1
measles 127–8
median nail dystrophy 119
melanocytic naevi 7, 10
melanoma
  acral lentiginous 2
  amelanotic 2–3
  malignant see malignant melanoma
  nodular 2
  prevention 3–4
  superficial spreading 2, 5
melasma 29, 32
microtia 173, 175
milia 45–6, 177–8, 198–9
moles 1, 5
molluscum contagiosum 45–7, 51–2
morphea 158
mouth ulcers 169–70
mucocoele 161
mumps 143–4
mycosis fungoides 17–19, 57, 59
naevus 7
nails 119–26, 196–7
  differential diagnosis 125
  involution 124–5
  Terry's half-and-half 121
  traumatized 123–6, 196–7
necrobiosis lipoidica 35–6
neurotic excoriations 96, 98
nickel dermatitis 173, 175
nipple 25–8, 192
  blood-stained discharge 25–6
  cracked 26–7
  discharge 25–6
  eczema 26
  galactorrhoea 25
  inverted 22–3, 26
  supernumerary 27
nodular basal cell carcinoma 36–7
nodular prurigo 95–6, 98
nose 183
onychogryphosis 123, 125
onycholysis 119–20
oral thrush 167–8
Paget's disease 23, 26–7
parapsoriasis 19–20
parasitophobia 97, 98
paronychia 124–5, 196–7
pearly penile papules 45–6
peau d'orange 21–2
periungual erythema 121–2
periungual warts 46
photosensitivity 185–7
pigmentation 185–7
pigmented basal cell carcinoma 9–10
pitted keratolysis 73–4
pityriasis alba 182
pityriasis amiantacea 152
pityriasis rosea 57, 59, 63–4
  herald patch 113, 116
plantar pustular psoriasis 72–3
plaque psoriasis 55–9, 193
  aetiology 55

diagnosis 55–6
differential diagnosis 57
management 56–7
presentation 55
scalp 57
poikiloderma of Civatte 29, 32
polycystic ovarian syndrome 138, 140
post-inflammatory hyperpigmentation 31–2
prolactinoma 25
pruritus 97, 102
psoriasis 18, 55–9, 68–70, 72–3, 152–3, 183, 185, 188
genital 109–10
nails 119–20, 196
pterygium 62
pubic lice 107–8
puerperal mastitis 27
purpura 185–7
red faces 127–31, 197
red and spotty faces 133–6, 197
rhinophyma 139
ringworm 67, 151
rosacea 34–6, 139–41
roseola infantum 129–31
rubella see German measles
salivary calculus 143, 145–6
sarcoidosis 143, 146–7
scabies 101–3, 110, 195
aetiology 101
differential diagnosis 103, 110
scaly feet see keratoderma, feet
scarlet fever 128–30, 168
Schamberg's disease 30–2
sebaceous naevus 158
seborrhoeic warts 5–6, 45, 191
self trauma 96, 98
Sézary syndrome 18
shingles 50–1
spider naevus 34, 36
splinter haemorrhages 121
spots and vesicles, diagnosing 49–53, 193
squamous cell carcinoma 14–15, 158, 164, 191
ear 174–5
Stevens Johnson Syndrome 87, 185, 187–9
striae 182–3
subungual haematoma 124–5
sunburn 1
sycosis barbae 134–5, 197
syphilis 63–5
syringoma 177–8
telangiectasia 33–7, 139, 182, 192
atrophic disorders 35–6
Campbell de Morgan spots 33–4, 36
hereditary 33, 36, 164
idiopathic 33–4, 36
lichen sclerosus et atrophicus 35–6
necrobiosis lipoidica 35–6
physical damage 35–6
secondary disease 34, 36
spider naevus 34, 36
telogen effluvium 152–3
tinea capitis 151–2
tinea corporis 63–4, 113–17, 196
tinea cruris 67, 70, 115
tinea incognito 115, 181–2
tinea manuum 76, 194
tongue 167–71, 198
black hairy 168–9
cancer 171
contact dermatitis 170

discolouration 168
fissured 167–8
geographic 167–8
strawberry 168–9
topical steroids 91–2, 97
adverse reactions 181–4, 199
skin damage 182
trichotillomania 150–1
tumours, facial 143, 146
urticaria 81–6, 185, 187–8, 194–5
aetiology 81
aquagenic, 85
autoimmune ordinary 81
cholinergic 82–3, 85
chronic 83, 85
contact 83, 85
diagnosis 84
differential diagnosis 85, 88
idiopathic chronic ordinary 81
management 84–6
non-immunological 81
ordinary acute 85
papular 82–3, 85
physical 82
pigmentosa 84–5
pregnancy 84–5
presentation 81
pressure 82, 85
solar 82, 85
thermal 82, 85
urticarial vasculitis 83, 85
vaccination 43, 46
varicella see chickenpox; shingles
vasculitis 185–7
venous lake 9, 10, 164
verrucae 39
viral warts 39–41, 192–3
complications 39–40
genital 39–40
mosaic 39
periungual 40–1
plane 39
plantar 39
presentation 39
psychosocial problems 40
treatment 40–1
verrucae 39
see also genital warts; warts
vulval intraepithelial neoplasia 44
warts
facial 40
viral see viral warts
Wickham's striae 61
xanthelasma 178–9
xerostomia 168–9